AF412722

Food Allergy: Molecular Basis and Clinical Practice

Chemical Immunology and Allergy

Vol. 101

Series Editors

Johannes Ring Munich
Kurt Blaser Davos
Monique Capron Lille
Judah A. Denburg Hamilton, Ont.
Stephen T. Holgate Southampton
Gianni Marone Naples
Hirohisa Saito Tokyo

Food Allergy: Molecular Basis and Clinical Practice

Volume Editors

Motohiro Ebisawa Sagamihara

Barbara K. Ballmer-Weber Zurich

Stefan Vieths Langen

Robert A. Wood Baltimore, Md.

19 figures, 4 in color, and 56 tables, 2015

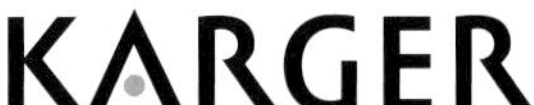

Basel · Freiburg · Paris · London · New York · Chennai · New Delhi · Bangkok · Beijing · Shanghai · Tokyo · Kuala Lumpur · Singapore · Sydney

Chemical Immunology and Allergy

Formerly published as 'Progress in Allergy' (founded 1939),
continued 1990–2002 as 'Chemical Immunology'
Edited by Paul Kallós 1939–1988, Byron H. Waksman 1962–2002

Motohiro Ebisawa, MD, PhD
Department of Allergy
Clinical Research Center for Allergology and
Rheumatology
Sagamihara National Hospital
Sagamihara, Kanagawa, Japan

Stefan Vieths, PhD
Paul-Ehrlich-Institut
Langen, Germany

Barbara K. Ballmer-Weber, MD
Allergy Unit
Department of Dermatology
University Hospital Zurich
Zurich, Switzerland

Robert A. Wood, MD
Division of Pediatric Allergy and Immunology
Johns Hopkins University School of Medicine and
Department of International Health
Johns Hopkins Bloomberg School of Public Health
Baltimore, Md., USA

Bibliographic Indices. This publication is listed in bibliographic services, including Current Contents® and PubMed/MEDLINE.

Disclaimer. The statements, opinions and data contained in this publication are solely those of the individual authors and contributors and not of the publisher and the editor(s). The appearance of advertisements in the book is not a warranty, endorsement, or approval of the products or services advertised or of their effectiveness, quality or safety. The publisher and the editor(s) disclaim responsibility for any injury to persons or property resulting from any ideas, methods, instructions or products referred to in the content or advertisements.

Drug Dosage. The authors and the publisher have exerted every effort to ensure that drug selection and dosage set forth in this text are in accord with current recommendations and practice at the time of publication. However, in view of ongoing research, changes in government regulations, and the constant flow of information relating to drug therapy and drug reactions, the reader is urged to check the package insert for each drug for any change in indications and dosage and for added warnings and precautions. This is particularly important when the recommended agent is a new and/or infrequently employed drug.

All rights reserved. No part of this publication may be translated into other languages, reproduced or utilized in any form or by any means electronic or mechanical, including photocopying, recording, microcopying, or by any information storage and retrieval system, without permission in writing from the publisher.

© Copyright 2015 by S. Karger AG, P.O. Box, CH-4009 Basel (Switzerland)
www.karger.com
Printed in Germany on acid-free and non-aging paper (ISO 9706) by Kraft Druck GmbH, Ettlingen
ISSN 1660–2242
e-ISSN 1662–2898
ISBN 978–3–318–02340–4
e-ISBN 978–3–318–02341–1

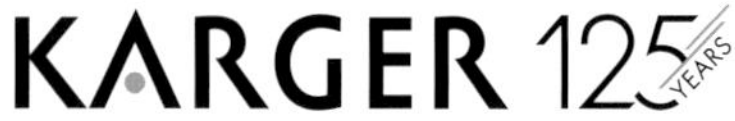

Contents

Clinical Aspects

Diagnosis and Management

87 Diagnostic Elimination Diets and Oral Food Provocation
Wood, R.A. (Baltimore, Md.)

96 Pharmacological Management of Acute Food-Allergic Reactions
Richards, S.; Tang, M. (Melbourne, Vic.)

106 Oral Immunotherapy and Potential Treatment
Sato, S.; Yanagida, N.; Ebisawa, M. (Sagamihara)

Allergen-Based Food Allergies

114 Cow's Milk Allergy in Children and Adults
Fiocchi, A.; Dahdah, L. (Rome); Albarini, M.; Martelli, A. (Milan)

124 Hen's Egg Allergy
Urisu, A.; Kondo, Y. (Nagoya); Tsuge, I. (Toyoake)

131 Peanut and Tree Nut Allergy
Cox, A.; Sicherer, S.H. (New York, N.Y.)

145   Grain and Legume Allergy

Ito, K. (Aichi)

152   Fish and Shellfish Allergy

Thalayasingam, M.; Lee, B.-W. (Singapore)

Special Topics

Contents

Preface

Although food allergy was first described a long time ago, as outlined in the chapter 'Historical background, definitions, and differential diagnosis', only in recent times has it started to be recognized as one of the major allergic diseases. In the past 50 years since the discovery of IgE by Dr. K. Ishizaka, we have experienced a steep increase in the prevalence of allergic diseases. The prevalence of food allergy around the world has not yet been clarified in detail. It is quite obvious that we have faced a rapid increase in patients with food allergy in both childhood and adulthood in most developed countries in the past 3 decades. The number of publications on food allergy reached 100/year in 1971 based on a PubMed search, and it went up to 500/year at the beginning of the 21st century and finally to more than 1,200/year in 2014. It is clear that food allergy research is currently a very hot topic among academics and that issues related to food allergy attract a lot of attention. We have collaborated with distinguished, world-class professionals on food allergy research and practice to put this book together. The topics are very practical and applicable to your practice. We hope that this book on food allergy will help clinicians, academics, and paramedics to better understand current food allergy practice and research.

Motohiro Ebisawa, Sagamihara
Barbara K. Ballmer-Weber, Zurich
Stefan Vieths, Langen
Robert A. Wood, Baltimore, Md.

Ebisawa M, Ballmer-Weber BK, Vieths S, Wood RA (eds): Food Allergy: Molecular Basis and Clinical Practice.
Chem Immunol Allergy. Basel, Karger, 2015, vol 101, pp 1–7 (DOI: 10.1159/000371644)

Historical Background, Definitions and Differential Diagnosis

Hugh A. Sampson

Division of Allergy and Immunology, Department of Pediatrics, Jaffe Food Allergy Institute, Icahn School of
Medicine at Mount Sinai, New York, N.Y., USA

Abstract

Although awareness that food can cause adverse symptoms and even death in some individuals has been present since the times of Hippocrates, it was not until the seminal experiment of Prausnitz that the investigation of food allergy had a more scientific basis. In the first half of the 20th century, there were periodic reports in the medical literature describing various food allergic reactions. Until the studies of Charles May and colleagues in the mid- to late '70s, there was a great deal of skepticism in the medical world about the relevance of food allergy and how to diagnose it, since standard skin testing was known to correlate poorly with clinical symptoms. With the introduction of the double-blind, placebo-controlled oral food challenge by May, the study of food allergy has become evidence based, and tremendous strides have been made in the study of basic immunopathogenic mechanisms and natural history as well as in the diagnosis and management of food allergies. Today, various IgE- and non-IgE-mediated food allergic disorders have been well characterized, and efforts to reverse these allergies using various immunotherapeutic strategies are well under way.

© 2015 S. Karger AG, Basel

Historical Background

While the first account of food allergy is attributed to Hippocrates, the Chinese emperors Shen Nong (2,735 BC) and Huang Di (2,698–2,598 BC) provided advice in 'Shi Jin-Jing' ('Interdictions concerning food') for pregnant women to avoid certain foods, e.g. shrimp, chicken and meats, and for individuals with certain skin lesions (possibly eczematous lesions) to avoid certain foods [1]. In the writings of Hippocrates (460–377 BC), he referred to the presence of 'hostile humors' in some men that made them 'suffer badly' following the ingestion of cheese [1]. One might interpret this hostile humor to be IgE. An often quoted line from a poem of Titus Lucretius Cato (98–55 BC), 'What is food to one, to another is rank poison' [1], strongly suggests an understanding of adverse reactions to foods over 2,000 years ago. Case reports of food-hypersensitivity reactions were recorded in the 17th century [1]: Jean Baptiste van Helmont reported asthmatic attacks following the ingestion of fish in *Oriatrike*, which was published in 1662, and Robert Willan, in his *Trea-*

tise on Dermatology (a multi-volume publication; 1798–1808), described urticaria following the ingestion of almonds, mushrooms, fish, crab, lobsters and mussels as well as 'urticaria febrilis' (fatal anaphylaxis) following the ingestion of mussels and lobsters.

While various reports of reactions to foods occurred periodically in the medical literature, it was not until 1921 that the classic experiment of Prausnitz initiated the scientific investigation of food allergy and established the immunologic basis of allergic reactions [2]. In his experiment, Prausnitz injected sera from a fish-allergic patient, named Kustner, and from a nonallergic control subject into his own skin, and on the following day, he injected fish extract into the same areas. A positive local reaction (Prausnitz-Kustner test) proved that sensitivity could be transferred by a factor in serum (IgE antibodies) from an allergic to a nonallergic individual.

Long before IgE antibodies were identified, studies of food allergy focused on radiologic changes associated with immediate hypersensitivity reactions. In one of the first of these reports on a patient with a wheat allergy, hypertonicity of the transverse and pelvic colon and hypotonicity of the cecum and ascending colon were noted following the ingestion of wheat by the allergic patient [3]. In a later study by Rowe and colleagues [4], fluoroscopy was used to compare the effect of barium contrast material containing food allergens with the effect of standard barium contrast material in 12 food-allergic children. The investigators noted prolonged gastric hypotonia and retention of the allergen test meal, prominent pylorospasm, and increased or decreased peristaltic activity of the intestines.

In an elegant series of experiments over 70 years ago, Walzer and his colleagues in New York utilized sera from food-allergic patients to passively sensitize volunteers and demonstrate that 'immunologically' intact antigens can cross the gastrointestinal mucosal barrier and rapidly disseminate throughout the body. The investigators

passively sensitized skin on the arms of a large series of adults with serum from a fish-allergic patient and of a large series of children with serum from an egg-allergic patient, as well as with nonallergic control serum [5, 6]. Twenty-four hours later, the adults and children were fed fish or eggs, respectively, and within about 90 min, nearly 90% of the study subjects developed a large wheal and flare response at the site on their arm that had been sensitized with 'allergic sera', but not at the site that had been sensitized with 'non-allergic control sera'. Using a similar approach, colonic mucosa from patients who had previously undergone an ileocolostomy was sensitized with serum from food-allergic patients or normal controls [7]. Sera from allergic patients were injected at the distal site of the ileocolostomy opening. Twenty-four hours later, the study subjects ingested the food allergen, and within 10–15 min, they developed hyperemia at the sensitized, distal colonic site that was followed shortly thereafter by pallor and edema and by prolonged, copious mucus secretion and petechiae at the site. Walzer's group also studied the effects of stomach acidity on food allergen uptake. They demonstrated that increased stomach acidity and the presence of other food in the gut decreased antigen absorption, while decreased stomach acidity, such as from today's H2-blockers and proton pump inhibitors, and ingestion of alcohol increased antigen absorption [8].

In the late 1930s, the rigid gastroscope was used to observe reactions in the stomachs of allergic patients. One study compared 6 patients with gastrointestinal food allergy or wheezing that were exacerbated by the ingestion of a food allergen with control subjects [9]. Thirty minutes after a food allergen was placed on the gastric mucosa, patients with a gastrointestinal food allergy developed markedly hyperemic and edematous patches with overlying thick, gray mucus and scattered petechiae at the site where the allergen was placed, similar to findings reported earlier by Walzer and colleagues on passively sensitized intestinal mucosal sites [8]. Only mild hyperemia of the gastric mucosa was noted in patients with wheezing provoked by food ingestion. A subsequent study by Reimann and Lewin evaluated 30 patients with a gastrointestinal food allergy, which confirmed these earlier observations and established an IgE-mediated mechanism for the reactions [10]. These investigators demonstrated that food-allergic patients had significant food-specific IgE antibodies and increased numbers of intestinal mast cells in the gastric mucosa prior to the laparoscopic placement of food on the gastric mucosa when compared with normal controls. They also found significant decreases in stainable mast cells and tissue histamine content following a positive response to the food allergen.

In 1912, Schloss introduced the concept of using chemically extracted protein from foods for scratch testing in the diagnosis of food allergy [1], but by then, there were already calls for curbing the growing practice of 'scratching the skin with a few food tests and putting the patient on a weird and impracticable diet which usually accomplishes no result…' [1]. In 1950, Loveless, in her report of the first blinded, placebo-controlled food trials in patients with milk allergy, demonstrated that the patient's history and presence of food-specific IgE antibodies were often insufficient to diagnose food allergy [11]. In a later report of 89 children being evaluated for milk allergy, Goldman and colleagues suggested that the diagnosis of food allergy could only be considered established when withdrawal of the food (milk) from the diet led to complete resolution of symptoms and when three successive challenges with the food (milk) duplicated the presenting symptoms [12]. Due to the potential severity of the reactions that developed during food challenges, this approach was not widely accepted. Following reports of work by Charles May and colleagues in the mid-70s [13], double-blind, placebo-controlled oral food challenge emerged as the accepted standard for the diagnosis of food allergy, and most recently, a consensus document attempting to standardize

double-blind, placebo-controlled oral food challenge was published by the American Academy of Allergy and Immunology and the European Academy of Allergy and Clinical Immunology [14].

Even before Prausnitz's classic experiment demonstrating that a transferable factor, i.e. IgE, was likely involved in the pathogenesis of food allergy, physicians began experimenting with immunotherapeutic approaches to treat food allergy. The first report of successful oral immunotherapy (OIT) was published in the *Lancet* in 1908 and described the successful treatment of a child with egg-induced anaphylaxis [15]. A few scattered case reports followed, including a report by Keston that reported very limited details on a '…*method as outlined above has been effective in desensitizing about fifty patients with allergic symptoms*' [16] and reports by Edwards [17] and Unger [18] that were equally sparse on results, e.g. '*Twelve of thirteen patients attempted have been successfully desensitized by the oral method*' [17]. In 1998, Patriarca and colleagues described a protocol used to desensitize a small cohort of children with food allergy [19] and noted that '…*although further studies (such as a randomized trial) are needed to reinforce the conclusions of this paper, oral desensitization may represent an alternative and safe approach in children with food allergy…*' [20]. In the past decade, over three dozen studies evaluating the effects of OIT, as well as other forms of immunotherapy, have been published, but most authorities agree that OIT is not yet ready for general use in the clinic [21].

Definitions and Differential Diagnosis

Some of the confusion in the minds of patients and general practitioners regarding food allergies likely stems from the use of disparate terms when referring to food-hypersensitivity reactions. This is somewhat complicated by the fact that the terminology used by investigators in the field of food allergy differs slightly in different parts of the world. The following represents the current terminology in the United States [21]. An *adverse food reaction* is a generic term indicating any untoward reaction that occurs following the ingestion of a food or food additive and may be the result of *toxic* or *nontoxic reactions*. *Toxic reactions* occur in any individual who is exposed to a sufficient quantity of the offending agent, whereas *nontoxic reactions* depend on individual susceptibilities and may be immune-mediated (food allergy or food hypersensitivity) or nonimmune-mediated (food intolerance). *Food intolerances* are responsible for most adverse food reactions and are categorized as *enzymatic, pharmacologic,* or *idiopathic* food intolerances. Secondary lactase deficiency, an enzymatic intolerance resulting in bloating, nausea, abdominal cramping, gas and diarrhea, affects the vast majority of adults throughout the world, whereas most other enzyme deficiencies are rare, inborn errors of metabolism and thus primarily affect infants and children. Pharmacologic food intolerances are present in individuals who are unusually reactive to substances such as vasoactive amines, which are normally present in some foods (e.g. tyramine in aged cheeses). Confirmed adverse food reactions for which the physiologic mechanism is not known are generally classified as idiopathic intolerances. *Food allergies* are usually characterized as IgE-mediated ('immediate') or non-IgE-mediated ('delayed'); the latter are presumed to be cell-mediated. IgE-mediated food allergies may provoke a variety of typical allergic symptoms, as noted in table 1. In general, food allergies are categorized according to the target organs that are affected and the mechanisms that are presumed to be responsible, as outlined in table 2.

The differential diagnosis of food allergy can be quite broad and depends upon the involved organ systems. With the onset of acute symptoms, many factors need to be considered in order to exclude the role of environmental allergens, e.g. pollens, animal dander, bee stings, etc.,

or medications in provoking immediate hypersensitivity reactions. A thorough clinical history generally provides guidance for the further evaluation of a potential food allergic reaction and helps to differentiate reactions provoked by nonallergic causes. In addition to the general medical history of a patient, including their age and atopic status, the clinical history should include the following information when evaluating a patient for food allergy: (1) the food suspected of provoking the reaction and the quantity and form of the food that was ingested, e.g.

Table 1. Symptoms associated with food-allergic reactions

Cutaneous	Pruritus
	Erythema/flushing
	Urticaria
	Angioedema
Ocular	Pruritus
	Tearing
	Conjunctival injection
	Periorbital edema
Respiratory	
Upper	Pruritus
	Nasal congestion
	Rhinorrhea
	Sneezing
	Hoarseness
	Laryngeal edema
Lower	Cough
	Wheezing
	Dyspnea
	Chest tightness/pain
Gastrointestinal	Oral pruritus
	Oral angioedema (lips, tongue, or palate)
	Pharyngeal pruritus/tightness
	Colicky abdominal pain
	Nausea
	Vomiting
	Diarrhea
Cardiovascular	Tachycardia
	Dizziness
	Hypotension
	Loss of consciousness/fainting
Miscellaneous	Metallic taste in mouth
	Uterine cramping/contractions
	Sense of impending doom

IgE-mediated	Mixed IgE- and non-IgE-mediated	Non-IgE mediated (cellular)
Skin		
Urticaria	Atopic dermatitis	Dermatitis herpetiformis
Angioedema		Contact dermatitis
Erythematous morbilliform rash		
Flaring		
Respiratory		
Allergic rhinoconjunctivitis	Asthma	Food-induced pulmonary hemosiderosis
Acute bronchospasm		(Heiner's syndrome)
Gastrointestinal		
Oral allergy syndrome		
Acute gastrointestinal spasm	Eosinophilic esophagitis	Food protein-induced enterocolitis syndrome
	Eosinophilic gastritis	Food protein-induced proctocolitis syndrome
	Eosinophilic gastroenteritis	Food protein-induced enteropathy syndrome
		Celiac disease
Cardiovascular		
Dizziness and fainting		
Anaphylaxis		
Food-associated, exercise-induced anaphylaxis		
Miscellaneous		
Uterine cramping and contractions		
Feeling of 'pending doom'		

cooked or raw, (2) the time between ingestion of the suspected food and the development of symptoms, (3) the types of symptoms elicited by the ingestion, (4) whether the patient has ingested the suspected food in the past and experienced similar symptoms on those occasions, (5) whether other inciting factors, such as exercise, alcohol or NSAIDs, may have been involved, and (6) the period of time since the last reaction to the food occurred. It is also important to know whether the patient was experiencing a viral illness at the time, which may induce rashes or urticaria and exacerbate symptoms similar to allergic rhinoconjunctivitis and asthma. Although very uncommon, a number of disorders, such as systemic mastocytosis, mast cell activation syndrome, hereditary or acquired angioedema syndrome, and pheochromocytoma, can mimic anaphylaxis provoked by food allergy. Table 3 lists a number of nonallergic disorders that may need to be considered in the evaluation of a food-allergic patient, the majority of which involve gastrointestinal symptoms.

Recent History and the Future

In the past 35 years, we have witnessed remarkable changes in our basic understanding of food-allergic disorders, which have elevated food allergy from a collection of unsubstantiated anecdotes that were largely discounted by investigators and clinicians to a science annually generating hundreds of publications in high-impact scientific journals, as will be summarized in subsequent chapters. This increase has paralleled an

Table 3. Nonallergic adverse reactions to foods

Condition	Symptoms	Mechanism
Cutaneous		
Auriculo-temporal syndrome (Freye syndrome)	Facial flush in trigeminal nerve distribution associated with spicy foods	Neurogenic reflex, frequently associated with birth trauma to the trigeminal nerve (forceps delivery)
Respiratory		
Gustatory rhinitis	Profuse, watery rhinorrhea associated with spicy foods	Neurogenic reflex
Gastrointestinal		
Lactose intolerance	Bloating, abdominal pain, diarrhea (dose-dependent)	Lactase deficiency
Fructose intolerance	Bloating, abdominal pain, diarrhea (dose-dependent)	Fructose deficiency
Pancreatic insufficiency	Malabsorption	Deficiency of pancreatic enzymes
Gallbladder/liver disease	Malabsorption	Deficiency of liver enzymes
Food poisoning	Pain, fever, nausea, emesis, diarrhea	Bacterial toxins in food
Scombroid fish poisoning	Flushing, angioedema, hives, abdominal pain	In spoiled fish, histidine is metabolized to histamine
Caffeine	Tremors, cramps, diarrhea	Pharmacologic effects of caffeine in susceptible individuals
Cardiovascular		
Vasovagal response	Fainting	Neurogenic response
Panic disorder	Subjective reactions, fainting upon smelling or seeing the food	Psychological

apparent increase in the prevalence of food allergy, from 0.2 to 0.3% of the pediatric population to about 10% of children today [22]. Severe food-allergic reactions were rare 35 years ago, but these reactions now represent the single-leading cause of anaphylaxis treated in emergency departments in the United States. Certain potential pathogenic factors, such as the gut microbiota, were barely discussed 3 decades ago, whereas today, new technologies have enabled investigators to focus on this new frontier. Although many of the same diagnostic tools that were utilized 30 years ago are still used to diagnose food allergy today, these tools have been refined. Thirty-five years ago, skin tests and patient history were used by most allergists to diagnose food allergy, in vitro, food-specific IgE measurements were rarely utilized, and few allergists performed oral food challenges, whereas today, oral food challenges are the accepted 'gold standard', and efforts have been made to standardize the procedure worldwide [14]. The management of

food allergy today is not much different from how it was 30 years ago, when food labels were not very informative, but self-injectable epinephrine was not typically prescribed, unlike today. Until recently, it was believed that strict allergen avoidance was the only hope for 'outgrowing' food allergies, and the concept of patients with different allergic phenotypes, i.e. reacting differently to conformational and sequential epitopes, was not known [21]. Although the first case of OIT was published in 1908, no immunotherapeutic approaches to treat food allergy were being pursued 35 years ago. Today, many investigators are evaluating OIT and other immunotherapeutic strategies. However, 35 years ago, there were no specific recommendations for trying to prevent food allergies. In the 1980s, mothers were told to eliminate major food allergens from their diets during pregnancy and lactation and to withhold major allergens from their newborns to prevent food allergies, whereas recent studies suggest that early introduction of food allergens may actually prevent the development of allergies. Clearly, tremendous progress has been made in the diagnosis and management of food allergy over the past $3^1/_2$ decades, and new information has dramatically altered our concept of food allergy. However, many more questions remain regarding the immunopathogenesis, diagnosis, management and prevention of food allergies and will likely keep investigators occupied for at least the next 30 years [21].

References

1 Cohen SG: Food allergens: landmarks along a historic trail. J Allergy Clin Immunol 2008;121:1521–1524.

2 Prausnitz C, Kustner H: Studies on supersensitivity. Centrabl Bakteriol 1921; 86:160–169.

3 Eyermann C: X-ray demonstration of colonic reaction in food allergy. J Missouri Med Assoc 1927;24:129–132.

4 Rowe AH: Roentgen studies of patients with gastro-intestinal food allergy. JAMA 1933;100:394–400.

5 Brunner M, Walzer M: Absorption of undigested proteins in human beings: the absorption of unaltered fish protein in adults. Arch Intern Med 1928;42: 173–179.

6 Wilson SJ, Walzer M: Absorption of undigested proteins in human beings. IV. Absorption of unaltered egg protein in infants. Am J Dis Child 1935;50:49–54.

7 Gray I, Harten M, Walzer M: Studies in mucous membrane hypersensitiveness. IV. The allergic reaction in the passively sensitized mucous membranes of the ileum and colon in humans. Ann Intern Med 1940;13:2050–2056.

8 Walzer M: Allergy of the abdominal organs. J Lab Clin Med 1941;26:1867–1877.

9 Pollard H, Stuart G: Experimental reproduction of gastric allergy in human beings with controlled observations on the mucosa. J Allergy 1942;13:467–473.

10 Reimann HJ, Lewin J: Gastric mucosal reactions in patients with food allergy. Am J Gastroenterol 1988;83:1212–1219.

11 Loveless MH: Allergy for corn and its derivatives: experiments with a masked ingestion test for its diagnosis. J Allergy 1950;21:500–509.

12 Goldman AS, Anderson DW, Sellers WA, Saperstein A, Kniker WT, Halpern SR: Milk allergy. I. Oral challenge with milk and isolated milk proteins in allergic children. Pediatrics 1963;32:425–443.

13 May CD: Objective clinical and laboratory studies of immediate hypersensitivity reactions to food in asthmatic children. J Allergy Clin Immunol 1976;58: 500–515.

14 Sampson HA, Gerth vWR, Bindslev-Jensen C, Sicherer S, Teuber SS, Burks AW, Dubois AE, Beyer K, Eigenmann PA, Spergel JM, Werfel T, Chinchilli VM: Standardizing double-blind, placebo-controlled oral food challenges: American Academy of Allergy, Asthma & Immunology-European Academy of Allergy and Clinical Immunology PRACTALL consensus report. J Allergy Clin Immunol 2012;130:1260–1274.

15 Schofield AT: A case of egg poisoning. Lancet 1908;1:716.

16 Keston BM, Waters I, Hopkins JG: Oral desensitization to common foods. J Allergy 1935;6:431–436.

17 Edwards HE: Oral desensitization in food allergy. Can Med Assoc J 1940;43: 234–236.

18 Unger L: Food desensitization in bronchial asthma. Ill Med J 1923;44:40–46.

19 Patriarca G, Schiavino D, Nucera E, Schinco G, Milani A, Gasbarrini GB: Food allergy in children: results of a standardized protocol for oral desensitization. Hepatogastroenterology 1998;45: 52–58.

20 Patriarca G, Nucera E, Pollastrini E, Roncallo C, De Pasquale T, Lombardo C, Pedone C, Gasbarrini G, Buonomo A, Schiavino D: Oral specific desensitization in food-allergic children. Dig Dis Sci 2007;52:1662–1672.

21 Boyce JA, Assa'ad A, Burks AW, Jones SM, Sampson HA, Wood RA, Plaut M, Cooper SF, Fenton MJ, Arshad SH, Bahna SL, Beck LA, Byrd-Bredbenner C, Camargo CA Jr, Eichenfield L, Furuta GT, Hanifin JM, Jones C, Kraft M, Levy BD, Lieberman P, Luccioli S, McCall KM, Schneider LC, Simon RA, Simons FE, Teach SJ, Yawn BP, Schwaninger JM: Guidelines for the diagnosis and management of food allergy in the United States: report of the NIAID-sponsored expert panel. J Allergy Clin Immunol 2010;126:S1–S58.

22 Sicherer SH, Sampson HA: Food allergy: epidemiology, pathogenesis, diagnosis, and treatment. J Allergy Clin Immunol 2014;133:291–307.

Prof. Hugh A. Sampson, MD
Division of Allergy and Immunology, Department of Pediatrics
Jaffe Food Allergy Institute, Icahn School of Medicine at Mount Sinai
One Gustave L. Levy Place
New York, NY 10029 (USA)
E-Mail hugh.sampson@mssm.edu

Ebisawa M, Ballmer-Weber BK, Vieths S, Wood RA (eds): Food Allergy: Molecular Basis and Clinical Practice.
Chem Immunol Allergy. Basel, Karger, 2015, vol 101, pp 8–17 (DOI: 10.1159/000371646)

Immunological Basis of Food Allergy (IgE-Mediated, Non-IgE-Mediated, and Tolerance)

Edwin H. Kim · Wesley Burks

Division of Rheumatology, Allergy and Immunology, Department of Medicine, University of North Carolina
at Chapel Hill, Chapel Hill, N.C., USA

Abstract

Food allergy includes a number of diseases that present with adverse immunological reactions to foods and can be IgE-mediated, non-IgE-mediated, or a combination of both mechanisms. IgE-mediated food allergy involves immediate hypersensitivity through the action of mast cells, whereas non-IgE-mediated food allergy is most commonly cell-mediated. These food allergies are thought to occur as a result of a breakdown in oral tolerance and, more specifically, from an aberrant regulatory T-cell response. Ongoing studies of experimental treatments for food allergy strive to induce oral tolerance and to teach us more about the pathogenesis of food allergy.

© 2015 S. Karger AG, Basel

Introduction

The term food allergy is used colloquially to describe a broad range of reactions that are associated with food ingestion. These reactions can include those that are immune-mediated or nonimmune-mediated. As the term allergy implies the involvement of an immune response, food allergy is more properly defined as an adverse health effect from a specific immune response that reproducibly occurs upon exposure to a given food [1].

Nonimmune-mediated reactions to foods are far more common than immune-mediated food allergies and can occur from food poisoning and other toxic reactions, host gastrointestinal disorders, food intolerances, and psychological reactions (table 1). Similar to food allergy, some of these reactions can be reproducible, e.g. as for certain food intolerances, but others could potentially be life threatening, e.g. as for toxic reactions. However, the majority of these nonimmune-mediated food reactions would be expected to be intermittent and mild in severity.

Immune-mediated food allergy can be broadly divided into IgE-mediated, non-IgE-mediated, and mixed-immune reactions (table 2). The following section will review the mechanisms underlying these types of reactions in the context of representative food allergy diseases. The section will conclude with a review of oral tolerance and a discussion of the recent advances in the quest to induce oral tolerance in food-allergic persons.

Table 1. Examples of nonimmunologic food reactions

Toxic reactions
    Scombroidosis
    Food poisoning (*S. aureus, B. cereus, Salmonella*)
Host gastrointestinal diseases
    Lactase deficiency
    Fructose malabsorption
    Sucrose-isomaltase deficiency
    Gastroesophageal reflux
    Pancreatic insufficiency
    Gall bladder/liver disease
Food intolerances
    Histamine (tomato, strawberry, chocolate, alcohol)
    Tyramine (aged cheeses)
    Caffeine
    Monosodium glutamate
Psychological reactions
    Food aversion
    Food phobias

IgE-Mediated Food Allergy

In 1963, Gell and Coombs defined 4 distinct types of immune-mediated hypersensitivity reactions. Type 1 reactions, described as immediate hypersensitivity reactions, are the mechanistic basis behind IgE-mediated food allergy reactions. Peanut allergy, which has been in the public eye because of its steady increase in prevalence [2] as well as its potential for life-threatening reactions [3], is a classic example of an IgE-mediated food allergy.

The allergic process begins with an initial exposure to peanut antigen. This exposure typically does not result in significant clinical symptoms but triggers B-cells to mature into plasma cells that then secrete IgE molecules specific to various epitopes within the peanut protein. This peanut-specific IgE then binds through its Fc portion to mast cells in the skin and basophils in the circulation via the high-affinity IgE receptor. Interestingly, in clinical practice, it is often unknown when this initial sensitization has occurred, as many patients describe symptoms with their first known exposure to peanut [4]. This, in part, has led to investigations regarding sensitization and the transfer of peanut proteins through the placenta while in utero [5] or postnatally through breastfeeding [6]. Thus far, although evidence suggests that food proteins indeed pass through the placenta and are present in breast milk, the causation of food allergy remains unclear [7].

Re-exposure of the sensitized patient to peanut results in binding of the peanut antigen to IgE molecules on the surfaces of mast cells and basophils. Cross-linking of IgE on these cells leads to a signaling cascade that triggers the release of inflammatory mediators that are responsible for the allergic response. Different characteristics of the effector cells and mediators are responsible for the acute-phase reaction and the late-phase reaction that makes up the overall allergic response. Mast cells are tissue-dwelling cells that contain numerous granules filled with various preformed mediators, such as histamine, tryptase, and heparin (fig. 1). Basophils reside in the circulation and similarly contain granules, although these almost exclusively contain histamine. It is these preformed mediators that primarily account for the acute phase reaction, with most symptoms occurring within minutes of exposure. Histamine is the best recognized of these mediators and causes vasodilation and vasopermeability, bronchospasm, increased mucus, gastric smooth muscle constriction and increased gastric acid, and intense pruritus. These effects result in the clinical symptoms commonly associated with anaphylaxis, including hives and flushing, wheeze and cough, rhinorrhea and congestion, abdominal pain and emesis, and hypotension. A second important preformed mediator that is found primarily in mast cells is tryptase. During an acute allergic reaction, the clinical effects of tryptase are more limited than for histamine, with it playing a role mostly in bronchospasm [8]. However, it has been used as a helpful tool in diagnosing suspected allergic reactions. The β-tryptase form of tryptase peaks 1 hour after the initial insult and remains elevated for 6–8 hours [9], providing a laboratory means of confirming mast cell degran-

Table 2. Examples of immune-mediated food allergy

IgE-mediated	Non-IgE-mediated	Mixed
Anaphylactic food allergy Pollen-food allergy syndrome	Celiac disease Food-protein-induced enterocolitis syndrome Food-protein-induced enteropathy Food-protein-induced proctitis/proctocolitis Food-induced pulmonary hemosiderosis (Heiner syndrome)	Atopic dermatitis Eosinophilic esophagitis Eosinophilic gastroenteritis Eosinophilic colitis

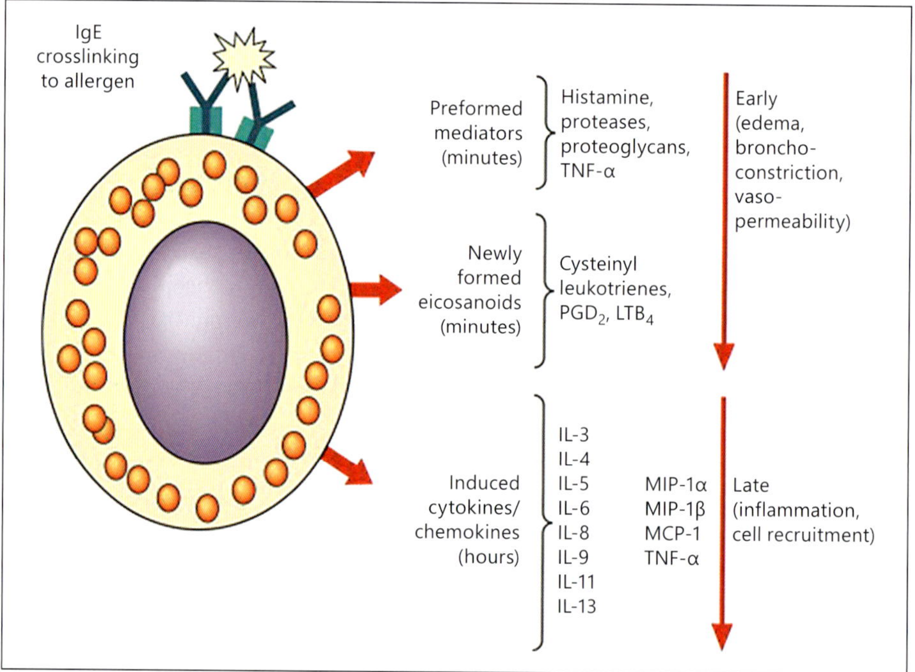

Fig. 1. The mast cell and its mediators. (Figure used with permission from Adkinson NF, Busse WW, Bochner BS, Holgate ST, Simons ER, Lemanske RF: Middleton's Allergy Principles and Practice, ed 7. Philadelphia, PA, Mosby/Elsevier, 2009, pp 319–323, Copyright Elsevier 2009.)

ulation. Interestingly, for food allergy, an increase in tryptase is often not seen after an acute allergic reaction. A greater role for basophils, which release minimal tryptase, as well as the possibility of localized mast cell degranulation or slower diffusion of tryptase from mucosal mast-cell sites, has been hypothesized [10].

In addition to the release of preformed mediators, mast cells and basophils synthesize pro-inflammatory molecules de novo as part of the allergic response. These molecules include products of the arachidonic acid pathway, such as the leukotrienes and prostaglandins, as well as various cytokines (fig. 1). Some of these newly formed

Birch pollen	Ragweed	Mugwort
Peach	Banana	Celery
Apple	Cantaloupe	Carrot
Pear	Honeydew	Green pepper
Plum	Watermelon	Onion
Cherry	Cucumber	Garlic
Carrot	Zucchini	
Celery		
Peanut		
Soybean		
Hazelnut		
Almond		

mediators, such as LTB_4, LTC_4, cysteinyl leukotrienes, and PGD_2, are rapidly synthesized and released within minutes and thereby contribute to the acute-phase reaction [11]. In contrast, cytokines and chemokines act more slowly and, through their direct action and the recruitment of other leukocytes, are responsible for the late-phase reaction [12]. Symptoms of the late-phase reaction involve more chronic edema and smooth muscle constriction and typically occur hours after initiation of the allergic response.

Whereas peanut allergy involves the recognition of proteins specific only to peanut by IgE, another type of IgE-mediated food allergy, called pollen-food allergy syndrome (oral-allergy syndrome), involves the recognition of proteins common to multiple foods. Patients with pollen-food allergy syndrome have IgE antibodies to certain aeroallergens, such as birch tree pollen and ragweed pollen, as part of their allergic rhinitis. These IgE antibodies target certain allergens, such as Bet v1 within birch pollen, that have been found to cross-react with proteins that are commonly found in many fruits and vegetables as well as in certain nuts and spices [13] (table 3). Mast cells localized to the mouth and oropharynx are primarily involved and cause itching, tingling and occasional swelling of the lips, tongue, palate, throat and ears. Other target organs are rarely involved, causing some to think of pollen-food allergy syndrome as a form of contact dermatitis rather than a systemic disease. Symptoms are typically transient and mild, although they can increase in intensity during the corresponding pollen season (spring for birch pollen, fall for ragweed pollen, etc.). Raw forms of the food are typically implicated, as cooking of the foods has been found to disrupt the binding epitopes, usually allowing for the safe ingestion of the foods [14]. An important exception to this phenomenon is seen with peanuts and tree nuts, as roasting seems to enhance the allergenicity of these foods.

An interesting exception to the immediate nature of IgE-mediated reactions has recently been described. Patients in the southern United States have reported allergic reactions after the ingestion of mammalian meats such as beef, pork, and lamb. IgE specific to a carbohydrate, galactose-alpha-1,3-galactose, that is present on the tissues of nonprimate mammals have been implicated [15]. These patients develop typical symptoms of histamine release such as flushing, hives, abdominal pain, emesis, cough, and wheeze; however, these symptoms typically do not present for up to 3–6 hours after ingestion. A relation to tick bites, specifically *Amblyomma americanum* (The Lone Star tick), has been suggested to explain the regional predilection [16]. The reasons for the delayed onset of reaction remain unclear, although the involvement of lipid absorption and chylomicrons has been proposed [17].

Non-IgE-Mediated Food Allergy

Non-IgE-mediated food allergies are more heterogeneous than IgE-mediated food allergies but are generally thought to involve cell-mediated immunity. One well-described example of this type of food allergy is celiac disease or gluten-sensitive enteropathy. With celiac disease, genetically susceptible people with the MHC Class II alleles HLA-DQ2 and HLA-DQ8 undergo activation of T-cells after the ingestion of gluten. These T-cells in turn release IFN-γ and other cytokines that cause tissue damage, resulting in the villous atrophy and crypt hypertrophy that are classically found upon endoscopy [18]. Clinically, these events lead to the malabsorption, watery diarrhea, and weight loss that are typical for celiac disease. With strict avoidance of gluten, the inflammatory response subsides, and the symptoms resolve.

Additional examples of non-IgE-mediated food allergy are food-protein induced gastrointestinal disorders. Food protein-induced enterocolitis syndrome (FPIES) is the most severe form of these disorders and affects infants in the first few months of life. Most commonly, with the introduction cow's milk or soy formula to the infant, these children develop recurrent emesis and diarrhea, with severe cases even leading to dehydration and hypotension. FPIES is thought to result from an inflammatory response in the gut, leading to increased intestinal permeability and fluid shift [19]. IgE testing is nearly always negative. Instead, FPIES has been presumed to be due to a cell-mediated T-cell response, perhaps through an overproduction of TNF-α and a deficiency of TGF-β [20]. However, at this time, definitive studies continue to be lacking. As with celiac disease, with strict avoidance, the symptoms promptly resolve and the child returns to normal.

Some clinicians, researchers, and laboratories have promoted the idea of food allergy driven by IgG molecules specific to foods. At this stage, the role of food-specific IgG is not entirely clear; however, there have been no definitive studies demonstrating a negative allergic response triggered by food-specific IgG. As such, the use of IgG testing for the diagnosis of food allergy has been strongly discouraged [1, 21]. In contrast, food-specific IgG is thought to represent prior exposure and tolerance to the food, with examples of this having been seen in studies of oral immunotherapy for food allergy [22].

Mixed-Immune Food Reactions

A third class of immune-mediated food reactions involves a mix of IgE-mediated and non-IgE-mediated responses. Atopic dermatitis and eosinophilic esophagitis (EoE) are two examples of mixed-immune food allergy. Atopic dermatitis is a chronic inflammatory skin disease that affects mostly children, although it can affect patients of all ages. It presents with extremely dry skin and itch that leads to scratching and a characteristic lichenified rash. An inflammatory response ensues, worsening the dry skin and continuing the itch-scratch cycle. A mixed-immune response involving IgE specific to foods and/or environmental allergens and excessive T_H2 signaling has classically been thought to cause the impaired barrier function seen in atopic dermatitis [23]; however, more recent studies have suggested that deficiencies of certain barrier proteins, such as filaggrin, may instead be the initial insult causing the barrier dysfunction [24]. With this new theory, the inherent, increased permeability of the skin permits allergen exposure to the immune system and the development of an IgE and T-cell response. This inflammatory response is then thought to exacerbate the barrier dysfunction, leading to what has been called the outside-inside-outside cycle [25]. The frequency of food allergy in atopic dermatitis patients has been shown to be increased, and avoidance has frequently led to improvement of the disease [26]. In addition, exacerbations of atopic dermatitis have been demonstrated during food challenges [27]; however, with this new paradigm, the exact role of foods is less clear.

Eosinophilic gastrointestinal diseases are another example of mixed-immune food allergic diseases, with EoE being the most recognized. EoE typically presents with abdominal pain, recurrent vomiting and food aversion in children and dysphagia and food impaction in adults. Endoscopies in these patients demonstrate increased eosinophils (>15 eos/hpf) and often other inflammatory changes [28]. A complex interplay between cell-mediated and IgE-mediated responses is thought to be responsible for these changes. The T_H2 response seems to play the major role in the pathogenesis of EoE, ultimately leading to the recruitment and maintenance of eosinophils in the esophagus [29]. Supporting a role for IgE in this process, the involvement of mast cells has been demonstrated [30], and clinical studies have shown symptomatic and histologic improvement with avoidance of skin test-identified food triggers [31]. However, like atopic dermatitis, much remains to be learned about this complex disease.

Oral Tolerance

The term tolerance is used to indicate a state of immunologic unresponsiveness to a stimulus. For food allergy, tolerance is typically used more specifically in reference to oral tolerance. All food antigens are foreign to the human immune system; however, the vast majority of foods do not cause symptoms upon ingestion due to oral tolerance. A defect in oral tolerance is thought to be the underlying cause of food allergy [32]. When food is ingested, mechanical digestion and the action of gastric acid and enzymes act as a first line of defense by breaking down food proteins. Secretory IgA also protects against potentially harmful food proteins by binding them and thereby preventing absorption. The remaining food proteins are then taken up by intestinal epithelial cells and dendritic cells through direct sampling or by specialized M cells in Peyer's patches and then presented to the immune system (fig. 2). Professional antigen-presenting cells then transport the antigen to the mesenteric lymph nodes, where tolerance is often induced. Depending on the dose of antigen, tolerance is achieved by two means, anergy or clonal deletion for high-dose exposures or suppression by regulatory T-cells for low-dose exposures

[33] (fig. 3). Anergy occurs when a T-cell interacts with an antigen-presenting cell without the appropriate co-stimulatory signals, while clonal deletion occurs via Fas-mediated apoptosis. Different subsets of regulatory T-cells, including the classical CD4+CD25+FoxP3+ regulatory T cell, the T_H3 cell and the T_R1 cell, have been described. These cells act to maintain tolerance by direct cell-to-cell contact, as in the case of the CD4+CD25+FoxP3+ regulatory T cell or through the secretion of pro-tolerogenic cytokines such as IL-10 by the T_R1 cell and TGF-β by the T_H3 cell. In addition to regulatory T-cells, suppressive CD8+ T-cells have been found to promote tolerance. A defect in this T-cell-induced suppression is suspected to result in the development of food allergy [34].

Recently, the use of food protein, in flour form, that is ingested (oral immunotherapy) and protein extract, in liquid form, that is held under the tongue (sublingual immunotherapy) has been investigated as potential treatments for food allergy. Similar to subcutaneous immunotherapy, which is used for allergic rhinitis and asthma, these therapies attempt to use a buildup and maintenance-dosing protocol to desensitize and ultimately induce tolerance. The preliminary results of these studies suggest that desensitization is possible, as demonstrated by the significant increase in the threshold of food allergen that is required to trigger a reaction while on the treatment [35–39]. This clinical improvement has been associated with the suppression of basophils, decrease in specific IgE and increase in specific IgG4 as well as the induction of regulatory T-cells [37, 38]. However, the exact mechanisms of the therapies remain unclear. In addition, the potential for these treatments to induce true immunological tolerance is unclear. Some food allergy research centers have described a small subset of patients who are able to successfully pass a blinded food challenge up to 3 months after discontinuing immunotherapy (unpublished data). Although this has been deemed by some to rep-

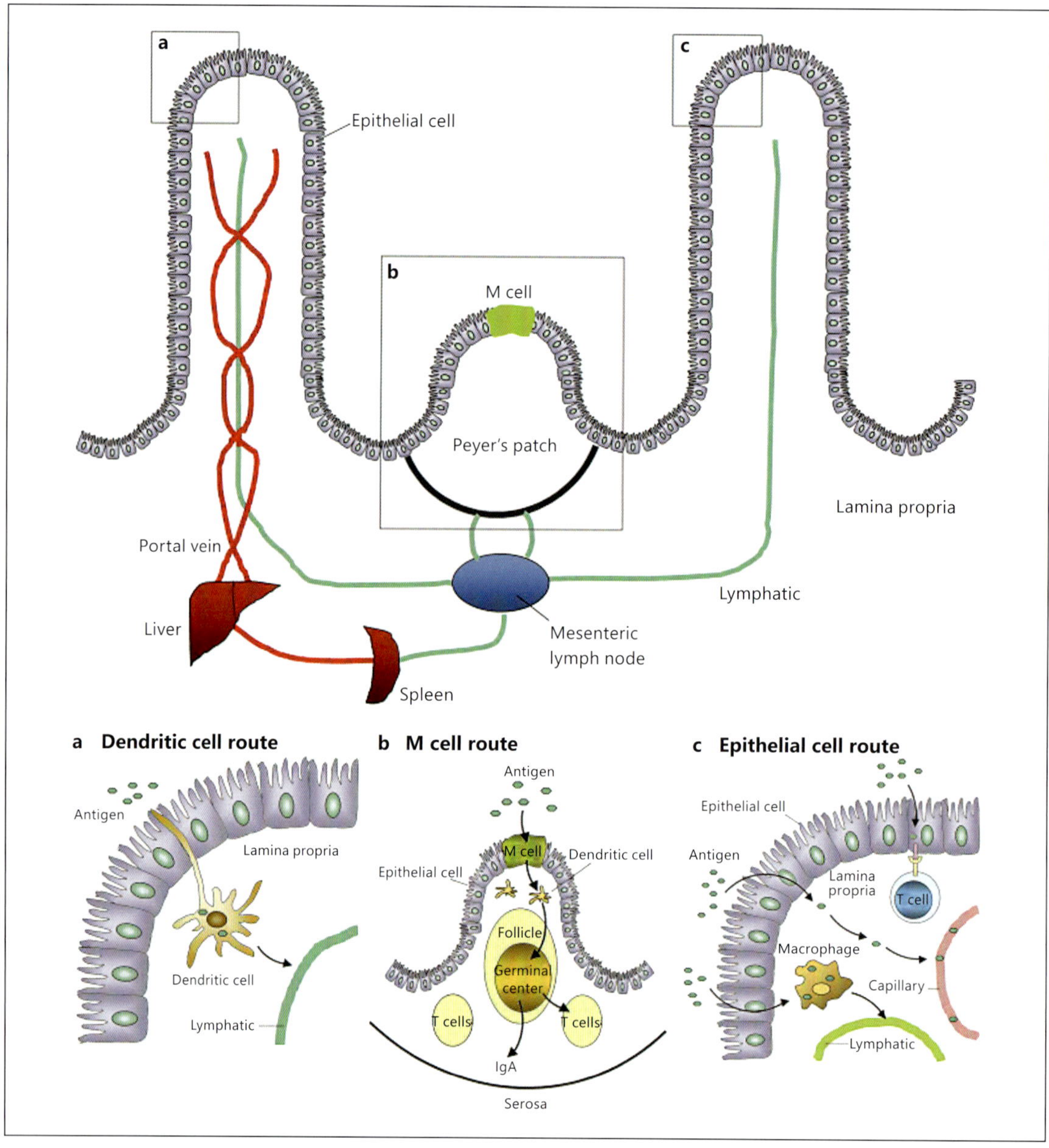

Fig. 2. Antigen uptake in the intestinal lumen. (Reprinted from Chehade M, Mayer L: Oral tolerance and its relation to food hypersensitivities. J Allergy Clin Immunol 2005;115:3–12, with permission from Elsevier.)

resent 'clinical tolerance', this is far from a cure, as important questions remain: What biomarkers define a tolerant state? How is a prolonged desensitized state differentiated from a truly tolerant state?

Conclusion

Although foods can cause a wide variety of reactions, the term food allergy is used to describe an abnormal immunological reaction to the inges-

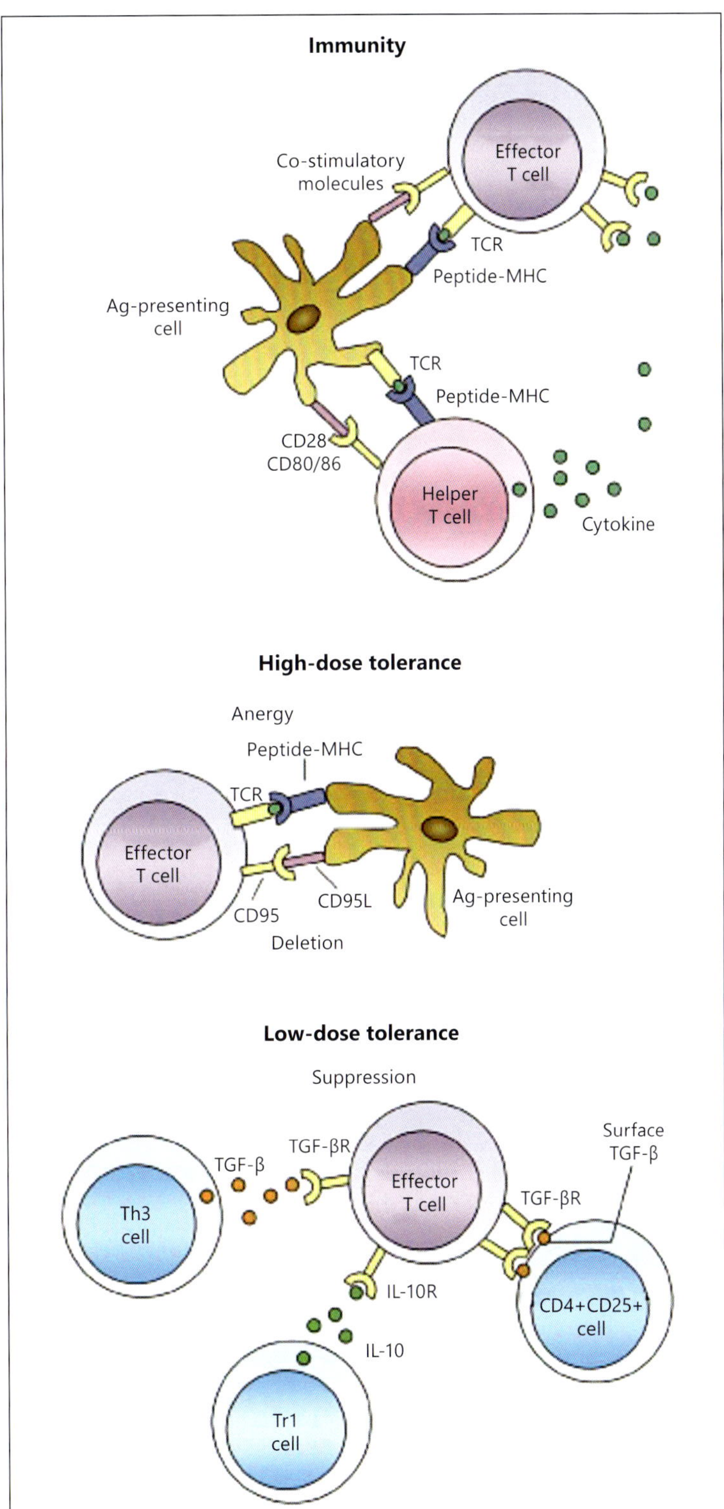

Fig. 3. Dose-dependent mechanisms of tolerance induction. (Reprinted from Chehade M, Mayer L: Oral tolerance and its relation to food hypersensitivities. J Allergy Clin Immunol 2005;115:3–12, with permission from Elsevier.)

tion of food. These reactions can be IgE-mediated, non-IgE-mediated, or a mixture of both. IgE-mediated reactions occur through the involvement of mast cells and their mediators, while non-IgE-mediated reactions are more heterogeneous but typically involve a delayed T-cell response. The pathogenesis of mixed reactions is frequently unclear but seems to revolve around a chronic T-cell inflammatory response with acute, IgE-driven exacerbations. All of these food allergy diseases likely stem from a breakdown of oral tolerance, which is the process by which humans can safely ingest foods. Current studies are seeking to artificially induce oral tolerance, but further work remains to be done.

References

1 Boyce JA, Assa'ad A, Burks AW, Jones SM, Sampson HA, Wood RA, Plaut M, Cooper SF, Fenton MJ, Arshad SH, Bahna SL, Beck LA, Byrd-Bredbenner C, Camargo CA Jr, Eichenfield L, Furuta GT, Hanifin JM, Jones C, Kraft M, Levy BD, Lieberman P, Luccioli S, McCall KM, Schneider LC, Simon RA, Simons FE, Teach SJ, Yawn BP, Schwaninger JM: Guidelines for the diagnosis and management of food allergy in the United States: report of the NIAID-sponsored expert panel. J Allergy Clin Immunol 2010;126(6 suppl):S1–S58.

2 Sicherer SH, Munoz-Furlong A, Godbold JH, Sampson HA: US prevalence of self-reported peanut, tree nut, and sesame allergy: 11-year follow-up. J Allergy Clin Immunol 2010;125:1322–1326.

3 Bock SA, Munoz-Furlong A, Sampson HA: Further fatalities caused by anaphylactic reactions to food, 2001–2006. J Allergy Clin Immunol 2007;119:1016–1018.

4 Hourihane JO, Dean TP, Warner JO: Peanut allergy in relation to heredity, maternal diet, and other atopic diseases: results of a questionnaire survey, skin prick testing, and food challenges. BMJ 1996;313:518–521.

5 Lopez-Exposito I, Song Y, Jarvinen KM, Srivastava K, Li XM: Maternal peanut exposure during pregnancy and lactation reduces peanut allergy risk in offspring. J Allergy Clin Immunol 2009; 124:1039–1046.

6 Vadas P, Wai Y, Burks W, Perelman B: Detection of peanut allergens in breast milk of lactating women. JAMA 2001; 285:1746–1748.

7 Kramer MS, Kakuma R: Maternal dietary antigen avoidance during pregnancy or lactation, or both, for preventing or treating atopic disease in the child. Cochrane Database Syst Rev 2012; 9:CD000133.

8 Caughey GH: Roles of mast cell tryptase and chymase in airway function. Am J Physiol 1989;257:L39–L46.

9 Schwartz LB, Yunginger JW, Miller J, Bokhari R, Dull D: Time course of appearance and disappearance of human mast cell tryptase in the circulation after anaphylaxis. J Clin Invest 1989;83:1551–1555.

10 Jarvinen KM: Food-induced anaphylaxis. Curr Opin Allergy Clin Immunol 2011;11:255–261.

11 Boyce JA: Mast cells and eicosanoid mediators: a system of reciprocal paracrine and autocrine regulation. Immunol Rev 2007;217:168–185.

12 Galli SJ, Tsai M, Piliponsky AM: The development of allergic inflammation. Nature 2008;454:445–454.

13 Katelaris CH: Food allergy and oral allergy or pollen-food syndrome. Curr Opin Allergy Clin Immunol 2010;10: 246–251.

14 Hofmann A, Burks AW: Pollen food syndrome: update on the allergens. Curr Allergy Asthma Rep 2008;8:413–417.

15 Commins SP, Satinover SM, Hosen J, Mozena J, Borish L, Lewis BD, Woodfolk JA, Platts-Mills TA: Delayed anaphylaxis, angioedema, or urticaria after consumption of red meat in patients with IgE antibodies specific for galactose-alpha-1,3-galactose. J Allergy Clin Immunol 2009;123:426–433.

16 Commins SP, James HR, Kelly LA, Pochan SL, Workman LJ, Perzanowski MS, Kocan KM, Fahy JV, Nganga LW, Ronmark E, Cooper PJ, Platts-Mills TA: The relevance of tick bites to the production of IgE antibodies to the mammalian oligosaccharide galactose-alpha-1,3-galactose. J Allergy Clin Immunol 2011; 127:1286–1293.e6.

17 Commins SP, Platts-Mills TA: Delayed anaphylaxis to red meat in patients with IgE specific for galactose alpha-1,3-galactose (alpha-gal). Curr Allergy Asthma Rep 2013;13:72–77.

18 Kagnoff MF: Celiac disease: pathogenesis of a model immunogenetic disease. J Clin Invest 2007;117:41–49.

19 Caubet JC, Nowak-Wegrzyn A: Current understanding of the immune mechanisms of food protein-induced enterocolitis syndrome. Expert Rev Clin Immunol 2011;7:317–327.

20 Chung HL, Hwang JB, Park JJ, Kim SG: Expression of transforming growth factor beta1, transforming growth factor type I and II receptors, and TNF-alpha in the mucosa of the small intestine in infants with food protein-induced enterocolitis syndrome. J Allergy Clin Immunol 2002;109:150–154.

21 Stapel SO, Asero R, Ballmer-Weber BK, Knol EF, Strobel S, Vieths S, Kleine-Tebbe J, Force ET: Testing for IgG4 against foods is not recommended as a diagnostic tool: EAACI Task Force Report. Allergy 2008;63:793–796.

22 Jones SM, Pons L, Roberts JL, Scurlock AM, Perry TT, Kulis M, Shreffler WG, Steele P, Henry KA, Adair M, Francis JM, Durham S, Vickery BP, Zhong X, Burks AW: Clinical efficacy and immune regulation with peanut oral immunotherapy. J Allergy Clin Immunol 2009;124:292–300.e1–e97.

23 Leung DY, Soter NA: Cellular and immunologic mechanisms in atopic dermatitis. J Am Acad Dermatol 2001; 44(1 suppl):S1–S12.

24 Palmer CN, Irvine AD, Terron-Kwiatkowski A, Zhao Y, Liao H, Lee SP, Goudie DR, Sandilands A, Campbell LE, Smith FJ, O'Regan GM, Watson RM, Cecil JE, Bale SJ, Compton JG, DiGiovanna JJ, Fleckman P, Lewis-Jones S, Arseculeratne G, Sergeant A, Munro CS, El Houate B, McElreavey K, Halkjaer LB, Bisgaard H, Mukhopadhyay S, McLean WH: Common loss-of-function variants of the epidermal barrier protein filaggrin are a major predisposing factor for atopic dermatitis. Nat Genet 2006;38: 441–446.

25 Elias PM, Schmuth M: Abnormal skin barrier in the etiopathogenesis of atopic dermatitis. Curr Opin Allergy Clin Immunol 2009;9:437–446.

26 Sicherer SH, Sampson HA: Food hypersensitivity and atopic dermatitis: pathophysiology, epidemiology, diagnosis, and management. J Allergy Clin Immunol 1999;104:S114–S122.

27 Breuer K, Heratizadeh A, Wulf A, Baumann U, Constien A, Tetau D, Kapp A, Werfel T: Late eczematous reactions to food in children with atopic dermatitis. Clin Exp Allergy 2004;34:817–824.

28 Prasad GA, Talley NJ, Romero Y, Arora AS, Kryzer LA, Smyrk TC, Alexander JA: Prevalence and predictive factors of eosinophilic esophagitis in patients presenting with dysphagia: a prospective study. Am J Gastroenterol 2007;102: 2627–2632.

29 Straumann A, Bauer M, Fischer B, Blaser K, Simon HU: Idiopathic eosinophilic esophagitis is associated with a T(H)2-type allergic inflammatory response. J Allergy Clin Immunol 2001; 108:954–961.

30 Abonia JP, Blanchard C, Butz BB, Rainey HF, Collins MH, Stringer K, Putnam PE, Rothenberg ME: Involvement of mast cells in eosinophilic esophagitis. J Allergy Clin Immunol 2010;126:140–149.

31 Spergel JM, Brown-Whitehorn TF, Cianferoni A, Shuker M, Wang ML, Verma R, Liacouras CA: Identification of causative foods in children with eosinophilic esophagitis treated with an elimination diet. J Allergy Clin Immunol 2012;130: 461–467.e5.

32 Burks AW, Laubach S, Jones SM: Oral tolerance, food allergy, and immunotherapy: implications for future treatment. J Allergy Clin Immunol 2008;121: 1344–1350.

33 Friedman A, Weiner HL: Induction of anergy or active suppression following oral tolerance is determined by antigen dosage. Proc Natl Acad Sci U S A 1994; 91:6688–6692.

34 Bennett CL, Christie J, Ramsdell F, Brunkow ME, Ferguson PJ, Whitesell L, Kelly TE, Saulsbury FT, Chance PF, Ochs HD: The immune dysregulation, polyendocrinopathy, enteropathy, X-linked syndrome (IPEX) is caused by mutations of FOXP3. Nat Genet 2001; 27:20–21.

35 Buchanan AD, Green TD, Jones SM, Scurlock AM, Christie L, Althage KA, Steele PH, Pons L, Helm RM, Lee LA, Burks AW: Egg oral immunotherapy in nonanaphylactic children with egg allergy. J Allergy Clin Immunol 2007;119: 199–205.

36 Skripak JM, Nash SD, Rowley H, Brereton NH, Oh S, Hamilton RG, Matsui EC, Burks AW, Wood RA: A randomized, double-blind, placebo-controlled study of milk oral immunotherapy for cow's milk allergy. J Allergy Clin Immunol 2008;122:1154–1160.

37 Varshney P, Jones SM, Scurlock AM, Perry TT, Kemper A, Steele P, Hiegel A, Kamilaris J, Carlisle S, Yue X, Kulis M, Pons L, Vickery B, Burks AW: A randomized controlled study of peanut oral immunotherapy: clinical desensitization and modulation of the allergic response. J Allergy Clin Immunol 2011;127:654–660.

38 Kim EH, Bird JA, Kulis M, Laubach S, Pons L, Shreffler W, Steele P, Kamilaris J, Vickery B, Burks AW: Sublingual immunotherapy for peanut allergy: clinical and immunologic evidence of desensitization. J Allergy Clin Immunol 2011; 127:640–646.e1.

39 Fleischer DM, Burks AW, Vickery BP, Scurlock AM, Wood RA, Jones SM, Sicherer SH, Liu AH, Stablein D, Henning AK, Mayer L, Lindblad R, Plaut M, Sampson HA, Consortium of Food Allergy Research (CoFAR): Sublingual immunotherapy for peanut allergy: a randomized, double-blind, placebo-controlled multicenter trial. J Allergy Clin Immunol 2013;131:119–127.e1–e7.

Edwin H. Kim, MD
Division of Rheumatology, Allergy and Immunology
Department of Medicine
University of North Carolina at Chapel Hill
3300 Thurston Bldg., CB#7280
Chapel Hill, NC 27599 (USA)
E-Mail edwinkim@med.unc.edu

Ebisawa M, Ballmer-Weber BK, Vieths S, Wood RA (eds): Food Allergy: Molecular Basis and Clinical Practice.
Chem Immunol Allergy. Basel, Karger, 2015, vol 101, pp 18–29 (DOI: 10.1159/000371647)

Food Allergens: Molecular and Immunological Aspects, Allergen Databases and Cross-Reactivity

Anne-Regine Lorenz · Stephan Scheurer · Stefan Vieths

Paul-Ehrlich-Institut, Langen, Germany

Abstract

The currently known food allergens are assigned to a relatively small number of protein families. Food allergens grouped into protein families share common functional and structural features that can be attributed to the allergenic potency and potential cross-reactivity of certain proteins. Molecular data, in terms of structural information, biochemical characteristics and clinical relevance for each known allergen, including isoforms and variants, are mainly compiled into four open-access databases. Allergens are designated according to defined criteria by the World Health Organization and the International Union of Immunological Societies Allergen Nomenclature Sub-committee. Food allergies are caused by primary sensitisation to the disease-eliciting food allergens (class I food allergen), or they can be elicited as a consequence of a primary sensitisation to inhalant allergens and subsequent IgE cross-reaction to homologous proteins in food (class II food allergens). Class I and class II allergens display different clinical significance in children and adults and are characterised by different molecular features. In line with this, high stability when exposed to gastrointestinal digestion and heat treatment is attributed to many class I food allergens that frequently induce severe reactions. The stability of a food allergen is determined by its molecular characteristics and can be influenced by structural (chemical) modifications due to thermal processing. Moreover, the immunogenicity and allergenicity of food allergens further depends on specific T cell and B cell epitopes. Although the T cell epitope pattern can be highly diverse for individual patients, several immuno-prominent T cell epitopes have been identified. Such conserved T cell epitopes and IgE cross-reactive B cell epitopes contribute to cross-reactivity between food allergens of the same family and to clinical cross-reactivity, similar to the birch pollen-food syndrome.

© 2015 S. Karger AG, Basel

Molecular Features of Food Allergens

Allergen Families

Only a small number of proteins to which humans are exposed via the inhalative, ingestive or cutaneous route are known as allergens. In order to attribute the allergenic potency of a certain protein to molecular features, known allergens have been grouped into protein families according to common structural features [1].

Currently, more than a thousand allergens are included in the AllFam (http://www.meduniwien.ac.at/allergens/allfam/) database. The protein families in AllFam refer to those of the Pfam database (http://pfam.sanger.ac.uk/), which is a large collection of protein families. Proteins generally comprise one or more functional domains, and identifying the domains present in a protein can provide insights into the function of that protein. The Pfam 27.0 (March 2013) database contains 14,831 protein families and includes about 80% of all sequence entries in the UniProt Knowledgebase. The majority of allergens in the AllFam database belong to a restricted number of 186 protein families, and the current AllFam database includes 399 food allergens that are grouped into 71 protein families. Remarkably, the majority of food allergens (>60%, n = 257) are assigned to only 10 protein families:

1. Prolamin superfamily (n = 65).
2. Cupin superfamily (n = 41).
3. EF-hand domain protein family (n = 37).
4. Tropomyosins (n = 35).
5. Profilins (n = 25).
6. Bet v 1-like proteins (n = 18).
7. Alpha/beta caseins (n = 10).
8. Hevein-like proteins (n = 9).
9. Thaumatins (n = 9).
10. Class I chitinases (n = 8).

The prolamin superfamily derives its name from the alcohol soluble proline- and glutamine-rich storage proteins of cereals. Members of this family are characterised by the presence of a conserved pattern of six or eight cysteine residues that form three or four intra-molecular disulphide bonds and the presence of an alpha-helical globular domain. Members of the prolamin superfamily include, among others, cereal proteins such as glutenin and gliadin, the non-specific lipid transfer proteins (nsLTPs) (e.g. Pru p 3 from peach, Hel a 3 from sunflower seed) and the 2S albumins, which are seed-storage proteins (e.g. Sin a 1 from yellow mustard, Ber e 1 from Brazil nut, Jug r 1 from English walnut, Cor a 14 from hazelnut, and Ara h 2 and Ara h 6 from peanut). Cupins are a large superfamily of proteins that have a common origin and immensely diverse functions. Allergenic cupins comprise the 7/8S globulins (vicilins) (e.g. Ara h 1 from peanut, Jug r 2 from walnut) and the 11S globulins (legumins) (e.g. Ara h 3 from peanut, Fag e 1 from buckwheat). Proteins with EF-hand domains include calcium-binding proteins such as parvalbumins, which are allergens from fish (e.g. Sal s 1 from salmon) and amphibians (e.g. Ran e 1 and 2 from edible frog), as well as troponin C and sarcoplasmic calcium-binding protein in crustaceans (e.g. Hom a 6 from lobster and Cra c 4 from shrimp, respectively). Tropomyosins have been identified as food allergens in crustaceans (e.g. Pen a 1 from shrimp, Cha f 1 from crab) and molluscs (e.g. Hel as 1 from snail, Tod p 1 from squid). Interestingly, vertebrate tropomyosins seem to be non-allergenic. Profilins are ubiquitous in all eukaryotic cells and therefore constitute a pan-allergenic structure. However, allergenic profilins are found almost exclusively in plants. Bet v 1-like proteins belong to the pathogenesis-related PR-10 protein family and are known as birch pollen-related food allergens (e.g. Mal d 1 from apple, Cor a 1.04 from hazelnut, Dau c 1 from carrot, Gly m 4 from soybean, and many others). The allergens from the alpha/beta caseins include milk allergens from cow, sheep and goat. Hevein-like proteins are characterised by a hevein-like domain, which is thought to be involved in the recognition or binding of chitin subunits (e.g. the hevein-like domain is the N-terminus of the major latex allergen prohevein (Hev b 6.01)). A number of plant and fungal proteins contain one or more copies of the hevein-like domain (e.g. wheat allergen Tri a 18, which contains four hevein-like domains). Thaumatin-like proteins in plants are pathogenesis-related proteins of the PR-5 family that are induced during ripening (e.g. Cup a 1 from bell pepper, Pru av 2 from cherry). Class I chitinases catalyse the hydrolysis of chitin polymers and function in the plant's defence against fungal and insect pathogens by destroying their chitin-containing cell wall (e.g. Mus a 2 from banana, Cas s 5 from chestnut, and Pers a 1 from avocado). Noteworthy, class I chitinases contain an N-terminal hevein-like domain that is homologous to latex hevein. Consequently, the above-mentioned class I chitinases also belong to the group of hevein-like domains.

In addition to allocating allergens to protein families, Radauer and colleagues classified allergens by their structural and functional features [1]. Using the Structural Classification of Proteins database, allergens with known 3-dimensional structure were grouped into 138 structural families, representing only 5% of all known families in the Structural Classification of Proteins database. Functional features were assigned to allergens according to the Gene Ontology (GO) database, which discriminates the functions of protein families by hierarchical order. Radauer and colleagues [1] assigned many but not all of the allergens to 351 different GO terms, such as (1) Molecular function, (2) Biological process and (3) Cellular component, which are three heading GO terms that contain many of the allergens. Within these three major GO terms are subcategories containing food allergen families. Examples of such further GO terms and assigned protein families are the following: (1) Molecular function, e.g. calcium ion-binding (sarcoplasmic calcium-binding proteins, parvalbumins, troponin C), nsLTPs, nutrient reservoir (prolamin and cupin superfamilies) or hydrolase activity (class I chitinases); (2) Biological process: e.g. transport (nsLTP, serum albumin, caseins); and (3) Cellular component: e.g. cytoskeleton (profilins). As allergen families without GO annotations, tropomyosins and thaumatin-like proteins, among others, were described by Radauer and colleagues.

Intrinsic immune-modulating properties similar to the MD2/TLR2-binding activity of the house dust mite allergen Der p 2 [2] have not yet been described for food allergens. However, few studies have investigated the influence of food allergens, e.g. milk proteins, on the tight junctions of intestinal epithelial cells that form a barrier against paraepithelial transport of ingestive proteins. The milk allergens β-lactoglobulin and bovine serum albumin have a stabilising effect on intestinal tight junctions, whereas hydrolysed peptides of the two allergens have an opposite effect on tight junctions [3]. Moreover, a peptide of cow's milk, derived from casein Bos d 10, enhanced epithelial barrier function [4].

Allergen Databases
Apart from the above-mentioned AllFam database, more open-access databases have compiled molecular and sometimes clinical data of allergens. The Allergen Nomenclature database represents the official list of allergens that have been approved by the World Health Organization and the International Union of Immunological Societies (WHO/IUIS) Allergen Nomenclature Subcommittee (http://www.allergen.org/). The Allergen Nomenclature system was founded in 1986 and was revised in 1994. This database lists all allergens based on an official denomination that has been approved by the Allergen Nomenclature Subcommittee. The criteria for official acceptance are that the allergen binds to specific IgE antibodies from the sera of at least 5 patients and that the prevalence of IgE reactivity is at least 5% in the respective patient collective. The allergen needs to be characterised by amino acid or DNA sequence and by additional molecular characteristics such as molecular weight or post-translational modifications. Two (or more) members of

the Executive Committee of the Allergen Nomenclature Subcommittee will review the submission and assess whether the allergen fulfils the molecular and immunological requirements for inclusion into the Allergen Nomenclature database. The allergen's official name is assigned according to the taxonomic name of the source organism (used by UniProt and NCBI), in Latin, and consists of the genus (3–4 letters) and the species (1–2 letters) as well as a subsequent numbering that usually indicates a certain protein family. Example: The first birch (*Betula verrucosa*) pollen allergen to be characterised according to the criteria of the Allergen Nomenclature Subcommittee has been named Bet v 1. Additionally, the Allergen Nomenclature database contains isoallergens that are of the same molecular weight, have identical biological function, belong to the same protein family and share an amino acid sequence identity of at least 67%. An important prerequisite for acceptance is demonstration of the IgE-binding activity of isoallergens, which are characterised by the subsequent two numbers, e.g. Bet v 1.01 and Bet v 1.02. Allergen sequences with closely related amino acid sequences (≥97% amino acid identity) are called isovariants and are designated by two additional numbers, e.g. Bet v 1.0201 and Bet v 1.0202 (the first two numbers characterise the isoallergen, and the last two numbers identify the isovariant). The Allergen Nomenclature database represents a uniform system of characterisation and denomination of allergens and is widely accepted in the field of allergology. The database from March 2014 comprises 771 allergens, of which 264 are food allergens.

The database 'Allergome – The Platform for Allergen Knowledge' (http://www.allergome.org) provides comprehensive information on allergenic sources and single allergens, including various aspects such as biochemistry, structure, function, molecular biology, immunochemistry, allergenicity, genetics, and epidemiology, and provides information on source tissues, route of exposure and isoallergens. Links are given to sequence databases, and pictures of the allergen sources are presented. Allergome started in 2002 but actually contains data from back to 1987 and (with gaps) even data from the early sixties of the last century, thus providing approximately 7,000 entries. Similar to the IUIS Database, Allergome focuses on molecules causing type I allergies. The information in Allergome is extracted from international, peer-reviewed scientific journals, other publications, and web-based sources. Allergome not only lists allergens that have been officially accepted by the IUIS Allergen Nomenclature Subcommittee but also additional molecules that have been reported as potential allergens. The Allergome database is usually updated several times per week. In contrast to the IUIS database, the scientific information in Allergome that has been extracted from the literature is not peer-reviewed by an independent expert panel.

The database 'Allfam – A Database of Allergen Families' (http://www.meduniwien.ac.at/aller gens/allfam/) is maintained by the Biochemistry and Bioinformatics group located in the Department of Pathophysiology and Allergy Research of the Medical University of Vienna, Austria [1]. AllFam groups allergens into protein families and tries to help answer questions such as the following: What makes a protein an allergen? Which allergens potentially facilitate IgE cross-reactivity? However, it has to be kept in mind that the vast majority of members of an allergen-containing protein family are usually not allergenic and that not all allergenic members of a protein family are cross-reactive. The sources of AllFam are the two databases Allergome and Pfam. In Pfam, allergens with known sequences are grouped into a protein family based on sequence alignments and hidden Markov models. Allergens that are multi-domain proteins are merged into a single AllFam family if the Pfam domain of these allergens occurs only in combination with a single other Pfam domain (e.g. propeptides of proteases that occur only with certain catalytic domains). Domains that are a part of proteins from different families represent separate AllFam families, e.g. the hevein-like domain. The actual update of the March 2014 AllFam is from 2011–09–12 and is based on Allergome version 2011–09–06 and Pfam 25.0 of March 2011 (the current version in March 2014 is Pfam 27.0 of March 2013). The actual version of the March 2014 AllFam contains 1,091 allergens, of which 995 are assigned into 186 protein families, and the 399 food allergens in AllFam are restricted to 71 protein families.

Allergen Online (http://www.allergenonline.org/) is a comprehensive allergen database that is maintained by the Food Allergy Research and Resource of the Department of Food Science and Technology at the University of Nebraska in Lincoln. AllergenOnline is intended for the identification of proteins that may present a potential risk of allergenic cross-reactivity, and it contains allergen sequences that have been peer-reviewed according to defined criteria. In Allergen Online, allergens are accepted only after a review process involving two international experts per allergen entry. According to the level of clinical information that is available for the respective protein sequences, potential allergens are classified as 'allergen', 'putative', or 'unproven'. The database is intended to compare the sequences of new proteins (in genetically modified crops or in a novel food) with known allergens as part of the safety assessment of, for example, genetically modified crop plants. Using the FASTA format, the database performs full-length alignments of newly identified allergens with allergens already existing in AllergenOnline. It is assumed that cross-reactivity is not likely for proteins with less than 50% identity over the entire protein sequence, but cross-reactivity is fairly common for those with higher than 70% identity. As a second option, AllergenOnline offers scans of each possible 80 amino acid segment of the target protein, looking for matches of at least 35% identity; this method has been suggested as a more reliable threshold for evaluating proteins in genetically modified

crops by a Codex Alimentarius publication in 2003. As a third option, eight identical consecutive amino acids have been suggested in a Food and Agriculture Organization (FAO)/WHO 2001 document to assess the allergenicity of genetically modified food, but this approach results in many false-positive hits. The project is funded by the agro-biotech industry. AllergenOnline is updated once a year, usually in February. The actual version, #14, is from 2014–01–20 and includes 1,706 sequences in 645 taxonomic groups.

Class I Food Allergens/Class II Food Allergens

Food allergies are allergic reactions that occur after ingestion of food. These allergic reactions are either caused by primary sensitisation to disease-eliciting food allergens, leading to symptoms upon secondary contact when ingesting the same allergen (class I food allergen), or can be elicited as a consequence of a primary sensitisation to inhalant allergens and subsequent IgE cross-reaction to homologous proteins in food (class II food allergens).

Class I Food Allergens

It is assumed that several food allergens act as a primary sensitising agent via the gut and elicit an allergic reaction upon ingestion of the food. These class I food allergens are also called 'classical', 'true' or 'complete' food allergens. There is some evidence that primary sensitisation to peanut may also occur by exposure to the skin [5]; however, urticaria elicited by skin contact with food proteins is not classified as a food allergy.

Examples of class I food allergens include the peanut allergens Ara h 1 and Ara h 2, the crustacean allergen tropomyosin, the bovine milk allergens β-lactoglobulin Bos d 5 and α-lactalbumin Bos d 4, the hen's egg allergens Gal d 1 and Gal d 2, soybean allergens (e.g. Gly m 5, Gly m 6), the fish allergen parvalbumin (e.g. Gad c 1 from codfish), and probably nsLTP allergens in plant-derived food (e.g. Pru p 3 from peach, Mal d 3 from apple). Food allergy in infants and small children is usually caused by class I food allergens. It has been reported that several class I food allergens display linear IgE epitopes (see the section on B cell epitopes), and the presence of linear epitopes has been associated with food allergies persisting after childhood [6]. Sensitisation to class I food allergens is often associated with severe and sometimes anaphylactic reactions and is thought to be related to the high stability of most of these allergens to digestive enzymes and high temperature.

Class II Food Allergens

Class II food allergens are considered to possess low immunogenicity upon ingestion. IgE reactivity to class II food allergens results from primary sensitisation to homologous allergens from a different source, particularly inhalant allergens such as weed, tree or grass pollen, and subsequent cross-reactivity of IgE antibodies with the respective food proteins from the same protein family. IgE cross-reactivity can develop upon primary sensitisation by a mechanism described as epitope spreading [7]. Class II food allergens are mainly involved in certain allergy syndromes, such as the birch-food syndrome (birch pollen-related food allergy), mugwort-celery/spices syndrome, plane tree pollen-food syndrome, bird-hen's egg syndrome, or latex-fruit syndrome. Several class II allergens are considered as pan-allergens and are highly conserved in many plant or animal species. Examples of class II allergens are food allergens from the Bet v 1 family (e.g. Mal d 1 and Cor a 1.04), Bet v 6-homologous proteins, profilins (e.g. Mal d 4 and Cor a 2), and serum albumins (e.g. Gal d 5 from hen's egg, which contributes to the bird-egg syndrome). In contrast to class I food allergens, sensitisation to class II food allergens is more prevalent in adolescents and adults. Sensitisation to class II food allergens is frequently associated with mild oral or mild systemic reactions, presumably due to the rela-

tively low stability of these allergens. A typical clinical symptom of pollen-related food allergy is the oral allergy syndrome.

Resistance to Food Processing and Digestion

Many class I food allergens are highly stable when exposed to gastrointestinal digestion and heat treatment. Stable allergens are presented to the immune system of the gut in a more or less intact form. Examples of such molecules are Ara h 2 and Ara h 6 from peanut or nsLTP allergens from several plant-derived foods. In contrast, class II food allergens, such as Bet v 1-related proteins or profilins, are relatively unstable when exposed to digestive enzymes and thermal processing. Nevertheless, the impact of the food matrix on the sensitisation capacity and properties eliciting allergic symptoms needs to be considered for both, class I and class II allergens.

Thermal Stability of Allergens

Heat treatment is the most important step in food processing, e.g. cooking, roasting, baking, sterilisation or pasteurisation, for increasing the storage stability of food products. Heat treatment results in denaturation of proteins, which is characterised by loss of tertiary structure and sometimes oligomerisation and crosslinking of proteins, and therefore a loss of conformational IgE epitopes. Other possible modifications of proteins during heating are alterations of the amino acid side-chains and reactions of the protein allergens with other molecules (proteins, carbohydrates and fatty acids) of the food matrix. Protein stability to thermal processing has been shown for several class I food allergens, e.g. the peanut allergens Ara h 1 and Ara h 2, nsLTPs in plant food, the hen's egg allergens Gal d 1 and Gal d 2, the bovine milk allergens casein, β-lactoglobulin, Bos d 5 and immunoglobulin Bos d 7, allergenic tropomyosin from crustaceae and other seafood, as well as the fish allergen parvalbumin. Molecular features enhancing the thermal stability of proteins include the following:

Intramolecular Disulphide Bonds. Prolamins (including 2S albumins and nsLTPs) are small, tightly packed, globular, alpha-helical proteins characterised by up to five intramolecular disulphide bonds that contribute to their high thermal resistance. In line with this, the 2S albumin-like peanut allergens Ara h 2 and Ara h 6 showed no change in secondary conformation when heated to 90°C [8]. Like prolamins, the β-lactoglobulins are globular proteins that are stabilised by two disulphide bonds, and their folding is not altered when heated to 65°C [9]. Likewise, the apple allergen nsLTP Mal d 3 was found to be very stable, and only intense heating led to the loss of one disulphide bond through oxidation and the decrease of IgE-binding activity and biological activity [10].

Ion-Binding. Parvalbumin, a protein with three EF-hands is considered to be stabilised by Ca^{2+}-binding, which is required for its structural integrity. Calcium depletion resulted in a change in its structure, as determined by circular dichroism spectroscopy [11]. This might explain why parvalbumin, despite it being cooked, retains the capacity to sensitise patients [12]. In contrast, it has been reported that no differences in thermal stability were found for the calcium-bound or calcium-depleted form of natural cod parvalbumin [13].

Protein Oligomerisation. It has been suggested that the tendency of certain parvalbumin isoforms to form oligomers might contribute to the maintenance of its allergenicity during heat processing [14]. Furthermore, the secondary structure of amandin, a hexameric major allergen of approximately 370 kDa from almond, was not affected by temperatures up to 90°C, whereas monomeric basic and acidic polypeptides showed lower thermal stability [15].

Chemical Modification. Among several chemical reactions that are triggered by thermal processing, glycation has been described to modulate the allergenicity of food proteins. Glycation, the reaction of reducing sugars with free amino groups on proteins, can take place during thermal processing or storage of food and is called the Maillard reaction. Glycation of proteins often impacts the tertiary structure of proteins and may consequently affect IgE-binding capacity, dendritic cell activation, and T cell reactivity. Studies have been performed using diverse allergens, such as the egg allergens ovalbumin (Gal d 2) and ovomucoid (Gal d 1) or allergens from peanut, milk (Bos d 5), soybean, seafood, hazelnut, apple, cherry and buckwheat. However, potential increase or decrease of allergenicity caused by the Maillard reaction cannot be predicted. Often, glycation of proteins induces a reduction of IgE-binding activity, but an increase in IgE binding or T cell reactivity has also been reported.

Usually, the heat stability of allergens is assessed by monitoring the integrity of their secondary structures using circular dichroism spectroscopy, their potential degradation by SDS-PAGE or chromatography, and their immune reactivity by IgE-binding assays with protein extracts or purified allergens. Thermal stability testing using this experimental setting has been shown to be strongly pH-dependent [16].

Influence of Digestion on Allergic Reaction to Food Allergens

Enzymatic digestion of food proteins takes place in the stomach, which secretes hydrochloric acid and pepsin and proceeds in the small intestine due to pancreatic enzymes, preferably trypsin and chymotrypsin. In order to assess the stability of food allergens to digestive enzymes, protein extracts or purified allergens were subjected to gastrointestinal fluids or purified enzyme preparations such as pepsin and trypsin, either separately or sequentially combined. Although food is frequently processed by heating, previous heating of allergens before simulating gastrointestinal digestion has not been performed in the majority of studies. However, heating is known to modify the digestibility of proteins. On the one hand, the accessibility of peptide bonds to proteases is enhanced by the unfolding of proteins upon heating. In line with this, the defolding of nsLTP Pru p 3 from peach results in enhanced enzymatic digestion by pepsin [17]. On the other hand, aggregates of allergens that are potentially formed after heating can display a reduced pepsin digestion rate, as reported for the legumin Ara h 3 from peanut and soy glycinin Gly m 6 [18].

In comparison to class I allergens, class II allergens often present reduced stability to digestive enzymes. Strong protein degradation upon pepsin treatment was reported for profilin (class II allergen) and Bet v 1-like (class II) allergens but was less pronounced for nsLTPs (class I allergens) [19, 20]. In line with this observation, the IgE reactivity of class II allergens upon digestion was diminished, whereas the allergenic potency of class I allergens, such as Ara h 2 from peanut, was retained [21, 22].

Influence of the Food Matrix on Digestion and Allergenicity of Food Allergens
The first studies demonstrated a potential impact of the food matrix, which mainly consists of other proteins, lipids and polysaccharides, on the digestibility or epithelial uptake of allergens and consequently on their stability, sensitisation capacity and allergenic potency. The pepsin digestion of kiwi allergen Act c 2, for example, is hampered by adding pectin from apple fruit [23]. Using representative class I (Bos d 5 and Cor a 8) and class II (Mal d 1) allergens, a delayed gastrointestinal degradation and epithelial transport of all three allergens was observed when in the presence of a protein-rich food matrix (here, hazelnut and peanut extracts) [24]. When heating egg white protein, e.g. ovomucoid together with wheat gluten, which mimics the baking process, the solubility of ovomucoid is reduced [25]. In addition, heating β-lactoglobulin results in the formation of intermolecular disulphide bonds

and subsequent binding to other food proteins, which was associated with a reduced allergenicity of β-lactoglobulin [26]. The Maillard reaction of ovalbumin with carbohydrates of the food matrix, enhances the T cell immunogenicity of ovalbumin [27].

Immunological Features of Food Allergens

T Cell and B Cell Epitopes of Food Allergens
The allergenicity of allergens is determined by the humoural and cellular immune responses as well as the reactivity of effector cells with allergen-specific epitopes. Epitopes are the specific binding sites of allergens for either IgE antibodies (B cell epitopes) or the T cell receptor on T lymphocytes (T cell epitopes).

T Cell Epitopes
T cell epitopes are short, linear peptides of 12–15 amino acids in length. Allergens are internalised by antigen-presenting cells (APCs), processed and presented to T cells, with MHC class II molecules, on the surface of APCs. The allergen-MHC II complexes on APCs are recognised by CD4$^+$ T helper cells via specific T cell receptors, which subsequently induce the maturation and expansion of B cells and the production of allergen-specific IgE. Multiple T cell epitopes have been identified on several food allergens, and numerous T cell epitopes on one food allergen can be recognised by individual patients [27]. Moreover, T cell epitope diversity has been reported between food-allergic subjects. Nevertheless, in several cases, immuno-dominant T cell epitopes were identified that were recognised by, for example, more than 50% of allergic individuals. Those allergen-specific T cell epitopes are important during the sensitisation phase and for the induction of peripheral tolerance. Rarely, an overlap between T cell and B cell epitopes has been found, as reported for Gal d 1 (chicken ovomucoid), a class I food allergen [28].

B Cell Epitopes

B cell epitopes are areas on the surface of allergens that bind to IgE antibodies. On many class I food allergens, consecutive amino acid stretches are found that bind IgE and have been termed sequential epitopes. Examples of allergens with sequential IgE-binding epitopes are Bos d 8 (caseins), Bos d 5 (β-lactoglobulin) and Bos d 4 (α-lactalbumin) in milk; Gal d 1 (ovomucoid) and Gal d 2 (ovalbumin) in eggs; Gad c 1 (parvalbumin) in cod; tropomyosins in shrimp species (Pen a 1, Cra c 1, Met e 1 and many more) and other seafood (lobster, crab, fish); and Ara h 1 (7S globulin vicilin), Ara h 2 (2S albumin conglutin) and Ara h 3 (11S globulin glycinin) in peanut. It remains unclear whether these short IgE-binding sequences present complete B cell epitopes and are able to fully account for the IgE-binding capacity of a given allergen or, in some cases, just represent substructures of conformational epitopes. The second type of B cell epitope is conformational, i.e. the amino acids involved in the contact with the antibody are located discontinuously in the protein sequence but are presented in the same area on the surface of a folded protein. Normally, 20 or more amino acids are involved and cover a relatively large part of the protein surface. The majority of B cell epitopes of food allergens is thought to be conformational.

Cross-Reactivity

Antibodies against a certain allergen potentially bind to other homologous allergens of the same protein family even though the subject has not been sensitised to the homologous allergen. This phenomenon is called cross-reactivity, and it increases the number of allergic sources against which a subject displays allergic reactions. For example, patients with allergy to tropomyosin from lobster (Hom a 1) may display allergic reactions to other foods containing highly similar tropomyosins, such as shrimps (Cha f 1, Cra c 1, Lit v 1, Met e 1, Pan b 1, Pen a 1, Pen I 1, Pen m 1, Por p 1) and other seafood, like lobster, fish and squid (Pan s 1, Ore m 4, Tod p 1) or garden snail (Hel as 1). However, cross-reactivity of food tropomyosins, in theory, is also possible with allergic tropomyosins from mites, such as German cockroach (Bla g 7), house dust mite (Der p 10, Der f 10) or other mites (Blo t 10, Chi k 10, Lep d 10, Per a 7, Tyr p 10), which are known elicitors of respiratory sensitisation. Another well-known example of IgE cross-reactivity occurs in allergic subjects sensitised against the major birch pollen allergen Bet v 1. The so-called Bet v 1 family comprises a large number of structurally related allergens in various food plants. Patients may develop clinical symptoms while consuming other foods containing Bet v 1-related allergens, such as apple (Mal d 1) and other *Rosaceae* fruit, kiwifruit (Act d 8), carrot (Dau c 1), celeriac (Api g 1), tomato (Sola l 4), peanut (Ara h 8) soybean (Gly m 4), hazelnut (Cor a 1.04) and several others (see table 1). It is very likely that sensitisation is caused by birch pollen via the respiratory route because it has been observed that, in most cases, (i) the pollen allergy precedes the food allergy, (ii) the food allergy against homologues of Bet v 1 without pollen sensitisation practically does not exist, and (iii) allergen-specific T cells proliferate more strongly upon stimulation by Bet v 1 compared to its food homologues. Apart from allergens of the Bet v 1 family, pollen-related food allergies can also be based on profilins, proteins of the Bet v 6 family, or nsLTPs (in Southern European countries). In addition, inhalation of pollen is known to cause sensitisation to particular cross-reactive carbohydrate determinants (CCDs) that are found on plant glycoproteins. The clinical relevance of IgE to CCDs is a subject of controversial discussion. It seems that CCD-specific IgE correlates only weakly with clinical food allergy. The plant species most clinically relevant to pollen-related food allergy in Europe are birch, mugwort and plane pollen. Latex is another non-pollen type of allergen source that causes food-related allergies of the so-called latex-

Table 1. Protein families containing cross-reactive food allergens

Protein family	Cross-reactivity possible between	Sources with potentially cross-reactive allergens*
Bet v 1-related family = pathogenesis-related PR-10 proteins	Food – Food	Food allergens in apple, cherry, apricot, pear, peach, raspberry, strawberry, kiwi, carrot, celery, tomato, hazelnut, peanut, soybean, mung bean, etc.
	Food – Inhalant (Pollen: 'Pollen-related food allergy', especially based on birch)	Inhalative allergens in pollen from birch, alder, hornbeam, oak, hazel tree, chestnut
Profilins	Food – Food	Food allergens in apples, sweet cherry, peach, pear, strawberry, orange, pineapple, kiwi, banana, melon, litchi, carrot, celery, tomato, bell pepper, mustard, peanut, soybean, hazelnut, almond, wheat, barley, rice, etc.
	Food – Inhalant (Pollen: 'Pollen-related food allergy', especially based on birch, ragweed and mugwort)	Inhalative allergens in pollen from birch, ragweed, mugwort, Bermuda grass, pellitory, timothy grass, annual mercury, lamb's quarters, Russian thistle, redroot pigweed, olive, date palm, hazel, sunflower, saffron crocus, rice, maize, etc.
	Food – Latex[1] ('Latex-fruit syndrome')	Latex
Lipid transfer proteins	Food – Food	Food allergens in peach, apricot, cherry, pear, apple, strawberry, plum, grape, mulberry, raspberry, orange, lemon, tangerine, kiwi, banana, celery, tomato, asparagus, lettuce, cauliflower, kidney bean, mustard, hazelnut, walnut, almond, sunflower seeds, peanut, maize, wheat, chestnut, etc.
	Food – Inhalant (Pollen: 'Pollen-related food allergy')	Inhalative allergens in pollen from ragweed, mugwort, pellitory, olive and, plane tree
	Food – Latex[1] ('Latex-fruit syndrome')	Latex
Bet v 6-related proteins	Food – Food	Food allergens in pear, carrot
	Food – Inhalant (Pollen: 'Pollen-related food allergy', based on birch)	Inhalative allergen in pollen from birch
Thaumatin-like proteins = PR-5	Food – Food	Food allergens in bell pepper, apple, cherry, peach, kiwi, banana
	Food – Inhalant (Pollen: 'Pollen-related food allergy')	Inhalative allergens in pollen from cypress, cedar

* The listed allergen sources contain allergens belonging to the respective allergen family. A cross-reactive reaction among the allergens of the same protein family is potentially possible but not inevitable. The food sources contain allergens that have been officially added to the IUIS list of official allergens.
[1] Latex can be an inhalant as well as a contact allergen.

fruit syndrome. However, due to the reduced use of latex derived products in hospitals, the importance of this syndrome is decreasing.

Cross-reactivity not only exists because of cross-reactive IgE antibodies but also on the T cell level. T cell cross-reactivity between Bet v 1 and the related food allergens Mal d 1 (apple) and Api g 1 (celeriac) occurs independently of IgE cross-reactivity. Remarkably, T cell-activating regions have been identified in corresponding homologous regions of all three allergens. In line with this, T cell cross-reactivity between Bet v 1 and the two food allergens Mal d 1 and Api g 1 could be demonstrated [29].

References

1   Radauer C, Bublin M, Wagner S, Mari A, Breiteneder H: Allergens are distributed into few protein families and possess a restricted number of biochemical functions. J Allergy Clin Immunol 2008;121: 847–852.
2   Trompette A, Divanovic S, Visintin A, Blanchard C, Hegde RS, Madan R, Thorne PS, Wills-Karp M, Gioannini TL, Weiss JP, Karp CL: Allergenicity resulting from functional mimicry of a Toll-like receptor complex protein. Nature 2009;457:585–588.
3   Hashimoto K, Takeda K, Nakayama T, Shimizu M: Stabilization of the tight junction of the intestinal Caco-2 cell monolayer by milk whey proteins. Biosc Biotech Biochem 1995;59:1951–1952.
4   Yatsumatsu H, Tanabe S: The casein peptide Asn-Pro-Trp-Asp-Gln enforces the intestinal tight junction partly by increasing occluding in Caco-2 cells. Br J Nutr 2010;104:9951–9956.
5   Fox AT, Sasieni P, du Toit G, Syed H, Lack G: Household peanut consumption as a risk factor for the development of peanut allergy. J Allergy Clin Immunol 2009;123:417–423.
6   Chatchatee P, Järvinen KM, Bardina L, Beyer K, Sampson HA: Identification of IgE- and IgG-binding epitopes on alpha(s1)-casein: differences in patients with persistent and transient cow's milk allergy. J Allergy Clin Immunol 2001; 107:379–383.
7   Gould HJ, Sutton BJ: IgE in allergy and asthma today. Nat Rev Immunol 2008;8: 205–217.
8   Lehmann K, Schweimer K, Reese G, Randow S, Suhr M, Becker WM, Vieths S, Rösch P: Structure and stability of 2S albumin-type peanut allergens: implications for the severity of peanut allergic reactions. Biochem J 2006;395:463–472.
9   Taheri-Kafrani A, Gaudin JC, Rabesona H, Nioi C, Agarwal D, Drouet M, Chobert JM, Bordbar AK, Haertle T: Effects of heating and glycation of beta-lactoglobulin on its recognition by IgE of sera from cow milk allergy patients. J Agric Food Chem 2009;57:4974–4982.
10   Sancho AI, Rigby NM, Zuidmeer L, Asero R, Mistrello G, Amato S, González-Mancebo E, Fernández-Rivas M, van Ree R, Mills EN: The effect of thermal processing on the IgE reactivity of the non-specific lipid transfer protein from apple, Mal d 3. Allergy 2005;60:1262–1268.
11   Griesmeier U, Bublin M, Radauer C, Vázquez-Cortés S, Ma Y, Fernández-Rivas M, Breiteneder H: Physicochemical properties and thermal stability of Lep w 1, the major allergen of whiff. Mol Nutr Food Res 2010;54:861–869.
12   Bugajska-Schretter A, Grote M, Vangelista L, Valent P, Sperr WR, Rumpold H, Pastore A, Reichelt R, Valenta R, Spitzauer S: Purification, biochemical, and immunological characterisation of a major food allergen: different immunoglobulin E recognition of the apo- and calcium-bound forms of carp parvalbumin. Gut 2000;46:661–669.
13   Ma Y, Griesmeier U, Susani M, Radauer C, Briza P, Erler A, Bublin M, Alessandri S, Himly M, Vàzquez-Cortés S, de Arellano IR, Vassilopoulou E, Saxoni-Papageorgiou P, Knulst AC, Fernández-Rivas M, Hoffmann-Sommergruber K, Breiteneder H: Comparison of natural and recombinant forms of the major fish allergen parvalbumin from cod and carp. Mol Nutr Food Res 2008; 52(suppl 2):S196–S207.
14   Cai QF, Liu GM, Li T, Hara K, Wang XC, Su WJ, Cao MJ: Purification and characterization of parvalbumins, the major allergens in red stingray (Dasyatis akajei). J Agric Food Chem 2010;58:12964–12969.
15   Albillos SM, Menhart N, Fu TJ: Structural stability of Amandin, a major allergen from almond (Prunus dulcis), and its acidic and basic polypeptides. J Agric Food Chem 2009;57:4698–4705.
16   Bublin M, Radauer C, Knulst A, Wagner S, Scheiner O, Mackie AR, Mills EN, Breiteneder H: Effects of gastrointestinal digestion and heating on the allergenicity of the kiwi allergens Act d 1, actinidin, and Act d 2, a thaumatin-like protein. Mol Nutr Food Res 2008;52: 1130–1139.
17   Toda M, Reese G, Gadermaier G, Schulten V, Lauer I, Egger M, Briza P, Randow S, Wolfheimer S, Kigongo V, Del Mar San Miguel Moncin M, Fötisch K, Bohle B, Vieths S, Scheurer S: Protein unfolding strongly modulates the allergenicity and immunogenicity of Pru p 3, the major peach allergen. J Allergy Clin Immunol 2011;128:1022–1030.
18   van Boxtel EL, Koppelman SJ, van den Broek LA, Gruppen H: Determination of pepsin-susceptible and pepsin-resistant epitopes in native and heat-treated peanut allergen Ara h 1. J Agric Food Chem 2008;56:2223–2230.
19   Scheurer S, Lauer I, Foetisch K, San Miguel Moncin M, Retzek M, Hartz C, Enrique E, Lidholm J, Cistero-Bahima A, Vieths S: Strong allergenicity of Pru av 3, the lipid transfer protein from cherry, is related to high stability against thermal processing and digestion. J Allergy Clin Immunol 2004;114:900–907.

20 Schimek EM, Zwölfer B, Briza P, Jahn-Schmid B, Vogel L, Vieths S, Ebner C, Bohle B: Gastrointestinal digestion of Bet v 1-homologous food allergens destroys their mediator-releasing, but not T cell-activating, capacity. J Allergy Clin Immunol 2005;116:1327–1333.

21 Sen M, Kopper R, Pons L, Abraham EC, Burks AW, Bannon GA: Protein structure plays a critical role in peanut allergen stability and may determine immunodominant IgE-binding epitopes. J Immunol 2002;169:882–887.

22 Untersmayr E, Jensen-Jarolim E: The role of protein digestibility and antacids on food allergy outcomes. J Allergy Clin Immunol 2008;121:1301–1308.

23 Polovic N, Blanusa M, Gavrovic-Jankulovic M, Atanaskovic-Markovic M, Burazer L, Jankov R, Cirkovic Velickovic T: A matrix effect in pectin-rich fruits hampers digestion of allergen by pepsin in vivo and in vitro. Clin Exp Allergy 2007;37:764.

24 Schulten V, Lauer I, Scheurer S, Thalhammer T, Bohle B: A food matrix reduces digestion and absorption of food allergens in vivo. Mol Nutr Food Res 2011;55:1484–1491.

25 Kato Y, Watanabe H, Matsuda T: Ovomucoid rendered insoluble by heating with wheat gluten but not with milk casein. Biosci Biotechnol Biochem 2000;64:198–201.

26 Thomas K, Herouet-Guicheney C, Ladics G, Bannon G, Cockburn A, Crevel R, Fitzpatrick J, Mills C, Privalle L, Vieths S: Evaluating the effect of food processing on the potential human allergenicity of novel proteins: international workshop report. Food Chem Toxicol 2007;45:1116–1122.

27 Bohle B: T-cell epitopes of food allergens. Clin Rev Allergy Immunol 2006;30:97–108.

28 Holen E, Bolann B, Elsayed S: Novel B and T cell epitopes of chicken ovomucoid (Gal d 1) induce T cell secretion of IL-6, IL-13, and IFN-gamma. Clin Exp Allergy 2001;31:952–964.

29 Jahn-Schmid B, Radakovics A, Lüttkopf D, Scheurer S, Vieths S, Ebner C, Bohle B: Bet v 1142-156 is the dominant T-cell epitope of the major birch pollen allergen and important for cross-reactivity with Bet v 1-related food allergens. J Allergy Clin Immunol. 2005;116:213–219.

30 Quirce S, Marañón F, Umpiérrez A, de las Heras M, Fernández-Caldas E, Sastre J: Chicken serum albumin (Gal d 5*) is a partially heat-labile inhalant and food allergen implicated in the bird-egg syndrome. Allergy 2001;56:754–762.

Stefan Vieths, PhD
Paul-Ehrlich-Institut
Paul-Ehrlich-Strasse 51–59
DE–63225 Langen (Germany)
E-Mail stefan.vieths@pei.de

Background

Ebisawa M, Ballmer-Weber BK, Vieths S, Wood RA (eds): Food Allergy: Molecular Basis and Clinical Practice.
Chem Immunol Allergy. Basel, Karger, 2015, vol 101, pp 30–37 (DOI: 10.1159/000371662)

Epidemiology: International Point of View, from Childhood to Adults, Food Allergens

Gary W.K. Wong

Department of Paediatrics and School of Public Health, Prince of Wales Hospital, Faculty of Medicine,
Chinese University of Hong Kong, Hong Kong, PR China

Abstract

Recent studies have suggested that the prevalence of food allergy is increasing in many parts of the world. However, many epidemiology studies have been based only on questionnaires without objective testing. The data from these studies do show that the pattern of food allergies is different across the world. In general, studies using objective testing reported a lower prevalence than those without objective testing. The most common food allergens are cow's milk, hen's egg, wheat, fish, shellfish, peanuts, and tree nuts. Recent evidence also suggested that some of these allergies might not persist longer than the childhood years. However, unlike milk and egg allergies, seafood allergy is more likely to persist into adulthood. Peanuts and tree nuts are some of the most common causes of anaphylaxis in developed countries, but these are rather rare in developing countries. Given the early evidence of an increasing prevalence of food allergies, continual monitoring of the changing prevalence and patterns in different countries should help us understand the true causes of food allergy.

© 2015 S. Karger AG, Basel

Epidemiology of Food Allergy

Food allergy is believed to be one of the most common allergic disorders, and recent evidence suggests that the prevalence of food allergy has increased in recent years [1, 2]. However, accurate documentation of the true prevalence of food allergy is very difficult. Most published epidemiological studies of food allergies have only used simple questionnaires, without objective testing, to document possible allergic symptoms [3]. Food allergy is more common in children, and its manifestation is very often the first step of the allergic march. Many conditions may cause symptoms that are mistaken as manifestations of food allergy; therefore, objective testing may be needed in order to confirm the diagnosis. Food allergy has been defined as an adverse health effect arising from a specific immune response that reproducibly occurs upon exposure to a given food [4]. The adverse effects of food allergy may be due to IgE-mediated or non-IgE-mediated reactions. However, most epidemiological studies have concentrated on studying the immediate types of food allergies that are mediated by IgE. It is very

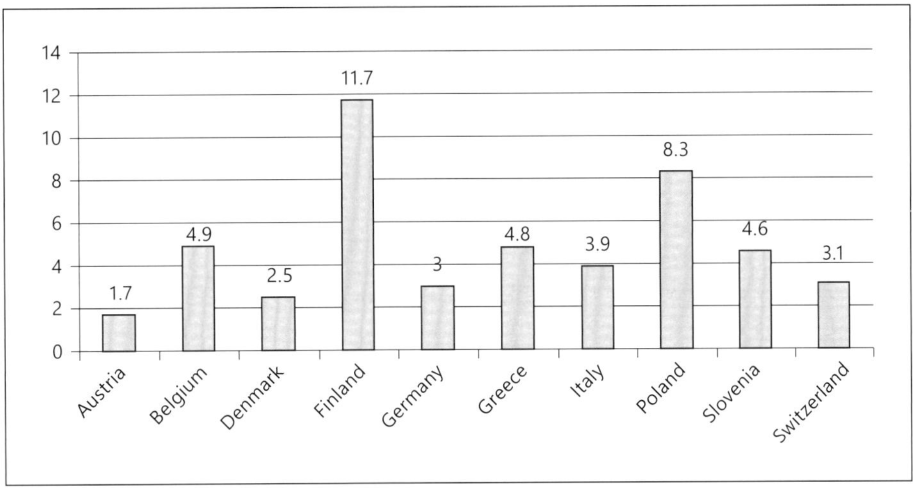

Fig. 1. Prevalence of perceived food allergy in children from 10 European nations, adapted from Steinke et al. [6].

difficult to conduct epidemiological studies on non-IgE-mediated food allergies; therefore, reliable data on non-IgE-mediated food allergy are rather limited. Among the published studies, there are marked variations in the prevalence of food allergies. A part of the differences may be due to the availability of different types of food sources and variations in local dietary practice. The lack of a standard definition of the diagnosis and proper validation of research methodologies are likely to be the most important reasons for such variations.

Reported Food Allergy and Epidemiology Study Methodology

Food allergy has been estimated to occur in 2–10% of the population [5]. However, it is very difficult to compare the prevalence rates reported by different studies, as there are marked variations in the methodologies and definitions of diagnosis. Food allergy is often the first manifestation of allergies among infants and young children. The majority of published epidemiology studies used simple questionnaires to ascertain the prevalence of various types of food allergies; however, the results of these questionnaires are likely to be overestimating the true occurrence of diseases. A number of recent epidemiological studies have used objective measurements, such as food challenge tests or serum-specific IgE measurements, to confirm or support the diagnosis of food allergy. A random-telephone survey conducted in 10 European nations to investigate the prevalence of possible food allergies in children reported a wide variation in the prevalence rates of suspected food allergies [6]. The target age group of this study was children under 18 years of age. The parents or guardians were interviewed to enquire about the possible food allergies of the subjects. The prevalence ranged from the highest of 11.7%, in Finland, to the lowest of 1.7%, in Austria. According to age groups, the highest rate of 7.2% was reported among children aged 2–3 years. The top five suspected offending foods were milk, fruits, eggs, vegetables, and fish. These reported rates most likely represent an overestimation, but such wide variation may be due to some true differences in the prevalence of food allergies (fig. 1).

A recent birth cohort study from Germany revealed an annual incidence of 4.7% during the first 2 years, and the incidence decreased to 1.2% by the 5th to 6th year of age [7]. A meta-analysis conducted by the EuroPrevall Research Consortium analyzed 51 epidemiology studies of food allergy and showed that there was marked heterogeneity in the prevalence of food allergy [3]. The prevalence of self-reported food allergy varied widely from 3 to 35%, with 12% of children under 16 years of age and 13% of adults being 'very high'. Not surprisingly, the overall prevalence of food allergy against any food was only 3%, as reported by studies that included history and objective testing. In order to obtain more reliable data and to improve our understanding for the prevention, diagnosis and treatment of food allergy, the EU-funded multidisciplinary Integrated Project, EuroPrevall, was initiated [8]. The primary aim of the EuroPrevall project is to evaluate the prevalence, basis and costs of food allergy in different European countries using the same standardized and validated methodology. Furthermore, non-European countries, including China, Russia and India, also participated and used the same standardized methodology [9].

Even standardized methodology and objective testing cannot overcome several difficulties that may hinder our interpretation of reported studies. First, the types of symptoms of the study subjects may not be clearly recorded, making it difficult to evaluate whether the symptoms may be truly due to an immune-mediated mechanism. Second, for those studies that included food challenges in the study protocol, the duration between the questionnaire assessment and the supervised food challenge may vary such that the suspected allergy may have resolved. Third, some subjects may have never ingested the particular food or may have actively avoided such food, resulting in underreporting of the adverse symptoms. Given all of these limitations, one must interpret the reported findings with caution, as many factors may have biased the results.

Prevalence of Common Food Allergies

Although it has been suggested that more than 170 foods could be associated with the development of allergy, most of the reported food allergies have been caused by a limited number of allergens. These food allergens are responsible for the majority of reported food allergies, and the subsequent sections will concentrate on the epidemiology of these food allergens, which include cow's milk, hen's egg, wheat, fish, shellfish, peanuts, and tree nuts. In addition, epidemiology of allergy to plant foods has also received some attention. This type of allergy often manifests as oral allergy syndrome, in which the primary sensitizers are pollen allergens, resulting in local symptoms due to cross-reactivity to plant or fruit antigens [10].

Cow's milk allergy (CMA) is one of the most common food allergies and commonly manifests within the first year of life. CMA can be due to IgE-mediated, non-IgE-mediated, or a mixture of both, resulting in different forms of manifestations. In non-Caucasian populations, lactose intolerance is rather common, and the associated symptoms may be mistaken as symptoms of food allergy. Similar to many other food allergies, CMA is more common in children than in adults. The prevalence of CMA in children has been reported to range from 0.3% to 3.5% according to different childhood studies. A prospective study of CMA in Danish infants during the first 3 years of life revealed that 6.7% were suspected to have CMA, but only 2.2% were confirmed to have CMA [11]. Another birth cohort from Norway, which followed children until 3 years of age, confirmed similar findings and showed that the prevalence of CMA and intolerance was estimated to be 1.1%, while 3.3% of the parents thought their children had an allergy or intolerance to cow's milk [12]. One should note that the remission rate was very high with increasing age. In a Danish study, 34 out of 39 subjects (87%) had recovered by 3 years of age and were able to tolerate milk by then. However, recent data from the US has suggested that the natural history may have changed in the recent decade. A hospital-based series of 807 children with confirmed CMA in the US reported that the resolution rate was only 42% by 8 years of age, but this may be a reflection of a selection bias of having more severe subjects followed up in this hospital [13].

In adults, CMA is rare when compared to that in children [14]. There have been quite a few studies on the prevalence rates of cow's milk sensitization, but most reported studies of CMA in adults were based primary on questionnaires only. The sensitization rates documented using either skin-prick tests (SPTs) or serum IgE measurements ranged from 0.1 to 1.1% [15]. A recent study from the US that was based on a telephone survey revealed a self-reported, doctor-diagnosed CMA rate of 1.1% [16]. Detailed information regarding how those doctors made the diagnosis of CMA was not available. It is highly likely that this represents an overestimation of the true prevalence in the studied population.

Together with cow's milk, hen's egg is also one of the most common food allergens, probably reflecting the wide availability of eggs in different parts of the world. It has been estimated that between 0.5 and 5% of infants and preschool children suffer from egg allergy. Much fewer data regarding the prevalence of egg allergy in older children and adults are available. The reported studies with objective assessment of true egg allergies revealed that egg allergy probably occurs in less than 0.5% of adults. A large, nationally representative US sample of children under 18 years of age revealed that 6.9% of the subjects were sensitized to egg, as shown by serum IgE measurement, while a cohort of high-risk infants (n = 620) from Australia revealed that 3.2% had egg allergy, as confirmed by SPTs and food challenge tests [16, 17]. Rancé et al. from France reported a study of 2,716 children aged 2–14 years that revealed that 0.8% had parent-reported egg allergy [18]. However, the self-reported, doctor-diagnosed egg allergy rate was only 0.3% in a large US study of 4,482 adults [14]. Osterballe et al. reported a study on 936 adults that used a questionnaire, SPTs, and serum-specific IgE and oral challenge tests to reveal that only 0.1% of the subjects were allergic to egg. It is quite clear that both the rate of sensitization and self-reported egg allergy were much higher than the actual rate of allergy that was confirmed by objective testing [19]. In line with the epidemiology of CMA, almost all follow-up studies evaluating the natural history of egg allergy were from children, and these children usually gradually developed tolerance to egg as they grew older [20–22]. A recent retrospective study of 881 pediatric cases of egg allergy in a US tertiary referral center revealed that resolution of the allergy occurred in 12% by the age of 6 years, in 37% by the age of 10 years, and in 68% by the age of 16 years [20]. These rates are rather low and slow when compared to previous studies, but this may be related to the more severe spectrum of diseases in the patients referred to the tertiary center [21]. Another study regarding the natural history of egg allergy has also been conducted on 58 Spanish children diagnosed with egg allergy before 2 years of age and followed for up to 86 months after diagnosis. Tolerance developed in 28% of the children at 24 months, 52% at 36 months, 57% at 48 months, and 66% at 60 months of follow-up [22]. Other factors, such as genetics as well as dietary habits, may contribute to the rate of resolution of egg allergy, and these factors may explain the differences reported in various studies of egg allergy in children.

Wheat allergy is a commonly suspected condition, but research studies have suggested that the prevalence is much lower than perceived by the subjects or their parents. Studies in Europe and America revealed that the prevalence of wheat allergy varies from 0.2 to 1.3%, with a higher prevalence noted in children. A large, nationwide study conducted in the United Kingdom revealed a self-reported prevalence of 0.9% [23]. In the same study, 20.4% of subjects reported that they had an allergy to a food; however, these reported rates were most likely over-estimates of the true prevalence. As patients with celiac disease would also have intolerance to gluten due to a non-IgE-mediated, immune-mediated mechanism, many of these patients would report symptoms after ingestion of wheat, but they did not actually have an IgE-mediated wheat allergy [24].

Although many studies have examined the natural history of CMA, very few studies have evaluated the natural history of wheat allergy. There have only been two pediatric studies to evaluate the natural history of wheat allergy. In a study of 28 children with challenge-proven wheat allergy presenting between 6 and 75 months of age, follow-up revealed that 59, 69, 84, and 96% tolerance was achieved by age 4, 6, 10, and 16 years, respectively [25]. In another study of 103 US children, a similar trend of gradual increase in tolerance was observed, but the rates were slightly lower than that in the Finnish study. Sensitization to gliadin, with an SPT wheal greater than or equal to 5 mm, and high wheat serum IgE were associated with a slower course of recovery, but the majority of children recovered by the time they reached adolescence [26].

Seafood, including fish and shellfish, is one of the most common foods to cause adverse allergic reactions. Unlike allergy to cow's milk and egg, fish and shellfish allergies were found to be less common in children than in adults. This may partly reflect the fact that young children probably eat less fish and shellfish than adults in most populations. The differences in the epidemiology of seafood allergy may also be due to the wide differences in the availability of seafood to different populations across different regions. Nevertheless, with the improvement of fish farming and storage and efficient transportation, increasing exposure may result in seafood allergy in population groups in which seafood is not a part of their usual diet. In Scandinavia, Spain, and Portugal, where fish is a common food in the diet, fish allergy has been reported to be common. Among many Asian countries, including Thailand, Singapore, and China, shellfish allergy has also been reported to be common. A very large-scaled telephone survey of 14,948 US subjects revealed a prevalence of fish allergy of 0.4% and of shellfish allergy of 2.0% [27]. Interestingly, of those with a reported allergy to crustaceans, 38% of them reported to have reactions to more than one species, suggesting a high possibility of cross-reactivity. A recent comparative study of Asian children from Singapore showed that the prevalences of reported shellfish allergies were 1.19 and 5.23% in preschoolers and adolescents, respectively [28]. We have conducted a questionnaire survey of preschoolers from Hong Kong, which showed that the prevalence of parent-reported shellfish allergy and fish allergy were 1.28 and 0.32%, respectively [29]. A birth cohort study from Norway revealed that 3% of 3,623 children had reported adverse reactions to fish by the age of 2 years [12]. Our early results of the EuroPrevall-INCO study revealed that fish and seafood allergies were almost nonexistent in children recruited from two participating centers in India [9].

Unlike CMA and egg allergy, seafood allergy is usually considered to be life-long. However, there have been a couple of small series suggesting that fish and shellfish allergy could remit in only a very small number of affected subjects [30, 31]. Daul et al. examined, in a longitudinal follow-up study, 11 subjects with proven shrimp allergy for 24 months, and there were no changes in the level of serum-specific IgE to shrimp over the study period, suggesting a low likelihood of remission. However, these studies were rather small, and the follow-up period was short. Longer-term studies with larger numbers of subjects with mild to severe forms of seafood allergy are needed to clarify the natural history of this form of allergy [32].

Peanut and tree nut allergy represent some common forms of food allergy that frequently result in anaphylaxis. Similar to seafood allergy, remission is less unlikely to occur in subjects with a peanut or tree nut allergy. Sicherer et al. reported three studies that used telephone surveys conducted from 1997 to 2008 and examined the prevalence of self-reported peanut allergy in the US population [33–35]. In 1999, 0.6% of children and 1.6% of adults of the general population reported to have peanut allergy. By 2008, the prevalence remained stable at 1.3% for adults; however, the reported prevalence had increased significantly to 2.1% in children under 18 years of age. One must interpret these data with caution, as no objective testing was carried out. Furthermore, increased awareness and perception may result in such findings but not be due to a true increase in the prevalence of peanut allergy. One interesting study comparing the prevalence of peanut allergy in Jewish children 4–18 years of age from the UK and Israel used objective testing, including SPTs or IgE or food challenge tests, to confirm the diagnosis of allergy [36]. The results showed that the prevalence was 1.85% in UK children, while it was only 0.17% in children in Israel. Such a large difference documented by objective methods is very convincing. Early consumption of peanuts is rather common for Israel children, and this may be one of the factors contributing to the markedly lower prevalence in Israeli children, given the similar genetic background of the two studied populations. Further studies in these populations may reveal the possible environmental factors that protect against the development of peanut allergy. A recent questionnaire study of Asian children of two age groups compared with expatriate children living in Singapore revealed a convincing history of peanut allergy in 0.64% of Singaporean children 4–6 years and in 1.29% of expatriate children living in Singapore [28]; there were similar findings for 14–16-year-old children. Such findings may possibly be due to differences in genetic background as well as environmental exposure factors between the studied population groups.

Although it has been thought that patients with peanut allergy rarely outgrow the disease, large longitudinal, follow-up studies have revealed that up to 20% of affected patients may outgrow their peanut allergy over time. A series of 230 children with confirmed peanut allergy were followed in two referral centers in the United Kingdom. A total of 22 (9.6%) children were able to tolerate peanut oral challenge upon follow-up, and their median age was 5 years [37]. In another large series of subjects, consisting of 223 patients with an age of diagnosis ranging from 4 to 20 years, 48 patients (21.5%) were found to tolerate peanut by the time they reached adolescence or early adulthood. A low level of peanut-specific IgE (less than 2 kU/l) was associated with a higher chance of tolerance to peanut upon challenge. The exact factors resulting in subsequent tolerance to peanut remain unknown [38].

Similar to peanut allergy, tree nut is another common allergen resulting in anaphylaxis. In most studies, the prevalence of nut allergy is not as common as peanut allergy. In a recent large telephone survey conducted in the US, the overall reported prevalence of tree nut allergy was 0.6%, and among these subjects, 0.2% reported to have both a peanut and tree nut allergy. There was no clear difference in the prevalence rates between adults and children [39]. A recent meta-analysis revealed that the perceived allergy to tree nuts was reported to be between 0.4 and 1.4%, while it was between 0.2 and 0.3% in children under 6 years of age, possibly due to the increased exposure of adults to tree nuts [40]. The prevalence of tree nut sensitization, however, has been found to be quite common in European adults, based on the results of the EuroPrevall consortium. Excluding those with birch sensitization, the prevalence rates of walnut and hazelnut sensitization were 1.8 and 3.1%, respectively [41]. Similar to peanut allergy, tree nut allergy tends to persist, especially in those with high levels of specific IgE. A large study including 278 patients with confirmed tree nut allergy revealed that 9% of the subjects outgrew their allergy over time [42].

Changing Prevalence of Food Allergy

Food allergy has been described as the second wave of the allergy epidemic after the rise in the prevalence of asthma and allergic rhinitis [1]. Although a number of studies and anecdotal experiences suggest that the prevalence of food allergy may be increasing, it has been very difficult to obtain solid scientific evidence confirming the increase due to the methodological difficulties described earlier. The data are also conflicting with regards to the particular allergen. For example, the reported prevalence of perceived peanut allergy has increased in the US for children, but no such change has been observed for tree nut or peanut allergy in adults. Recent hospitalization data of food-induced anaphylaxis has suggested that the incidence rate has been increasing, especially in children under 4 years of age, in Australia [43]. An increasing failure rate of resolution of food allergy, such as that documented for egg allergy, is also a cause of worry [20]. The current scene of food allergy epidemiology research is similar to the situation of asthma epidemiology research 25 years ago. A variety of methodologies have been used in different studies, but most of these methodologies have not been validated properly. Furthermore, in these research studies, different definitions of food allergies were used, depending on what types of testing were performed. Very few studies used food challenge as the 'gold standard' for the diagnosis of food allergy. As discussed earlier, different types of food allergy will have different natural histories, such as age being an important factor affecting the results. The use of standardized methodology in large collaborative studies, such as the work of EuroPrevall, should be encouraged in order to come up with meaningful results for comparison in future epidemiology studies. Given what is known for other allergic conditions, environmental factors are likely to play important roles in the pathogenesis of food allergy. Longitudinal epidemiology studies with careful documentation of environmental exposures coupled with genetic analyses would be necessary to help us understand the true causes of food allergy [44].

References

1 Prescott S, Allen KJ: Food allergy: riding the second wave of the allergy epidemic. Pediatr Allergy Immunol 2011;22:155–160.
2 Osborne NJ, Koplin JJ, Martin PE, Gurrin LC, Lowe AJ, Matheson MC, et al: Prevalence of challenge-proven IgE-mediated food allergy using population-based sampling and predetermined challenge criteria in infants. J Allergy Clin Immunol 2011;127:668–676.
3 Rona RJ, Keil T, Summers C, Gislason D, Zuidmeer L, Sodergren E, et al: The prevalence of food allergy: a meta-analysis. J Allergy Clin Immunol 2007;120:638–646.
4 Boyce JA, Assa'ad A, Burks AW, Jones SM, Sampson HA, Wood RA, et al: Guidelines for the diagnosis and management of food allergy in the United States: report of the NIAID-sponsored expert panel. J Allergy Clin Immunol 2010;126(suppl):S1–S58.
5 Chafen JJ, Newberry SJ, Riedl MA, Bravata DM, Maglione M, Suttorp MJ, et al: Diagnosing and managing common food allergies: a systematic review. JAMA 2010;303:1848–1856.
6 Steinke M, Fiocchi A, Kirchlechner V, Ballmer-Weber B, Brockow K, Hischenhuber C, et al: Perceived food allergy in children in 10 European nations. A randomised telephone survey. Int Arch Allergy Immunol 2007;143:290–295.
7 Schnabel E, Sausenthaler S, Schaaf B, Schäfer T, Lehmann I, Behrendt H, et al: Prospective association between food sensitization and food allergy: results of the LISA birth cohort study. Clin Exp Allergy 2010;40:450–457.
8 Mills EN, Mackie AR, Burney P, Beyer K, Frewer L, Madsen C, et al: The prevalence, cost and basis of food allergy across Europe. Allergy 2007;62:717–722.
9 Wong GW, Mahesh PA, Ogorodova L, Leung TF, Fedorova O, Holla AD, et al: The EuroPrevall-INCO surveys on the prevalence of food allergies in children from China, India and Russia: the study methodology. Allergy 2010;65:385–390.
10 Katelaris CH: Food allergy and oral allergy or pollen-food syndrome. Curr Opin Allergy Clin Immunol 2010;10:246–251.
11 Høst A, Halken S: Clinical course in relation to clinical and immunological type of hypersensitivity reaction. Allergy 1990;45:587–596.
12 Eggesbø M, Halvorsen R, Tambs K, Botten G: Prevalence of parentally perceived adverse reactions to food in young children. Pediatr Allergy Immunol 1999;10:122–132.
13 Skripak JM, Matsui EC, Mudd K, Wood RA: The natural history of IgE-mediated cow's milk allergy. J Allergy Clin Immunol 2007;120:1172–1177.

14 Vierk KA, Koehler KM, Fein SB, Street DA: Prevalence of self-reported food allergy in American adults and use of food labels. J Allergy Clin Immunol 2007;119:1504–1510.

15 Venter C, Arshad SH: Epidemiology of food allergy. Pediatr Clin North Am 2011;58:327–349.

16 Branum AM, Lukacs SL: Food allergy among children in the United States. Pediatrics 2009;124:1549–1555.

17 Hill DJ, Hosking CS, Zhie CY, Leung R, Baratwidjaja K, Iikura Y, et al: The frequency of food allergy in Australia and Asia. Environ Toxicol Pharmacol 1997; 4:101–110.

18 Rancé F, Grandmottet X, Grandjean H: Prevalence and main characteristics of schoolchildren diagnosed with food allergies in France. Clin Exp Allergy 2005; 35:167–172.

19 Osterballe M, Hansen TK, Mortz CG, Høst A, Bindslev-Jensen C: The prevalence of food hypersensitivity in an unselected population of children and adults. Pediatr Allergy Immunol 2005; 16:567–573.

20 Savage JH, Matsui EC, Skripak JM, Wood RA: The natural history of egg allergy. J Allergy Clin Immunol 2007; 120:1413–1417.

21 Hattevig G, Kjellman B, Björkstén B: Clinical symptoms and IgE responses to common food proteins and inhalants in the first 7 years of life. Clin Allergy 1987; 17:571–578.

22 Boyano-Martínez T, García-Ara C, Díaz-Pena JM, Martín-Esteban M: Prediction of tolerance on the basis of quantification of egg white-specific IgE antibodies in children with egg allergy. J Allergy Clin Immunol 2002;110:304–309.

23 Young E, Stoneham MD, Petruckevitch A, Barton J, Rona R: A population study of food intolerance. Lancet 1994;343: 1127–1130.

24 Sapone A, Bai JC, Ciacci C, Dolinsek J, Green PH, Hadjivassiliou M, et al: Spectrum of gluten-related disorders: consensus on new nomenclature and classification. BMC Med 2012;10:13.

25 Kotaniemi-Syrjänen A, Palosuo K, Jartti T, Kuitunen M, Pelkonen AS, Mäkelä MJ: The prognosis of wheat hypersensitivity in children. Pediatr Allergy Immunol 2010;21:e421–e428.

26 Keet CA, Matsui EC, Dhillon G, Lenehan P, Paterakis M, Wood RA: The natural history of wheat allergy. Ann Allergy Asthma Immunol 2009;102:410–415.

27 Sicherer SH, Muñoz-Furlong A, Sampson HA: Prevalence of seafood allergy in the United States determined by a random telephone survey. J Allergy Clin Immunol 2004;114:159–165.

28 Shek LP, Cabrera-Morales EA, Soh SE, Gerez I, Ng PZ, Yi FC, et al: A population-based questionnaire survey on the prevalence of peanut, tree nut, and shellfish allergy in 2 Asian populations. J Allergy Clin Immunol 2010;126:324–331.

29 Leung TF, Yung E, Wong YS, Lam CW, Wong GW: Parent-reported adverse food reactions in Hong Kong Chinese pre-schoolers: epidemiology, clinical spectrum and risk factors. Pediatr Allergy Immunol 2009;20:339–346.

30 Tsabouri S, Triga M, Makris M, Kalogeromitros D, Church MK, Priftis KN: Fish and shellfish allergy in children: review of a persistent food allergy. Pediatr Allergy Immunol 2012;23:608–615.

31 Dannaeus A, Inganäs M: A follow-up study of children with food allergy. Clinical course in relation to serum IgE- and IgG-antibody levels to milk, egg and fish. Clin Allergy 1981;11:533–539.

32 Daul CB, Morgan JE, Lehrer SB: The natural history of shrimp hypersensitivity. J Allergy Clin Immunol 1990;86: 88–93.

33 Sicherer SH, Muñoz-Furlong A, Godbold JH, Sampson HA: US prevalence of self-reported peanut, tree nut, and sesame allergy: 11-year follow-up. J Allergy Clin Immunol 2010;125:1322–1326

34 Sicherer SH, Muñoz-Furlong A, Sampson HA: Prevalence of peanut and tree nut allergy in the United States determined by means of a random digit dial telephone survey: a 5-year follow-up study. J Allergy Clin Immunol 2003;112: 1203–1207.

35 Sicherer SH, Muñoz-Furlong A, Burks AW, Sampson HA: Prevalence of peanut and tree nut allergy in the US determined by a random digit dial telephone survey. J Allergy Clin Immunol 1999; 103:559–562.

36 Du Toit G, Katz Y, Sasieni P, Mesher D, Maleki SJ, Fisher HR, et al: Early consumption of peanuts in infancy is associated with a low prevalence of peanut allergy. J Allergy Clin Immunol 2008; 122:984–991.

37 Hourihane JO, Roberts SA, Warner JO: Resolution of peanut allergy: case-control study. BMJ 1998;316:1271–1275.

38 Skolnick HS, Conover-Walker MK, Koerner CB, Sampson HA, Burks W, Wood RA: The natural history of peanut allergy. J Allergy Clin Immunol 2001;107: 367–374.

39 de Silva IL, Mehr SS, Tey D, Tang ML: Paediatric anaphylaxis: a 5 year retrospective review. Allergy 2008;63:1071–1076.

40 Zuidmeer L, Goldhahn K, Rona RJ, Gislason D, Madsen C, Summers C, et al: The prevalence of plant food allergies: a systematic review. J Allergy Clin Immunol 2008;121:1210–1218.

41 Burney P, Summers C, Chinn S, Hooper R, van Ree R, Lidholm J: Prevalence and distribution of sensitization to foods in the European Community Respiratory Health Survey: a EuroPrevall analysis. Allergy 2010;65:1182–1188.

42 Fleischer DM, Conover-Walker MK, Matsui EC, Wood RA: The natural history of tree nut allergy. J Allergy Clin Immunol 2005;116:1087–1093.

43 Poulos LM, Waters AM, Correll PK, Loblay RH, Marks GB: Trends in hospitalizations for anaphylaxis, angioedema, and urticaria in Australia, 1993–1994 to 2004–2005. J Allergy Clin Immunol 2007;120:878–884.

44 Tezza G, Mazzei F, Boner A: Epigenetics of allergy. Early Hum Dev 2013; 89(S1):S20–S21.

Gary W.K. Wong, MD, FRCPC, FHKAM
Department of Paediatrics, Prince of Wales Hospital
Faculty of Medicine, Chinese University of Hong Kong
Shatin, NT, Hong Kong (PR China)
E-Mail wingkinwong@cuhk.edu.hk

Ebisawa M, Ballmer-Weber BK, Vieths S, Wood RA (eds): Food Allergy: Molecular Basis and Clinical Practice.
Chem Immunol Allergy. Basel, Karger, 2015, vol 101, pp 38–50 (DOI: 10.1159/000371666)

Food Allergy in Childhood (Infancy to School Age)

Marcel M. Bergmann · Philippe A. Eigenmann

Pediatric Allergy Unit, Department of Child and Adolescent, University Hospitals of Geneva, Geneva,
Switzerland

Abstract

Food allergy is a potentially life-threatening condition
affecting almost 10% of children, with an increasing incidence in the last few decades. It is defined as an immune reaction to food, and its pathogenesis may be IgE
mediated, mixed IgE and non-IgE mediated, or non-IgE
mediated. Potentially all foods can cause food allergy,
but a minority of foods are responsible for the vast majority of reactions reported. A good clinical history is crucial for an accurate diagnosis. Allergy tests, including the
skin prick test and measurement of specific IgE antibodies, are useful tools in the case of IgE-mediated or mixed
allergy but have not been shown to be of any help in
delayed allergic reactions to foods.

© 2015 S. Karger AG, Basel

Introduction

Food allergy (FA) affects 6–8% of children less
than 5 years of age and 4% of the general population, with an increasing incidence over the last
few decades [1, 2]. Its prevalence is higher in the
first 1–2 years of life and diminishes rapidly in
late childhood [3]. Several studies assessing children have shown an important difference between the rates of self-reported and proven FA
[3–5].

FA is defined as an immune response to foods.
It is distinct from other nonimmunological adverse food reactions, such as food intolerance,
toxin-mediated reactions, and pharmacologic reactions. The clinical manifestations are heterogeneous and relate to underlying immunological
pathways and the affected organs (see fig. 1).

Immediate reactions classically occur within
2 h of ingestion of the food and involve an IgE-
mediated mechanism. Nine foods, including
cow's milk, hen's egg, peanut, tree nuts, and
wheat, are responsible for 90% of IgE-mediated
FA in children. The clinical history is usually suggestive, and the FA is confirmed by allergy testing
for IgE-type sensitization.

Non-IgE-mediated FAs usually involve the
gastrointestinal (GI) tract. Clinical symptoms
and their severity vary according to the affected
site. In food protein-induced enterocolitis
(FPIES), the reaction is classically explosive, occurring 2 or more hours after ingestion of the
culprit food, with acute emesis or, later on, pro-

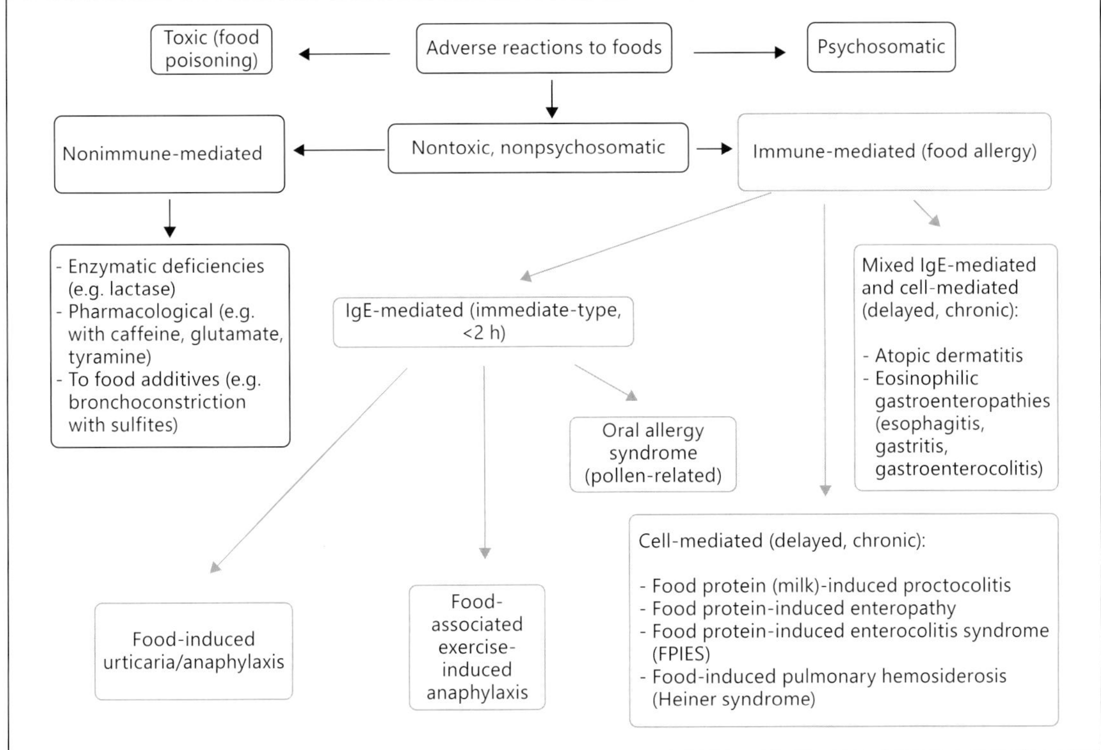

Fig. 1. Classification of adverse reactions to foods.

fuse diarrhea. Food protein-induced enteropathy is characterized by chronic symptoms, such as failure to thrive, relapsing emesis, and/or diarrhea. Infants affected by allergic proctocolitis have isolated bloody stool. Frequently, symptom overlaps exist in clinical practice, and no diagnostic test is yet available for this type of FA. Thus, accurate diagnosis of these particular forms of FA might be difficult to achieve. In addition, the exact immunological mechanisms are still undefined.

In some children affected by atopic dermatitis (AD) and eosinophilic gastroenteropathic disorders (EGIDs), an allergic trigger might be present, contributing to the inflammation that is present as the allergy-independent baseline of the disease. When present, this form of allergy may be due to both IgE- and non-IgE-mediated mechanisms.

IgE-Mediated (Immediate-Type) Food Allergy

Food-Induced Urticaria and Anaphylaxis
Immediate-type, IgE-mediated FA is rapid in onset and uniphasic and generally appears within 2 h after ingestion of the culprit food [6]. Biphasic reactions, with relapses usually seen within 1–5 h and up to 78 h have also been described, but they remain rare.

Potentially any food can trigger an allergic response. However, cow's milk, hen's egg, peanut, tree nuts, wheat, soy, crustaceans, and fish are responsible for the great majority of IgE-mediated allergic reactions in children. The list of incriminated foods is usually age dependent [7]. Major food allergens are water-soluble glycoproteins resistant to heat, although the allergenicity of both milk and egg can be significantly reduced by extensive heating.

Table 1. IgE-mediated food allergy syndromes in children

Clinical features	Urticaria/anaphylaxis	Food-associated exercise-induced anaphylaxis	Oral allergy syndrome (pollen-related)
Symptoms	*Nervous system:* anxiety, behavior changes *Cutaneous:* erythema, pruritus, urticaria (also contact urticaria), angioedema, other type of rashes *Gastrointestinal:* oral pruritus, abdominal pain, nausea, vomiting, diarrhea *Upper respiratory tract:* acute nasal congestion, sneezing, ocular hyperemia, tearing *Lower respiratory tract:* acute cough, laryngeal tightness, hoarseness, stridor, wheezing, dyspnea *Cardiovascular:* tachycardia, dizziness, blood pressure drop, collapse		Oral pruritus, tingling, erythema, mild edema in and around the mouth (7% beyond, 1–2% systemic symptoms) Exacerbation possible during pollen season Systemic reactions (rare)
Chronology	<2 h from food intake	Food ingestion followed by exercise	Directly after food ingestion
Incriminated foods	Potentially all foods *Major food allergens:* cow's milk, hen's egg, wheat, tree nuts, peanut, fish, shellfish, soy	Mainly wheat, shellfish, celery (the last more common in adults)	Exclusively raw fruits and vegetables (e.g. birch-related)

Recent studies have shown that some children tolerate baked milk or eggs while reacting to the raw form [8, 9]. These children usually achieve natural tolerance more rapidly, and it appears that the acquisition of tolerance may be enhanced by exposure to extensively heated forms of these foods.

The clinical characteristics of immediate IgE-mediated allergy are listed in table 1. Skin manifestations are most common, occurring in about 74% of patients with an immediate allergic reaction to a food, of which about 30% only involve the skin [10].

Direct skin contact with food can also lead to urticarial lesions.

In recent reviews on FA, some authors classified reactions involving only the skin as a different entity, distinct from more severe, multisystemic reactions (anaphylaxis). This kind of distinction can be useful but needs to be interpreted carefully in clinical practice. In fact, a child experiencing a mild cutaneous allergic reaction can, in the case of further exposure, experience a more severe, potentially life-threatening reaction [11].

Acute GI food reactions can include oral itching, nausea, vomiting, and/or abdominal pain that can appear rapidly after food intake. Diarrhea might also be present, typically after 2–6 h.

Although not life threatening, upper respiratory symptoms are rarely isolated. They are present in about 40% of reactions and usually are part of a systemic reaction [12]. Lower respiratory symptoms are also common components of systemic reactions. These, however, can be severe, and it is important to recognize that respiratory failure is the most common cause of death among fatal reactions.

It has been proposed that the severity of clinical symptoms can be graded on a scale from 1 to 5, with grade 4 and 5 reactions involving the lower respiratory tract and/or the cardiovascular system [13]. In grade 4 and 5 reactions, epinephrine should be administered without delay, as this can clearly improve the outcome and reduce mortality [14]. In children, severe reactions with cardiovascular compromise are rare overall [15]. Interestingly, increased airway reactivity measured by methacholine inhalation challenge have been found in half of challenged patients, even in the

Table 2. Risk factors for severe immediate allergic reactions to food

The concomitant presence of asthma (although the severity of asthma does not appear to be a factor)
Past allergic reactions to extremely small amounts of food
A history of a previous food-induced anaphylactic reaction of any severity (most victims of fatal reactions have had relatively mild reactions in the past)
Allergy to peanuts, tree nuts, fish, or shellfish

absence of clinically manifested respiratory symptoms [16]. Several risk factors for fatal food-induced anaphylaxis have been defined and are listed in table 2.

The severity of allergic reactions may depend on many factors, including the food itself, the amount and preparation (raw or cooked) of the food, co-ingestion of other foods, the patient's age, comorbid conditions such as asthma, and cofactors such as exercise or concomitant viral illness [5]. In Germany and the United States, peanuts and tree nuts are the most frequent foods causing severe anaphylactic reactions, followed by shellfish and fish [17]. Milk and hen's egg have also been reported as causing severe anaphylactic reactions in children [18]. Regional differences in culprit foods, depending on the local diet, have to be taken into account. In a recent German population-based study [15], elevated specific IgE antibody levels, a young age, and a history of AD were associated with a positive challenge outcome in cow's milk- and hen's egg-allergic patients. In the same study, cow's milk and hen's egg tended to induce more severe symptoms at a low dose compared with wheat and soy.

Various experts have established clinical criteria for the diagnosis of severe anaphylaxis, mainly based on the presence of skin symptoms in concomitance with other organ involvement [19, 20].

A retrospective study from Germany analyzing 1,843 consecutive oral food challenges (OFCs) has shown interesting data about differences in clinical symptoms depending on the culprit food [18]. All foods tested (cow's milk, hen's egg, peanut, hazelnut, wheat, and soy) had a similar prevalence of skin manifestations (between 80 and 100%). Angioedema was rare overall (among all foods), and urticaria was predominantly seen in peanut (85%), hen's egg (78%), hazelnut (69%), and cow's milk allergy, followed by wheat and soy allergy. Soy and wheat were clearly more prone to inducing AD flares (69 and 52%, respectively). Concerning other organs, OFC with hen's egg and peanut more often induced GI symptoms (44.4 and 45.7%, respectively), and peanut (41.3%) was most often associated with a higher rate of respiratory symptoms, followed by hen's egg (19.5%) and cow's milk (17.3%).

Although oral ingestion is the primary route of exposure, symptoms mainly of the upper and lower respiratory tracts may also occur following direct inhalation of aerosolized particles containing the culprit food [21, 22]. In our experience, these self-reported reactions are usually not severe and are often not confirmed, suggesting that anxiety may be a factor contributing to symptom reports.

IgE-mediated FA is strongly associated with a history of past or current AD [23]. Various studies have reported the presence of IgE-mediated immediate-type FA in children with AD [10, 24, 25]. This concept will be examined later on in this chapter.

Food-Dependent Exercise-Induced Anaphylaxis
Food-dependent exercise-induced anaphylaxis is a variant of food-induced anaphylaxis, in which exercise undertaken within a few hours after intake of a food triggers an IgE-mediated reaction [26]. No reactions to the culprit food occur in the absence of exercise and vice versa. Foods classically implicated are wheat, seafood or nuts, although this anaphylaxis can occur with a wide variety of foods.

Oral Allergy Syndrome
Oral allergy syndrome (OAS), or pollen-associated FA syndrome, is a common form of allergy mainly found in adolescents and adults that is related to pollen sensitization. Nevertheless, symptoms do often begin in childhood, although the exact prevalence has varied among pediatric studies [27, 28]. Sensitization to tree pollens, and specifically to birch pollens and less frequently to other pollens (grass pollen, ragweed, or mugwort), is strongly associated with OAS [29]. Sensitization to multiple pollens is also a risk factor for OAS [30]. Patients with clinically relevant pollen sensitization are at greater risk of developing OAS than asymptomatic but sensitized adult patients are [29].

The major pollen allergens involved in OAS belong to pathogenesis-related protein family 10, e.g. the major birch pollen allergen Bet v1. Numerous fruits and vegetables, mostly from the *Rosaceae*, *Umbelliferae*, and *Solanaceae* families, the most common being apple, hazelnut, carrot, and celery, cross-react with proteins from pathogenesis-related protein family 10 [31]. These allergens are sensitive to heat (cooking), and symptoms develop primarily after eating the food in its raw, uncooked form. The specific pollens and foods related to this condition vary geographically, depending mostly on the density of given plants and trees [32].

Clinical symptoms are usually limited to the oropharynx and are characterized by pruritus, tingling, erythema, and mild edema of the inner side of the mouth or the oropharynx shortly after ingestion of the causative food. Abdominal pain might also be present. Symptoms might be stronger during the pollen season due to seasonal allergen exposure.

More severe systemic symptoms, similar to classical anaphylaxis, have also been described for pollen-related foods [33]. Although rare, these reactions seem more frequent in patients without associated pollinosis [34]. Sensitivity to other families of allergens present in plants, such as lipid transfer proteins (LTPs), has been described in this group of patients [35]. These sensitizations also seem to be geographically restricted. In Europe, systemic reactions to peach have been widely described with sensitization to the allergen Pru p3 [35, 36]. Conversely, sensitization to the LTP family does not predict an allergic reaction [37].

Mixed IgE and Non-IgE-Mediated Food Allergy

Atopic Dermatitis and Food Allergy
AD (atopic eczema) is a common skin disease characterized by inflammatory, chronically relapsing pruritic eczematous flares affecting 10–30% of children [38, 39]. Its onset is typically in early childhood and often represents the first manifestation of the atopic march.

Several studies have shown that FA might aggravate the severity of the disease [24, 40]. In fact, associated FA has been shown to occur in 30–40% of children with treatment-refractory moderate-to-severe AD [41]. Cow's milk, hen's egg, peanut, tree nuts, wheat, soy, and fish are responsible of >90% of FA-triggered AD.

In older children and adolescents, pollen (birch)-related foods have also been described as potential triggers of AD [24, 42]. In contrast to the OAS discussed above, these delayed reactions might occur with cooked as well as raw foods.

Three different patterns of clinical reaction have been described after OFC in children with AD:
- *Immediate-type* (anaphylactic) *reactions* within 2 h of ingestion, with typical symptoms of anaphylaxis [10, 24, 25]. In addition, a delayed, nonspecific rash might also occur 6–10 h after OFC, considered as a late-phase IgE-mediated reaction [10].
- *Immediate-type reaction followed by an eczematous delayed-type reaction* has been described in 40% of children with a positive OFC [43].

– Exclusive *delayed-type reactions* (food-induced eczema) typically occur 6–48 h after OFC with eczematous flares at the predilection sites of AD, and affect up to 25% of children with FA-triggered AD [44].

It should be pointed out that in children with AD who have never experienced a history of immediate allergic reaction, optimal skin care should be performed prior to considering an allergy work-up or food elimination. In fact, as mentioned earlier, FA might aggravate the severity of flares only in a minority of children with refractory moderate-to-severe AD.

Eosinophilic Gastroenteropathies (Esophagitis, Gastritis, Enteritis, and Gastroenteritis)

EGIDs are a clinically heterogeneous group of diseases sharing a common histological feature, characterized by mucosal infiltration by eosinophils in the gut [45]. A mixed IgE-mediated and cellular (Th2-type) response is strongly suspected. EGIDs are usually responsive to oral steroid treatment.

A variety of clinical symptoms have been associated with EGIDs, depending on the segment of the gut affected: dysphagia, nausea, vomiting, and irritability have been reported in the case of proximal gut involvement, with the esophagus and/or the stomach being affected. Failure to thrive, abdominal pain, diarrhea, microcytic anemia, and even hypoalbuminemia are more typical of distal inflammation affecting the small and/or large intestine.

Eosinophilic esophagitis (EoE) is the most commonly reported EGID and was first described in 1966 [46]. Its incidence appears to have increased over the last few decades [47]. Currently, EoE affects between 40 and 55 individuals per 100,000 inhabitants [47]. EoE might affect individuals at any age [48]. Its prevalence in the pediatric population is not known.

EoE is not an allergic disease by itself. It can, however, be triggered by allergens, and particularly by a few allergenic foods. In relation to this,

Table 3. Symptoms suggestive of EoE in children

Food refusal
Failure to thrive
Abnormal eating patterns (excessive mastication, 'slow eating')
Decreased appetite
GERD-like symptoms (heartburn, reflux, coughing) refractory to therapy
Dysphagia (mainly with solid food)
Nausea, vomiting
Abdominal pain
Diarrhea
Throat pain
Food impaction

several clinical trials have reported significant improvement after various diets (adjusted elimination diet [49], 6-food elimination diet [50], and protein-free elemental diet [51]) when compared with standard topical medication.

Allergy testing should always be considered in children diagnosed with EoE. A recent retrospective analysis of children by Spergel et al. [49] showed a 77% improvement with a diet based on allergy testing (prick and epicutaneous testing), combined with a systematic cow's milk diet. Interestingly, this success rate was similar to that of an empiric 8-food elimination diet (lacking milk, soy, hen's egg, wheat, and various meats).

The clinical symptoms of EoE in children are nonspecific and age related, and slightly differ from symptoms in adults (table 3). Food refusal is the most common indirect symptom reported in neonates and infants with dysphagia [52]. Other frequent symptoms in children are therapy-refractory symptoms of gastroesophageal reflux disease (GERD); vomiting; abdominal pain; and, less frequently, failure to thrive and diarrhea [53]. Food impaction is more often reported at an older age, typically in adolescence and adulthood.

The diagnosis of EoE should be based on clinical symptoms as well as on endoscopic and histological findings [53]. The histology classically shows an increased number of eosinophils (>15 in at least one high-power field). This feature is generally required for the diagnosis of EoE [54]. Nevertheless, none of these endoscopic and histological findings is specific for EoE.

The differential diagnosis includes a variety of conditions, the most important being GERD. Similar symptoms are found in these two conditions, and a moderate number of eosinophils in the esophageal mucosa may be seen in association with GERD. Before diagnosing EoE, GERD should be excluded clinically; endoscopically; histologically; and, if necessary, with functional studies (pH monitoring). A good clinical response to proton-pump inhibitors is also strongly suggestive of GERD, although biopsies may be needed to confirm the apparent clinical response [55].

Eosinophilic gastritis, enteritis, and gastroenteritis compose a rare group of diseases potentially affecting all age groups, but mostly male adults in their third or fifth decade of life [56]. These diseases are characterized by the selective or diffuse infiltration of eosinophils into the stomach, small intestine, or large intestine.

Although these diseases are mostly not related to a specific trigger, food sensitivity seems to play a role in selected patients. In fact, food allergen-specific T cells have been found in patients with these diseases [57, 58]. Furthermore, complete resolution of symptoms has been achieved in some patients with an amino-acid-based elemental diet, with subsequent reintroduction of various foods under endoscopic control [59]. When the diseases are related to FA, cow's milk, soy, hen's egg, wheat, and fish are the most commonly implicated foods.

Symptoms are related to the depth of inflammation (mainly the mucosa but also the muscle and/or the subserosa) as well as to the magnitude of the eosinophilic infiltration in the gut [60]. In the case of mucosal involvement, the following symptoms have been described: abdominal pain, early satiety, nausea, vomiting, bloody diarrhea, iron-deficiency anemia, failure to thrive, protein-loss enteropathy, and malabsorption.

Non-IgE-Mediated Food Allergy

In this section, we will discuss a group of non-IgE-mediated food protein-induced syndromes affecting the GI tract, and primarily affecting infants (table 4).

Food Protein-Induced Enterocolitis Syndrome
FPIES is a non-IgE-mediated food hypersensitivity characterized by GI symptoms that typically affects young infants. A chronic form with mild digestive symptoms may occur when the food is regularly ingested. In acute FPIES, symptoms are explosive and typically occur after occasional ingestion of the culprit food.

Although initial reports of FPIES were published as early as in the 1960s and 1970s and although various case reports have established the syndrome [61, 62], it remains an under-diagnosed manifestation of FA.

In an Israeli birth cohort of 13,019 infants [63], an incidence of 0.34% by the age of 1 year was found for cow's milk-related FPIES, compared with 0.5% for IgE-mediated cow's milk allergy. The initial symptoms presented prior to 6 months of life in all infants, with a median age of 30 days.

The immunological mechanism of FPIES is not fully understood. Food allergen-specific local inflammation of the gut involving T cells, with increased intestinal permeability and fluid shift, is postulated [64, 65].

Cow's milk and soy are the most common food triggers of classical FPIES [66]. Although initially suspected, cross-reactivity between these two foods has not been confirmed [63]. Cases of

Table 4. Non-IgE-mediated food allergy syndromes in children

Clinical features	Food protein-induced enterocolitis syndrome (FPIES)	Food protein (milk)-induced proctocolitis	Food protein-induced enteropathy	Heiner syndrome
Age of onset	Days to 1 year (later onset possible for solid food)	Days to 6 months	2–24 months	Mostly infants
Clinical symptoms	*Chronic symptoms (food regularly ingested):* failure to thrive, intermittent vomiting and diarrhea, rectorrhagia *Acute symptoms (food occasionally eaten):* Profuse vomiting or diarrhea after 1–4 and 5–8 h, respectively, lethargy, pallor (CAVE: cardiovascular shock in 15–20%)	Isolated bloody stool	Failure to thrive, malabsorption, intermittent emesis, moderate diarrhea, rare bloody stool or edema, anemia	Failure to thrive, iron-deficiency anemia, cough, recurrent fever, wheezing, nasal congestion, recurrent otitis media, hemoptysis, dyspnea, colic, anorexia, vomiting, diarrhea, hematochezia
Diagnosis	Clinical history, OFC (elevation of PMNs >3,500 G/L after a positive challenge) Typically negative specific IgE tests	Clinical history, OFC Negative specific IgE tests Occasional blood eosinophilia	Clinical history, OFC Negative specific IgE tests	Suggestive clinical history Chest X-ray: pulmonary infiltrates Precipitating antibodies Possibly positive specific IgE tests
Prognosis	For milk: spontaneous resolution in 64% by the age of 10 months and in 100% by the age of 24 months Later resolution for solid foods	Spontaneous resolution by the age of 12 months	Generally resolves after 24 months of age	Generally resolves by the age of 36 months
Incriminated food(s)	Mostly cow's milk *Other foods:* soy, grains (rice, oats, barley), meat and poultry (beef, chicken, turkey), vegetables and fruit (sweet potato, squash, string beans, banana), legumes (peas, lentils), fish, and the probiotic *Saccharomyces boulardii*	Cow's milk (through breastfeeding), soy(-milk)	Mainly cow's milk Also hen's egg, rice, poultry, fish, or shellfish (typically after an episode of gastroenteritis)	Cow's milk

PMNs = Polymorphonuclear cells.

cow's milk-related FPIES in exclusively breastfed infants have been described [67], but such observations remain uncommon. Recently, FPIES due to various solid foods, and predominantly rice [68] but also grains (wheat, barley, and oats), corn, poultry (chicken and turkey), legumes (green peas, lentils, string beans, and peanuts), hen's egg, potato, fish, and shellfish, and even due to orange juice has been described.

As mentioned earlier, FPIES may present independently or sequentially in two phases (see table 5) [63, 69]. The chronic phase, while food is regularly ingested, is usually characterized by intermittent vomiting, failure to thrive, weight loss, diarrhea, bloody stool, and lethargy. Symptoms resolve after elimination of the culprit food.

The symptoms of acute FPIES, typically occurring upon exposure to the causative food on an intermittent basis, are explosive and characterized by acute profuse vomiting (onset within 1–4 h after food intake) and/or diarrhea (onset within 5–8 h after food intake). The child appears acutely ill and lethargic. Dehydration can lead to potentially severe hypotension and shock [61].

Table 5. Clinical symptoms of food protein-induced enterocolitis syndrome (FPIES)

Chronic FPIES	Acute FPIES
Failure to thrive	Acute profuse vomiting (onset within 1–4 h after eating)
Weight loss	Diarrhea (onset within 5–8 h)
Intermittent vomiting	Lethargy
Diarrhea	Acute dehydration
Blood in the stool	Pallor
Microcytic anemia	Hypothermia
Dehydration	Hypotension
Lethargy	Cardiovascular shock (sepsis-like presentation in child)

The diagnosis is exclusively based on the clinical history and on the improvement of symptoms after avoidance of the culprit food. IgE allergy testing (skin prick and specific IgE testing) is typically negative. A small proportion of patients may, however, present positive specific IgE tests, suggestive of a mixed IgE-mediated and non-IgE-mediated pattern. Subsequent naturally acquired tolerance rates are lower in this particular group of patients [70].

Recently, the following diagnostic criteria for FPIES have been proposed [71]:
- Less than 9 months of age when symptoms initially present
- GI symptoms after repeated exposure to a given food
- Absence of symptoms suggestive of IgE-mediated FA
- Resolution of symptoms after initiation of an eviction diet
- Recurrence of typical symptoms within 4 h of an OFC

Treatment consists of avoidance of the culprit food. The resolution of FPIES seems to be population dependent, particularly for cow's milk and soy allergy [63, 66, 72]. The majority of patients with FPIES related to milk become tolerant by the age of 3 years [61]. A recent Korean publication describing 27 children with cow's milk-related FPIES has shown that 64% tolerated cow's milk at 10 months and that 92% tolerated soy at the same age [72]. Solid food-related FPIES tends to appear later in life and might relate to protracted resolution [62, 63, 66, 69].

Food Protein-Induced Proctocolitis
Food protein-induced proctocolitis, or allergic proctocolitis, is a major cause of rectal bleeding in young infants. This benign disorder is characterized by an inflammatory reaction to a food allergen limited to the rectum and distal sigmoid colon. It typically affects infants under 12 months of age.

The first descriptions of this syndrome were made as early as 1940 by Rubin et al. [73]. Later on, in a large prospective study, Lake et al. [74] showed that 88% of 95 breastfed infants presenting with bloody stool were found to have food-induced symptoms due to initial food consumption by the mother. The large majority of cases were attributable to cow's milk (65%), followed by hen's egg (19%) and, in a minority of cases, corn or soy. In a recent prospective population-based study following 13,019 Israeli children from birth, the prevalence of isolated rectal bleeding due to cow's milk was 0.16% [75].

The disease typically appears between 2 and 8 weeks of life but might be seen as early as in the first week of life [76]. Bloody stool and occasionally diarrhea, with or without mucus, are the major clinical features of allergic proctocolitis. A

Table 6. Clinical characteristics of allergic proctocolitis

Bloody stools ± diarrhea
Healthy-appearing infant
Normal growth pattern
First symptoms during the first 6 months of life
Cow's milk (breastfed or formula-fed infants) or soy(-milk) induced
Diagnosed based on a suggestive clinical history
Avoidance of the causative food leads to resolution of symptoms within 48–72 h
Natural tolerance acquired usually by 1 year of age

gradual onset and an increasing frequency of bloody stool until removal of the causative food are usually reported [74]. The infants are typically in good health, and no growth delay or poor weight gain is seen. Occasionally, these infants may have a slight associated anemia.

The main features of allergic proctocolitis are summarized in table 6.

Treatment consists of eliminating the suspected food (via a dairy-free diet for breastfeeding mothers or an extensively hydrolyzed formula milk for formula-fed infants), which leads to resolution of symptoms within 48–72 h. Natural resolution of the disease is usually seen by 1 year of age.

Food Protein-Induced Enteropathy
Food protein-induced enteropathy is characterized by chronic GI symptoms while the offending food is regularly ingested. It typically starts during the first months of life. Endoscopic findings might be similar to those of celiac disease, with diffuse or patchy villous injury and cellular infiltrates in the small bowel [77].

Cow's milk is the major allergen involved [78]. Clinical symptoms include recurrent vomiting, diarrhea, malabsorption, failure to thrive, anemia, and hypoalbuminemia. The diagnosis is based on clinical symptoms and on a biopsy showing villous injuries. Symptoms resolve upon strict avoidance of the offending food. Resolution of this form of allergy is usually achieved by the age of 2 years [78].

Heiner Syndrome (Milk-Induced Pulmonary Disease)
Unlike the syndromes described above, with involvement of the gut, Heiner syndrome (HS), or milk-induced pulmonary disease, is a rare condition typically affecting children under 30 months of age [79]. The name was given after Dr. Heiner's first description in the early 1960s.

The exact immunological mechanisms involved are not clearly established but seem to involve immune complex (type III) and type IV cell-mediated hypersensitivities (according to Gell and Coombs' classification) [80].

Children present with recurrent or chronic lower and sometimes upper respiratory symptoms, including a chronic cough, difficulty breathing, wheezing, tachypnea, nasal congestion, and recurrent acute otitis media. Pulmonary hemosiderosis is the major complication of HS and is characterized clinically by hemoptysis with subsequent anemia.

Anorexia, failure to thrive, recurrent fever, and GI symptoms (vomiting, diarrhea, and rectorrhagia) have also been described.

Milk-specific precipitating antibodies in the serum are a common laboratory finding strongly suggesting the diagnosis. A chest X-ray usually reveals patchy pulmonary infiltrates. Iron-laden macrophages are found in the bronchoalveolar lavage in patients with associated hemosiderosis. Positive specific IgE for cow's milk is found in nearly half of these patients [79].

Treatment mainly consists of strict avoidance of cow's milk, which leads to significant clinical and radiological improvement. The pulmonary hemosiderosis might completely resolve. The long-term evolution of HS is not known.

Conclusions

FA is a challenging diagnosis for clinicians. It may present with various clinical aspects, depending on the underlying immunological mechanism and the organ affected. The clinical history has a central role in the diagnosis of FA. In mixed and non-IgE-mediated FAs, usual allergy tests will not be helpful. Elimination diets followed by diagnostic OFC play a central role in the diagnosis. Avoidance of the causative food will improve the disease. A follow-up is mandatory, as the majority of children will naturally outgrow their FA.

References

1 Sicherer SH, Sampson HA: Food allergy. J Allergy Clin Immunol 2010;125:S116–S125.
2 Branum AM, Lukacs SL: Food allergy among children in the United States. Pediatrics 2009;124:1549–1555.
3 Young E, Stoneham MD, Petruckevitch A, Barton J, Rona R: A population study of food intolerance. Lancet 1994;343:1127–1130.
4 Roehr CC, Edenharter G, Reimann S, Ehlers I, Worm M, Zuberbier T, et al: Food allergy and non-allergic food hypersensitivity in children and adolescents. Clin Exp Allergy 2004;34:1534–1541.
5 Boyce JA, Assa'ad A, Burks AW, Jones SM, Sampson HA, Wood RA, et al: Guidelines for the diagnosis and management of food allergy in the United States: summary of the NIAID-Sponsored Expert Panel Report. J Allergy Clin Immunol 2010;126:1105–1118.
6 Sampson HA, Munoz-Furlong A, Bock SA, Schmitt C, Bass R, Chowdhury BA, et al: Symposium on the definition and management of anaphylaxis: summary report. J Allergy Clin Immunol 2005;115:584–591.
7 Sicherer SH, Sampson HA: 9. Food allergy. J Allergy Clin Immunol 2006;117:S470–S475.
8 Lemon-Mule H, Sampson HA, Sicherer SH, Shreffler WG, Noone S, Nowak-Wegrzyn A: Immunologic changes in children with egg allergy ingesting extensively heated egg. J Allergy Clin Immunol 2008;122:977–983.e1.
9 Nowak-Wegrzyn A, Bloom KA, Sicherer SH, Shreffler WG, Noone S, Wanich N, et al: Tolerance to extensively heated milk in children with cow's milk allergy. J Allergy Clin Immunol 2008;122:342–347, 347.e1–e2.
10 Sampson HA: The evaluation and management of food allergy in atopic dermatitis. Clin Dermatol 2003;21:183–192.
11 Ewan PW, Clark AT: Long-term prospective observational study of patients with peanut and nut allergy after participation in a management plan. Lancet 2001;357:111–115.
12 Bock SA, Atkins FM: Patterns of food hypersensitivity during sixteen years of double-blind, placebo-controlled food challenges. J Pediatr 1990;117:561–567.
13 Sampson HA. Anaphylaxis and emergency treatment. Pediatrics 2003;111:1601–1608.
14 Sampson HA, Mendelson L, Rosen JP: Fatal and near-fatal anaphylactic reactions to food in children and adolescents. N Engl J Med 1992;327:380–384.
15 Rolinck-Werninghaus C, Niggemann B, Grabenhenrich L, Wahn U, Beyer K: Outcome of oral food challenges in children in relation to symptom-eliciting allergen dose and allergen-specific IgE. Allergy 2012;67:951–957.
16 James JM, Eigenmann PA, Eggleston PA, Sampson HA: Airway reactivity changes in asthmatic patients undergoing blinded food challenges. Am J Respir Crit Care Med 1996;153:597–603.
17 Hompes S, Kohli A, Nemat K, Scherer K, Lange L, Rueff F, et al: Provoking allergens and treatment of anaphylaxis in children and adolescents – data from the anaphylaxis registry of German-speaking countries. Pediatr Allergy Immunol 2011;22:568–574.
18 Ahrens B, Niggemann B, Wahn U, Beyer K: Organ-specific symptoms during oral food challenge in children with food allergy. J Allergy Clin Immunol 2012;130:549–551.
19 Sampson HA, Munoz-Furlong A, Campbell RL, Adkinson NF Jr, Bock SA, Branum A, et al: Second symposium on the definition and management of anaphylaxis: summary report–Second National Institute of Allergy and Infectious Disease/Food Allergy and Anaphylaxis Network symposium. J Allergy Clin Immunol 2006;117:391–397.
20 Muraro A, Roberts G, Clark A, Eigenmann PA, Halken S, Lack G, et al: The management of anaphylaxis in childhood: position paper of the European academy of allergology and clinical immunology. Allergy 2007;62:857–871.
21 Sicherer SH, Furlong TJ, DeSimone J, Sampson HA: Self-reported allergic reactions to peanut on commercial airliners. J Allergy Clin Immunol 1999;104:186–189.
22 Crespo JF, Pascual C, Dominguez C, Ojeda I, Munoz FM, Esteban MM: Allergic reactions associated with airborne fish particles in IgE-mediated fish hypersensitive patients. Allergy 1995;50:257–261.
23 Mattila L, Kilpelainen M, Terho EO, Koskenvuo M, Helenius H, Kalimo K: Food hypersensitivity among Finnish university students: association with atopic diseases. Clin Exp Allergy 2003;33:600–606.
24 Breuer K, Wulf A, Constien A, Tetau D, Kapp A, Werfel T: Birch pollen-related food as a provocation factor of allergic symptoms in children with atopic eczema/dermatitis syndrome. Allergy 2004;59:988–994.

25 Werfel T, Erdmann S, Fuchs T, Henzgen M, Kleine-Tebbe J, Lepp U, et al: Approach to suspected food allergy in atopic dermatitis. Guideline of the Task Force on Food Allergy of the German Society of Allergology and Clinical Immunology (DGAKI) and the Medical Association of German Allergologists (ADA) and the German Society of Pediatric Allergology (GPA). J Dtsch Dermatol Ges 2009;7:265–271.

26 Romano A, Di Fonso M, Giuffreda F, Papa G, Artesani MC, Viola M, et al: Food-dependent exercise-induced anaphylaxis: clinical and laboratory findings in 54 subjects. Int Arch Allergy Immunol 2001;125:264–272.

27 Zuidmeer L, Goldhahn K, Rona RJ, Gislason D, Madsen C, Summers C, et al: The prevalence of plant food allergies: a systematic review. J Allergy Clin Immunol 2008;121:1210–1218.e4.

28 Moller C: Effect of pollen immunotherapy on food hypersensitivity in children with birch pollinosis. Ann Allergy 1989;62:343–345.

29 Osterballe M, Hansen TK, Mortz CG, Bindslev-Jensen C: The clinical relevance of sensitization to pollen-related fruits and vegetables in unselected pollen-sensitized adults. Allergy 2005;60:218–225.

30 Ricci G, Righetti F, Menna G, Bellini F, Miniaci A, Masi M: Relationship between Bet v 1 and Bet v 2 specific IgE and food allergy in children with grass pollen respiratory allergy. Mol Immunol 2005;42:1251–1257.

31 Sicherer SH: Clinical implications of cross-reactive food allergens. J Allergy Clin Immunol 2001;108:881–890.

32 Asero R, Massironi F, Velati C: Detection of prognostic factors for oral allergy syndrome in patients with birch pollen hypersensitivity. J Allergy Clin Immunol 1996;97:611–616.

33 Ortolani C, Pastorello EA, Farioli L, Ispano M, Pravettoni V, Berti C, et al: IgE-mediated allergy from vegetable allergens. Ann Allergy 1993;71:470–476.

34 Fernandez-Rivas M, van Ree R, Cuevas M: Allergy to Rosaceae fruits without related pollinosis. J Allergy Clin Immunol 1997;100:728–733.

35 Pascal M, Munoz-Cano R, Reina Z, Palacin A, Vilella R, Picado C, et al: Lipid transfer protein syndrome: clinical pattern, cofactor effect and profile of molecular sensitization to plant-foods and pollens. Clin Exp Allergy 2012;42:1529–1539.

36 Cuesta-Herranz J, Lazaro M, de las Heras M, Lluch M, Figueredo E, Umpierrez A, et al: Peach allergy pattern: experience in 70 patients. Allergy 1998;53:78–82.

37 Rodriguez J, Crespo JF, Lopez-Rubio A, De La Cruz-Bertolo J, Ferrando-Vivas P, Vives R, et al: Clinical cross-reactivity among foods of the Rosaceae family. J Allergy Clin Immunol 2000;106:183–189.

38 Worldwide variation in prevalence of symptoms of asthma, allergic rhinoconjunctivitis, and atopic eczema: ISAAC. The International Study of Asthma and Allergies in Childhood (ISAAC) Steering Committee. Lancet 1998;351:1225–1232.

39 Roduit C, Frei R, Loss G, Buchele G, Weber J, Depner M, et al: Development of atopic dermatitis according to age of onset and association with early-life exposures. J Allergy Clin Immunol 2012;130:130–136.e5.

40 Sampson HA: Role of immediate food hypersensitivity in the pathogenesis of atopic dermatitis. J Allergy Clin Immunol 1983;71:473–480.

41 Eigenmann PA, Sicherer SH, Borkowski TA, Cohen BA, Sampson HA: Prevalence of IgE-mediated food allergy among children with atopic dermatitis. Pediatrics 1998;101:E8.

42 Reekers R, Busche M, Wittmann M, Kapp A, Werfel T: Birch pollen-related foods trigger atopic dermatitis in patients with specific cutaneous T-cell responses to birch pollen antigens. J Allergy Clin Immunol 1999;104:466–472.

43 Werfel T, Ballmer-Weber B, Eigenmann PA, Niggemann B, Rance F, Turjanmaa K, et al: Eczematous reactions to food in atopic eczema: position paper of the EAACI and GA2LEN. Allergy 2007;62:723–728.

44 Breuer K, Heratizadeh A, Wulf A, Baumann U, Constien A, Tetau D, et al: Late eczematous reactions to food in children with atopic dermatitis. Clin Exp Allergy 2004;34:817–824.

45 Rothenberg ME: Eosinophilic gastrointestinal disorders (EGID). J Allergy Clin Immunol 2004;113:11–28; quiz 29.

46 Kelley ML Jr, Frazer JP: Symptomatic mid-esophageal webs. JAMA 1966;197:143–146.

47 Hruz P, Straumann A, Bussmann C, Heer P, Simon HU, Zwahlen M, et al: Escalating incidence of eosinophilic esophagitis: a 20-year prospective, population-based study in Olten County, Switzerland. J Allergy Clin Immunol 2011;128:1349–1350.e5.

48 Kapel RC, Miller JK, Torres C, Aksoy S, Lash R, Katzka DA: Eosinophilic esophagitis: a prevalent disease in the United States that affects all age groups. Gastroenterology 2008;134:1316–1321.

49 Spergel JM, Brown-Whitehorn TF, Cianferoni A, Shuker M, Wang ML, Verma R, et al: Identification of causative foods in children with eosinophilic esophagitis treated with an elimination diet. J Allergy Clin Immunol 2012;130:461–467.e5.

50 Kagalwalla AF, Sentongo TA, Ritz S, Hess T, Nelson SP, Emerick KM, et al: Effect of six-food elimination diet on clinical and histologic outcomes in eosinophilic esophagitis. Clin Gastroenterol Hepatol 2006;4:1097–1102.

51 Markowitz JE, Spergel JM, Ruchelli E, Liacouras CA: Elemental diet is an effective treatment for eosinophilic esophagitis in children and adolescents. Am J Gastroenterol 2003;98:777–782.

52 Noel RJ, Putnam PE, Rothenberg ME: Eosinophilic esophagitis. N Engl J Med 2004;351:940–941.

53 Liacouras CA, Spergel JM, Ruchelli E, Verma R, Mascarenhas M, Semeao E, et al: Eosinophilic esophagitis: a 10-year experience in 381 children. Clin Gastroenterol Hepatol 2005;3:1198–1206.

54 Furuta GT, Liacouras CA, Collins MH, Gupta SK, Justinich C, Putnam PE, et al: Eosinophilic esophagitis in children and adults: a systematic review and consensus recommendations for diagnosis and treatment. Gastroenterology 2007;133:1342–1363.

55 Straumann A: Eosinophilic esophagitis: rapidly emerging disorder. Swiss Med Wkly 2012;142:w13513.

56 Talley NJ, Shorter RG, Phillips SF, Zinsmeister AR: Eosinophilic gastroenteritis: a clinicopathological study of patients with disease of the mucosa, muscle layer, and subserosal tissues. Gut 1990;31:54–58.

57 Jaffe JS, James SP, Mullins GE, Braun-Elwert L, Lubensky I, Metcalfe DD: Evidence for an abnormal profile of interleukin-4 (IL-4), IL-5, and gamma-interferon (gamma-IFN) in peripheral blood T cells from patients with allergic eosinophilic gastroenteritis. J Clin Immunol 1994;14:299–309.

58 Prussin C, Lee J, Foster B: Eosinophilic gastrointestinal disease and peanut allergy are alternatively associated with IL-5+ and IL-5(–) T(H)2 responses. J Allergy Clin Immunol 2009;124:1326–1332.e6.

59 Justinich C, Katz A, Gurbindo C, Lepage G, Chad Z, Bouthillier L, et al: Elemental diet improves steroid-dependent eosinophilic gastroenteritis and reverses growth failure. J Pediatr Gastroenterol Nutr 1996;23:81–85.

60 Chang JY, Choung RS, Lee RM, Locke GR 3rd, Schleck CD, Zinsmeister AR, et al: A shift in the clinical spectrum of eosinophilic gastroenteritis toward the mucosal disease type. Clin Gastroenterol Hepatol 2010;8:669–675; quiz e88.

61 Sicherer SH, Eigenmann PA, Sampson HA: Clinical features of food protein-induced enterocolitis syndrome. J Pediatr 1998;133:214–219.

62 Nowak-Wegrzyn A, Sampson HA, Wood RA, Sicherer SH: Food protein-induced enterocolitis syndrome caused by solid food proteins. Pediatrics 2003;111:829–835.

63 Katz Y, Goldberg MR, Rajuan N, Cohen A, Leshno M: The prevalence and natural course of food protein-induced enterocolitis syndrome to cow's milk: a large-scale, prospective population-based study. J Allergy Clin Immunol 2011;127:647–653.e1–e3.

64 Caubet JC, Nowak-Wegrzyn A: Food protein-induced enterocolitis to hen's egg. J Allergy Clin Immunol 2011;128:1386–1388.

65 Caubet JC, Nowak-Wegrzyn A: Current understanding of the immune mechanisms of food protein-induced enterocolitis syndrome. Expert Rev Clin Immunol 2011;7:317–327.

66 Sopo SM, Giorgio V, Dello Iacono I, Novembre E, Mori F, Onesimo R: A multicentre retrospective study of 66 Italian children with food protein-induced enterocolitis syndrome: different management for different phenotypes. Clin Exp Allergy 2012;42:1257–1265.

67 Tan J, Campbell D, Mehr S: Food protein-induced enterocolitis syndrome in an exclusively breast-fed infant-an uncommon entity. J Allergy Clin Immunol 2012;129:873; author reply 873–874.

68 Mehr SS, Kakakios AM, Kemp AS: Rice: a common and severe cause of food protein-induced enterocolitis syndrome. Arch Dis Child 2009;94:220–223.

69 Mehr S, Kakakios A, Frith K, Kemp AS: Food protein-induced enterocolitis syndrome: 16-year experience. Pediatrics 2009;123:e459–e464.

70 Murray KF, Christie DL: Dietary protein intolerance in infants with transient methemoglobinemia and diarrhea. J Pediatr 1993;122:90–92.

71 Leonard SA, Nowak-Wegrzyn A: Clinical diagnosis and management of food protein-induced enterocolitis syndrome. Curr Opin Pediatr 2012;24:739–745.

72 Hwang JB, Sohn SM, Kim AS: Prospective follow-up oral food challenge in food protein-induced enterocolitis syndrome. Arch Dis Child 2009;94:425–428.

73 Rubin M: Allergic intestinal bleeding in the newborn. Amer J Med Sci 1940;200:385.

74 Lake AM: Food-induced eosinophilic proctocolitis. J Pediatr Gastroenterol Nutr 2000;30(suppl):S58–S60.

75 Elizur A, Cohen M, Goldberg MR, Rajuan N, Cohen A, Leshno M, et al: Cow's milk associated rectal bleeding: a population based prospective study. Pediatr Allergy Immunol 2012;23:766–770.

76 Ravelli A, Villanacci V, Chiappa S, Bolognini S, Manenti S, Fuoti M: Dietary protein-induced proctocolitis in childhood. Am J Gastroenterol 2008;103:2605–2612.

77 Lyngkaran N: Severity and extend of upper bowel mucosal damage in cow's milk protein-sensitive enteropathy. J Pediatr Gastroenterol Nutr 1988;7:667.

78 Walker-Smith JA: Cow milk-sensitive enteropathy: predisposing factors and treatment. J Pediatr 1992;121:S111–S115.

79 Moissidis I, Chaidaroon D, Vichyanond P, Bahna SL: Milk-induced pulmonary disease in infants (Heiner syndrome). Pediatr Allergy Immunol 2005;16:545–552.

80 Stafford HA, Polmar SH, Boat TF: Immunologic studies in cow's milk-induced pulmonary hemosiderosis. Pediatr Res 1977;11:898–903.

Philippe A. Eigenmann, MD
Pediatric Allergy Unit
Department of Child and Adolescent
University Hospitals of Geneva
Rue Willy-Donze 6
CH–1211 Genève 14 (Switzerland)
E-Mail philippe.eigenmann@hcuge.ch

Clinical Aspects

Ebisawa M, Ballmer-Weber BK, Vieths S, Wood RA (eds): Food Allergy: Molecular Basis and Clinical Practice.
Chem Immunol Allergy. Basel, Karger, 2015, vol 101, pp 51–58 (DOI: 10.1159/000371669)

Food Allergy in Adolescence and Adulthood

Barbara K. Ballmer-Weber

Allergy Unit, Department of Dermatology, University Hospital Zurich, Zurich, Switzerland

Abstract

In young children, food allergy is usually acquired via the gastrointestinal tract and directed toward egg and milk. Adolescent and adult patients, however, mainly acquire food allergy via primary sensitization to inhalant allergens on the basis of cross-reactivity between proteins in inhalant sources and in food. This type of food allergy is frequently mediated by sensitization to broadly represented allergens, or so-called panallergens. Food allergic reactions in adult patients – similar to those in children – range in severity from very mild and local symptoms, as in contact urticaria of the oral mucosa, to systemic symptoms involving distal organs, to a fatal outcome. Plant foods, such as fruits, nuts, and vegetables, are the most prevalent allergenic foods in this age group.

© 2015 S. Karger AG, Basel

Introduction

Up to 30% of the general population perceives food allergy as a major health problem for them, although only part of the claims can be confirmed after a full clinical evaluation, including controlled oral challenges. Recent population surveys have provided some insight into the prevalence of food allergy. According to these investigations, food allergy is estimated to affect at least 1–4% of the general population. In the adult population, however, the prevalence is very likely underestimated. In infancy, food allergy is most frequently the result of primary sensitization to food allergens via the gastrointestinal tract, directed toward digestion-resistant food allergens. Even though the majority of food-allergic children lose their food allergy, particularly to egg and milk, with increasing age, a subgroup of these young patients are affected by persistent food allergy, especially to legumes, nuts, fish, or crustaceans. In adults, however, newly acquired food allergy is often the result of primary sensitization to inhalant allergens, and particularly pollen, with subsequent sensitization to cross-reactive allergens in food. Within the 'European Community Respiratory Health Survey', sensitization to aeroallergens was assessed in 18,102 adult patients, and the overall sensitization to birch pollen by skin testing was 6%. In Central and Northern Europe, however, this figure increased up to 22% [1]. A Danish study investigated the probability of a clinical reaction to foods among 936 pollen-sensitized patients. Sensitization to birch pollen or combined sensitization to birch and grass or mugwort pollen has been associated with food allergy in 25–

50% of cases [2]. Taking into account these results and the rate of sensitization to birch pollen, we are most likely confronted with up to 5–10% of adults who suffer from a pollen-related food allergy, at least in some parts of Europe. Furthermore, a yet-unknown proportion of adults suffer from food intolerances, such as intolerance to lactose, fructose, or gluten, with symptoms that are sometimes difficult to distinguish from food allergy. Thus, adverse reactions to foods in adults can be a consequence of persistent or newly acquired primary food allergy, due to an inhalant allergen-mediated cross-reactive food allergy, or can be due to intolerance reactions to food ingredients or psychological diseases. Consequently, the management of an adult patient presenting with food-induced symptoms is an enormous challenge for the responsible allergist.

Food Allergies Due to Cross-Reaction with Inhalant Allergens

A hallmark of adult food allergy is a high prevalence of secondary food allergy, in which the primary sensitization is directed toward an inhalant allergen (i.e. pollen). The food allergen is recognized by inhalant allergen-specific IgEs due to a high structural homology between the food and the inhalant allergen on the basis of cross-reaction [3, 4].

Fruits, vegetables, and nuts are some of the most important elicitors of food allergy in adults and adolescents. Recently, a review of 36 studies, covering data from over 250,000 children and adults with respect to plant food allergy, was published. In most studies, allergy was not confirmed by challenges, but 6 studies revealed a prevalence rate for vegetable allergies of 1.4%. Furthermore, according to this recent analysis, the prevalence of fruit allergy, as confirmed by food challenges, ranged from 0.1 to 4.3% [5]. Among tree nuts, the highest prevalence was over 4%, for hazelnuts. In another investigation, sera from a random sample of young adults (n = 4,522) living in 13 countries and assessed within the 'European Community Respiratory Health Survey' were analyzed for IgE against 24 foods. The sensitization rates among fruits were highest for peach (5.4%), apple (4.2%), and kiwifruit (3.6%); among vegetables, for carrot (3.6%) and celeriac (3.5%); and among nuts, for hazelnut (7.2%) [6]. The majority of allergic reactions against these plant foods are highly associated with several pollen allergies.

Birch Pollen-Mediated Food Allergy
Birch pollen-related food allergies are mainly mediated by cross-reactions between either the PR-10-protein Bet v 1, the major allergen in birch pollen, or, less frequently, the profilin Bet v 2 and homologous proteins in plant food [3, 4]. Whereas the clinical relevance of sensitization to Bet v 1-homologous food proteins is well established, the clinical implication of profilin sensitization is still a matter of controversy. Sensitization to birch profilin was demonstrated to result in a broad pattern of sensitization to plant foods, without being translated into the same spectrum of clinical food allergies. IgE antibodies specific for the major birch pollen allergen Bet v 1 have been shown to cross-react with homologous proteins identified in different stone and pip fruits, e.g. apple (Mal d 1), cherry (Pru av 1), and pear (Py r c 1), as well as in hazelnut (Cor a 1), celeriac (Api g 1), carrot (Dau c 1), legumes such as soybean (Gly m 4) and peanut (Ara h 8), kiwi (Act d 8), and many other plant foods. Table 1 summarizes the most prevalent birch pollen-related food allergies. Food allergies associated with birch pollen or related tree pollen (i.e. alder pollen) are most important in Northern and Central Europe, but they are also observed in the U.S. and in Japan [7].

Usually, birch pollen-related food allergies induce mild allergic symptoms often restricted to the oral cavity (so-called oral allergy syndrome, OAS). Food challenge studies on hazelnut, apple, and cherry allergy support this observation [8–

Table 1. Examples of potential food allergies in patients with sensitization to inhalant allergens

Pollen	Food
Birch pollen	apple, pear, cherry, peach, nectarine, apricot, plum, kiwi, hazelnut, almond, walnut, celeriac, carrot, peanut, soy, raw potato
Mugwort pollen	celeriac, carrot, spices (caraway, coriander seeds, paprika, pepper), sunflower seeds, honey, melon, lychee, mango, peach, pistachio, cashew nut, grape, tomato, paprika, cucumber, chamomile, parsley, fennel, aniseed, garlic, onion, mustard, broccoli, cabbage, cauliflower
Ragweed pollen	melon, zucchini, cucumber, banana
Plane pollen	hazelnut, peach, apple, melon, kiwi, peanut, corn, chickpea, lettuce, green bean
Latex	avocado, banana, kiwi, chestnut, papaya, fig, passion fruit, pineapple, melon, peach, apple, carrot, celeriac, tomato, potato, paprika, zucchini
House dust mite	crustaceans, mollusks
Bird feathers and droppings	egg yolk
Cat epithelia	pork

10]. However, studies on celeriac and carrot allergy in pollen-allergic subjects have reported systemic reactions in up to 50% of the patients [11, 12]. Similarly, severe allergic reactions, including anaphylaxis, were first observed in birch pollen-mediated soy allergy by Kleine-Tebbe et al., particularly after intake of a soybean-containing dietary product. Shortly afterward, the Bet v 1-homologous protein Gly m 4 was detected as the responsible allergen in birch pollen-mediated soy allergy [13]. In rare cases, such severe reactions also occur after intake of fruits or freshly harvested hazelnuts. One hypothesis is that the high protein content of a food matrix can enhance the stability of an allergen against gastrointestinal degradation. Additionally, the intake of protein-rich soybean-containing products (dietary products, milk) or protein-rich hazelnuts, for instance, into an empty stomach, with a consequent rapid rise in the gastric pH that also hampers the degradation of proteins, may induce absorption of large amounts of Bet v 1-homologous food proteins, which can lead to severe systemic allergic reactions [14].

Since tree pollen-related allergens in food are heat labile, the majority of patients with a birch pollen-related food allergy tolerate the allergenic food after cooking. In highly sensitized patients, however, roasted hazelnuts [15] and cooked celeriac [16] are still able to evoke symptoms.

Mugwort Pollen-Mediated Food Allergy
About 20% of mugwort pollen-sensitized patients are estimated to suffer from an associated food allergy, mainly directed toward members of the Apiaceae family, such as celeriac, carrot, fennel, parsley, and aniseed, but also directed toward spices, fruits such as mango or peach, honey, mustard, and sunflower seeds [17]. The association between sensitization to mugwort, celeriac, and spices was first observed by Wüthrich et al. almost 30 years ago and published under the term 'celery-

mugwort-spice syndrome'. Most mugwort-associated food allergies have been described in case reports or small case series. Cross-reactive allergens have not been fully elucidated so far. Some of these food allergies, particularly to celeriac and carrot, also occur in association with birch pollen sensitization. Mugwort-related food allergies usually are associated with a more severe clinical manifestation, up to anaphylaxis, than birch pollen-associated food allergies are [11, 12]. Mugwort-associated peach allergy has been observed not only in the Mediterranean area but also in China, where a lipid transfer protein was reported to be the responsible cross-reactive allergen.

Grass, Ragweed, and Plane Pollen-Mediated Food Allergy
Sensitization to apple, peach, tomato, or peanut has been detected in grass pollen-allergic subjects. The cross-sensitization, however, was mainly mediated by profilin or so-called cross-reactive carbohydrate determinants, which are often not clinically relevant [18]. Thus, in Central and Northern Europe, grass pollen-mediated food allergy could not be confirmed to date. However, another situation might be encountered in the Mediterranean area, where patients show higher levels of IgE to grass profilin [12]. Ragweed pollen-associated food allergies to banana or melon have been described in small case series. More comprehensive studies that confirm these initial observations, however, are lacking. In Spain, an association between sensitization to plane pollen and food allergy has been observed [19].

Other Cross-Reactive Food Allergies
An association between sensitization to latex and foods such as chestnut, avocado, kiwi, and banana and many others have been observed and published under the term 'latex-fruit syndrome'. Among 137 patients with a latex allergy, 42% reported allergic reactions to different fruits [20]. Due to successful preventive strategies, the prevalence of latex allergy is decreasing in many countries. Accordingly, latex-associated food allergy is currently less frequently observed.

The muscle protein tropomyosin, present in arachnids such as house dust mites (mite tropomyosins Der p 10 and Der f 10) and in crustaceans (shrimp, crab, lobster, etc.) and mollusks (mussels, squid, etc.), is responsible for so-called 'crustacean-mite syndrome' [21]. Inhalant allergy to bird feathers or bird droppings might be accompanied by an allergy to egg yolk. This constellation is called 'bird-egg syndrome' [22]. Alpha-livetin (bird serum albumin, or Gad c 5 in egg yolk) has been identified as the responsible cross-reactive allergen.

Patients with sensitization to cat epithelium and associated pork meat allergy have been described using the term 'pork-cat syndrome' [23].

Allergic Reactions to Foods May Already Occur upon First Consumption
The presence of broadly cross-reacting allergens (so-called panallergens) in pollen and plant foods may lead to a phenomenon in which patients with sensitization to such allergens react upon first ingestion of a food containing these allergens. Thus, a subgroup of Swiss patients with pollen and/or food sensitization who had never been exposed to three exotic vegetables (water spinach, hyacinth bean, and Ethiopian eggplant) in the past responded with allergic symptoms upon provocation with these foods [24]. Danish pollen-sensitized patients recognized Nangai nut extract without having been previously exposed to this nut, and allergy to exotic fruits like jackfruit was observed in birch pollen-allergic patients due to the presence of Bet v 1 homologs in exotic fruits.

Sensitization to Galactose-Alpha-1,3-Galactose and Allergy to Red Meat

The overall prevalence of meat allergy is low. Recently, however, delayed-type reactions to mammalian meat were observed first in patients in the southeastern U.S. and later in other regions, such as Australia. In those patients, IgE antibodies directed toward an oligosaccharide, i.e. galactose-alpha-1,3-galactose (alpha-gal), present in beef, pork, lamb meat, and cat dander were observed. IgE to alpha-gal was first detected in patients from similar geographic regions suffering from immediate-type reactions to cetuximab, a recombinant chimeric anti-epidermal growth factor monoclonal antibody. IgE antibodies in these patients were directed toward the alpha-gal component of the Fab fragment of the cetuximab heavy chain. It was further observed that bites from the tick species *Amblyomma americanum* (lone star tick), found in the southeastern U.S., might precede hypersensitivity to alpha-gal. In an Australian study, allergy to red meat was reported together with a history of bites from other ticks. Clinical symptoms in alpha-gal-induced food allergy to meat are similar to the immediate-type reactions observed in other food allergies, although the symptoms usually occur with a delay of hours after ingestion of the culprit meat [25].

Clinical Symptoms

As in children, in adult and adolescent patients, food allergy symptoms usually occur within a few minutes up to two hours after ingestion of the culprit food, with manifestations involving one or more organ systems, such as the skin, the respiratory tract, the gastrointestinal tract, or the cardiovascular system.

Local Oral Symptoms
The most frequent clinical presentation of food allergy in adults occurs at the oropharyngeal mucosa and at the lips immediately after contact with the responsible food, comparable with contact urticaria of the skin. In the literature, this symptom has been mislabeled as a 'syndrome', i.e. OAS [8]. Within seconds to minutes, patients experience tingling and itching sensations on the oral mucosa, lips, tongue, throat, and ears that last for a few minutes, and occasionally for up to one hour. In some patients, short-lived blisters on the mucosa or redness of the oral mucosa, with slight swelling, is observed. Since pollen-related allergy to plant foods is often restricted to these local symptoms of the oral mucosa, 'OAS' is often used by mistake as a synonym for pollen-related food allergy. However, contact urticaria of the oral mucosa is as frequently reported by patients suffering from a primary food allergy, such as to peanut, egg, or shrimp. The symptoms of oral contact urticaria are self-limiting, particularly in pollen-related food allergy, but can be followed by systemic reactions, up to anaphylaxis.

Warning Signs for Impending Systemic Reactions
Contact urticaria of the oral mucosa or OAS might be a warning sign for impending more severe symptoms. Frequently, patients with food-mediated systemic allergy experience local oral symptoms as a first symptom at low amounts of the responsible food. With continuous intake of the food, i.e. increasing amounts, more severe systemic reactions occur. Other warning signs are tingling and itching sensations on the palms, soles, or capillitium; nausea; and cramps of the gastrointestinal tract. Generally, patients usually develop subjective symptoms of the involved organ systems before the more severe and objective symptoms occur (fig. 1). Thus, in our own studies, we observed that under provocation, 90% of peanut-allergic subjects presented local oral symptoms, which were followed by systemic, partly severe allergic symptoms with increasing doses of peanuts in 80% of challenged cases.

Food Allergy-Induced Systemic Reactions
Cutaneous symptoms such as flush, urticaria, or angioedema are the most prevalent systemic symptoms in food allergy. They are frequently observed in combination with symptoms of other target organs but may also be present as the sole manifestation. Contact urticaria (a local wheal-

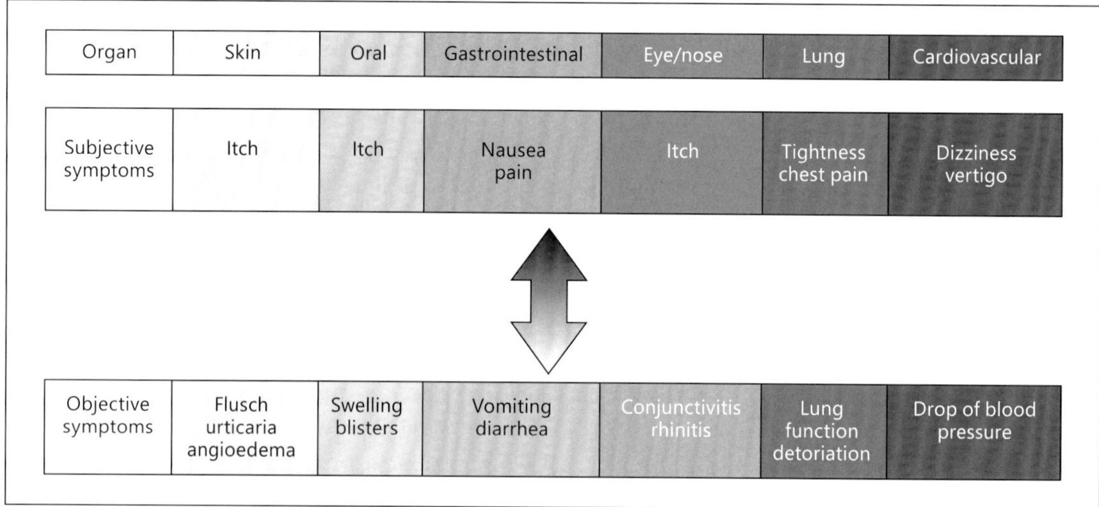

Fig. 1. Subjective symptoms observed during food allergic reactions that might be followed by objective symptoms of the same target organ.

and-flare reaction at the site of contact with the food) is rather commonly present. In adults, symptoms of the gastrointestinal tract, such as nausea, emesis, abdominal cramps, or diarrhea, rarely occur as an isolated manifestation but are commonly accompanied by symptoms from other organ systems. Symptoms from the upper and lower respiratory tract, such as rhinoconjunctivitis, laryngeal edema, or bronchospasm, are commonly observed mainly in relation to other allergic manifestations. Criteria for the diagnosis of anaphylaxis, a potentially life-threatening reaction, are discussed by Pesek and Jones (pp. 191–198).

Differential Diagnosis of Food Allergy in Adults

Various intolerance reactions to foods might mimic food allergy since they elicit symptoms similar to those observed during a food allergic reaction. A situation in which carbohydrates are inadequately digested and absorbed in the intestine and are again inadequately metabolized by bacteria in the colon, leading to symptoms, is called carbohydrate malabsorption. These symptoms consist of abdominal cramps, bloating, flatulence, nausea, and diarrhea. Carbohydrate malabsorption might be induced by different conditions, such as (1) genetically transmitted or acquired deficiency of intestinal enzymes that are needed for the digestion of carbohydrates, such as in lactose intolerance, or (2) ingestion of carbohydrates for which a physiologically defined and limited absorption capacity exists, such as for fructose or sorbitol. Recently, observational data have been published on patients reporting gluten sensitivity or intolerance in the absence of celiac disease or wheat allergy [26]. Apart from lactose intolerance, most other food-mediated intolerance reactions lack convincing evidence in terms of diagnosis and management.

In the following, carbohydrate malabsorption (lactose intolerance and fructose malabsorption, reviewed by [27]) and histamine intolerance are briefly summarized. After exclusion of IgE-mediated food allergy, such intolerance reactions have to be taken into account as a differential diagnosis in adult patients.

Lactose Intolerance
Primary lactase deficiency is the most frequently observed form of lactase deficiency in adulthood. Secondary lactase deficiency might be the consequence of extensive small bowel disease, such as celiac disease. Lactose is a disaccharide cleaved into glucose and galactose by lactase, which is located on enterocytes of the proximal small bowel. Glucose and galactose can be absorbed in the small bowel. A decrease in lactase activity or expression leads to accelerated intestinal transit and metabolism of lactose to short-chain fatty acids, hydrogen, and other metabolites by bacteria in the colon, leading to abdominal symptoms.

A single-nucleotide polymorphism 13,910 bp above the structural gene coding for lactase on the short arm of chromosome 2q.21–22 has been described. The polymorphism consists of a nucleotide switch of T for C, resulting in variants CC, CT, and TT-13910. CC is associated with lactase deficiency (reviewed by [27]).

Fructose Malabsorption
Fructose is a monosaccharide occurring in our diet in different forms: as a monosaccharide contained in many different fruits; as the disaccharide sucrose (glucose and fructose); and in polymerized forms, such as inulins, fructans, and fructooligosaccharide. High-fructose corn syrup was developed from cornstarch in the 1960s as a cheap sweetener added, for instance, to soft drinks or desserts. In the U.S., consumption of high-fructose corn syrup increased to around 17% of the total energy intake [27]. Fructose uptake occurs by passive diffusion facilitated by a carrier system, and the transport capacity is dependent on the presence of glucose. Thus, fructose malabsorption occurs after intake of foods in which fructose is in excess of glucose. Furthermore, sorbitol, a sugar alcohol used as a sweetener in sugar-free food products, reduces the capacity for fructose absorption. As described for lactose, nonabsorbed fructose reaches the colon and gets metabolized to short-chain fatty acids and other metabolites that induce abdominal symptoms. Since the normal capacity for fructose absorption in healthy individuals is not defined, the condition is difficult to diagnose [27].

Histamine Intolerance
Histamine intolerance is a scientifically not-yet-defined disease. It has been suggested that histamine intolerance is caused by an accumulation of histamine caused by inadequate degradation due to the impaired function or a low concentration of histamine-degrading enzymes, and particularly diamine oxidase. The accumulation of histamine leads to allergy-like symptoms, such as abdominal cramps, diarrhea, nausea, itching, flush or urticaria, wheezing, or hypotension and headache. The prevalence of this disease is not yet known but is suggested to be around 1% [28].

References

1 Bousquet PJ, Chinn S, Janson C, Kogevinas M, Burney P, Jarvis D; European Community Respiratory Health Survey I: Geographical variation in the prevalence of positive skin tests to environmental aeroallergens in the European Community Respiratory Health Survey I. Allergy 2007;62:301–309.

2 Osterballe M, Hansen TK, Mortz CG, Bindslev-Jensen C: The clinical relevance of sensitization to pollen-related fruits and vegetables in unselected pollen-sensitized adults. Allergy 2005;60: 218–225.

3 Vieths S, Scheurer S, Ballmer-Weber B: Current understanding of cross-reactivity of food allergens and pollen. Ann N Y Acad Sci 2002;964:47–68.

4 Steckelbroeck S, Ballmer-Weber BK, Vieths S: Potential, pitfalls, and prospects of food allergy diagnostics with recombinant allergens or synthetic sequential epitopes. J Allergy Clin Immunol 2008;121:1323–1330.

5 Zuidmeer L, Goldhahn K, Rona RJ, Gislason D, Madsen C, Summers C, Sodergren E, Dahlstrom J, Lindner T, Sigurdardottir ST, McBride D, Keil T: The prevalence of plant food allergies: a systematic review. J Allergy Clin Immunol 2008;121:1210–1218.

6 Burney P, Summers C, Chinn S, Hooper R, van Ree R, Lidholm J: Prevalence and distribution of sensitization to foods in the European Community Respiratory Health Survey: a EuroPrevall analysis. Allergy 2010;65:1182–1188.

7 Ballmer-Weber BK, Hoffmann-Sommergruber K: Molecular diagnosis of fruit and vegetable allergy. Curr Opin Allergy Clin Immunol 2011;11:229–235.

8 Mari A, Ballmer-Weber BK, Vieths S: The oral allergy syndrome: improved diagnostic and treatment methods. Curr Opin Allergy Clin Immunol 2005;5:267–273.

9 Ballmer-Weber BK, Scheurer S, Fritsche P, Enrique E, Cistero-Bahima A, Haase T, Wüthrich B: Component-resolved diagnosis with recombinant allergens in patients with cherry allergy. J Allergy Clin Immunol 2002;110:167–173.

10 Hansen KS, Ballmer-Weber BK, Sastre J, Lidholm J, Andersson K, Oberhofer H, Lluch-Bernal M, Ostling J, Mattsson L, Schocker F, Vieths S, Poulsen LK: Component-resolved in vitro diagnosis of hazelnut allergy in Europe. J Allergy Clin Immunol 2009;123:1134–1141.

11 Bauermeister K, Ballmer-Weber BK, Bublin M, Fritsche P, Hanschmann KM, Hoffmann-Sommergruber K, Lidholm J, Oberhuber C, Randow S, Holzhauser T, Vieths S: Assessment of component-resolved in vitro diagnosis of celeriac allergy. J Allergy Clin Immunol 2009;124:1273–1281.

12 Ballmer-Weber BK, Skamstrup Hansen K, Sastre J, Andersson K, Bätscher I, Ostling J, Dahl L, Hanschmann KM, Holzhauser T, Poulsen LK, Lidholm J, Vieths S: Component-resolved in vitro diagnosis of carrot allergy in three different regions of Europe. Allergy 2012;67:758–766.

13 Mittag D, Vieths S, Vogel L, Becker WM, Rihs HP, Helbling A, Wüthrich B, Ballmer-Weber BK: Soybean allergy in patients allergic to birch pollen: clinical investigation and molecular characterization of allergens. J Allergy Clin Immunol 2004;113:148–154.

14 Schulten V, Lauer I, Scheurer S, Thalhammer T, Bohle B: A food matrix reduces digestion and absorption of food allergens in vivo. Mol Nutr Food Res 2011;55:1484–1491.

15 Hansen KS, Ballmer-Weber BK, Lüttkopf D, Skov PS, Wüthrich B, Bindslev-Jensen C, Vieths S, Poulsen LK: Roasted hazelnuts – allergenic activity evaluated by double-blind, placebo-controlled food challenge. Allergy 2003;58:132–138.

16 Ballmer-Weber BK, Hoffmann A, Wüthrich B, Lüttkopf D, Pompei C, Wangorsch A, Kästner M, Vieths S: Influence of food processing on the allergenicity of celery: DBPCFC with celery spice and cooked celery in patients with celery allergy. Allergy 2002;57:228–235.

17 Egger M, Mutschlechner S, Wopfner N, Gadermaier G, Briza P, Ferreira F: Pollen-food syndromes associated with weed pollinosis: an update from the molecular point of view. Allergy 2006;61:461–476.

18 Guilloux L, Morisset M, Codreanu F, Parisot L, Moneret-Vautrin DA: Peanut allergy diagnosis in the context of grass pollen sensitization for 125 patients: roles of peanut and cross-reactive carbohydrate determinants specific IgE. Int Arch Allergy Immunol 2009;149:91–97.

19 Enrique E, Cisteró-Bahíma A, Bartolomé B, Alonso R, San Miguel-Moncín MM, Bartra J, Martínez A: Platanus acerifolia pollinosis and food allergy. Allergy 2002;57:351–356.

20 Brehler R, Theissen U, Mohr C, Luger T: 'Latex-fruit syndrome': frequency of cross-reacting IgE antibodies. Allergy 1997;52:404–410.

21 Ayuso R, Reese G, Leong-Kee S, Plante M, Lehrer SB: Molecular basis of arthropod cross-reactivity: IgE-binding cross-reactive epitopes of shrimp, house dust mite and cockroach tropomyosins. Int Arch Allergy Immunol 2002;129:38–48.

22 Szépfalusi Z, Ebner C, Pandjaitan R, Orlicek F, Scheiner O, Boltz-Nitulescu G, Kraft D, Ebner H: Egg yolk alpha-livetin (chicken serum albumin) is a cross-reactive allergen in the bird-egg syndrome. J Allergy Clin Immunol 1994;93:932–942.

23 Drouet M, Boutet S, Lauret MG, Chène J, Bonneau JC, Le Sellin J, Hassoun S, Gay G, Sabbah A: The pork-cat syndrome or crossed allergy between pork meat and cat epithelia. Allerg Immunol (Paris) 1994;26:166–168.

24 Gubesch M, Theler B, Dutta M, Baumer B, Mathis A, Holzhauser T, Vieths S, Ballmer-Weber BK: Strategy for allergenicity assessment of 'natural novel foods': clinical and molecular investigation of exotic vegetables (water spinach, hyacinth bean and Ethiopian eggplant). Allergy 2007;62:1243–1250.

25 Commins SP, Satinover SM, Hosen J, Mozena J, Borish L, Lewis BD, Woodfolk JA, Platts-Mills TA: Delayed anaphylaxis, angioedema, or urticaria after consumption of red meat in patients with IgE antibodies specific for galactose-alpha-1,3-galactose. J Allergy Clin Immunol 2009;123:426–433.

26 Aziz I, Hadjivassiliou M, Sanders DS: Does gluten sensitivity in the absence of coeliac disease exist? BMJ 2012;30:345.

27 Hammer HF, Hammer J: Diarrhea caused by carbohydrate malabsorption. Gastroenterol Clin North Am 2012;41:611–627.

28 Maintz L, Novak N: Histamine and histamine intolerance. Am J Clin Nutr 2007;85:1185–1196.

Prof. Barbara K. Ballmer-Weber, MD
Allergy Unit, Department of Dermatology
University Hospital Zurich
Gloriastrasse 31
CH–8091 Zurich (Switzerland)
E-Mail barbara.ballmer@usz.ch

Ebisawa M, Ballmer-Weber BK, Vieths S, Wood RA (eds): Food Allergy: Molecular Basis and Clinical Practice.
Chem Immunol Allergy. Basel, Karger, 2015, vol 101, pp 59–67 (DOI: 10.1159/000371674)

Hints for Diagnosis

Lars K. Poulsen

Laboratory of Medical Allergology, Allergy Clinic, Copenhagen University Hospital at Gentofte, Copenhagen,
Denmark

Abstract

The diagnosis of food allergy requires responses to two important questions: Does the patient have a food allergy? If so, which foods will elicit allergic symptoms? The first question will most often have to be answered following a physical examination and an interview with the patient and/or caretakers. Based on this, a provisional decision to pursue a food allergy diagnosis may be made after carefully considering other possible reasons for an adverse reaction to a food: aversion, infection, intoxication, or an underlying metabolic disease. To respond to the next question, the anamnesis is highly important in selecting which tests and, ultimately, oral food challenges the patient should undergo to reach the final diagnosis. For the diagnosing doctor, it is important to know and consider the regional pattern of inhalation and food allergies, the food consumption patterns in the local community, and the selection of patients – in terms of both age groups and symptoms – visiting the center.

© 2015 S. Karger AG, Basel

The Purpose of the Diagnosis

The purpose of diagnosing food allergy is ideally to explain the symptoms and complaints previously experienced by the patient and to ensure that he or she may live a future life with a manyfold reduced or no risk of food allergic reactions. Since treatments for food allergies, such as immunotherapy or anti-IgE treatment, are still mainly in the experimental stage, the patient must avoid not only the primary offending foods but also foods that may elicit clinically proven cross reactions. Thus, a thorough knowledge of which foods may cause allergic reactions and at approximately which dosages and of how to avoid getting exposed should be the goal for the patient and/or caretakers. In addition, aims should include knowledge of modifying risk factors, early-warning symptoms, and emergency treatment of reactions.

Is It Food Allergy?

As described in previous chapters, the symptomatology of food allergy is quite variable, and the fact that most people ingest large amounts and perhaps even high numbers of foods every day makes the diagnostic process more complicated. Depending on the affected organs and the symptoms, many inflammatory and other disease states may have to be excluded before a food al-

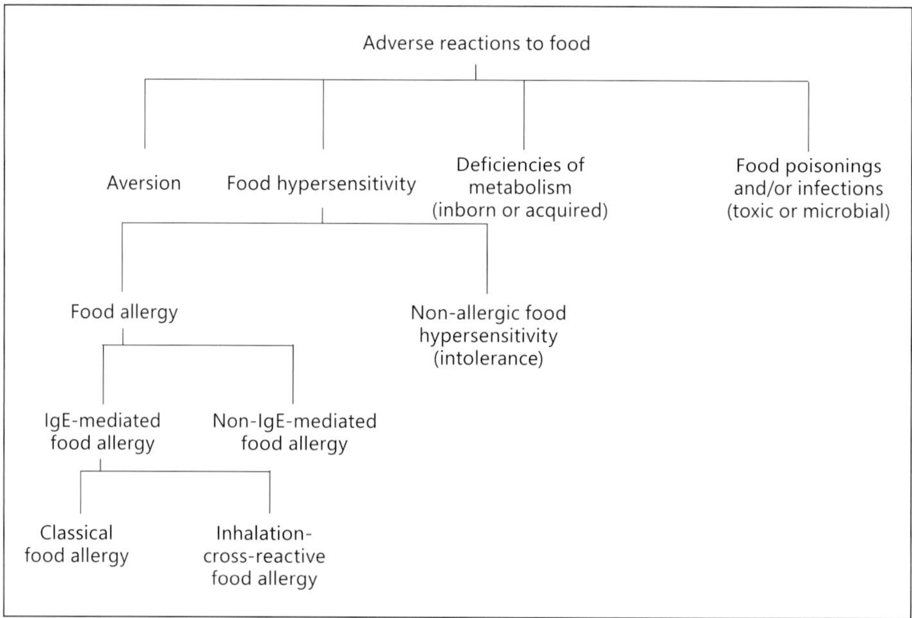

Fig. 1. Classification of food allergy as a subcategory of adverse reactions to food. Expanded and modified from [8].

lergy diagnosis can be considered. If the anamnesis suggests a link between food or drink intake and symptoms, it may be helpful to consider food allergy as only a subgroup of adverse reactions to foods (fig. 1).

It is important to first exclude *food poisonings or infections*, i.e. if more than a single person has reacted to the same food exposure, it is likely to be due to a mechanism other than allergy. In this respect, it is important to remember that allergy-like symptoms may also be a part of the pattern of food-borne poisoning, such as for scombroid poisoning (a dramatic example of an outbreak is given in [1], where the active substance was histamine stemming from decarboxylation of the amino acid histidine, e.g. in fish during putrefaction).

Another differential diagnosis comprises *genetic or acquired deficiencies in metabolism*, of which lactase deficiency [2] is probably the most common. In adult and adolescent patients, alcohol intolerance may be another important diagnosis in this respect, but alcohol could also be a co-factor in eliciting food allergy by reducing the threshold dose to which the patient reacts.

Physiological and pathophysiological reactions may be mediated via taste [3], and this may lead to conditional behavior, such as *aversion*, in which stimulation of taste receptors initiates a central nervous reflex [4] that may ultimately lead to reactions that could be misinterpreted as food allergy. This phenomenon – in combination with a patient's potential psychological fear of ingesting a food believed to have previously caused a severe reaction – is the main reason for employing double-blind, placebo-controlled challenges in the diagnosis of food allergy. It should be noted that recent research in this area [5] has suggested that taste receptors are not limited to the oral cavity but may also be found in the gastrointestinal system.

If the consideration and exclusion of the above-mentioned differential diagnoses lead to the tentative conclusion that the patient reacts to amounts of food that would be tolerated by most individuals in the population, the diagnosis of *food hypersensitivity* may be reached. Such a diagnosis can be strongly supported by a positive challenge with the offending food, but it is important to emphasize that a positive challenge alone rarely suggests the disease mechanism. By definition, *food allergy* is a food hypersensitivity that has an immunological background, whereas non-immunological food hypersensitivity – formerly described as food intolerance – depends on other, not necessarily known mechanisms. Since the latter disease states are not well described in terms of pathophysiology, it is mandatory to establish a clinically proven diagnosis of food hypersensitivity and to not only rely on laboratory or other paraclinical tests [6, 7].

This definition of food allergy [8] (see [9] for a discussion and references to further guidelines for classification) leads to the inclusion of diseases, such as celiac disease or rare conditions including food-induced nickel allergy (systemic contact dermatitis) [10], besides IgE-mediated food allergy. While the symptomatology may be suggestive of the disease mechanism, the ultimate diagnosis lies in the demonstration of a pathophysiological immune response that may explain the symptoms. Here, we cite the use of anti-trans-aminase antibodies for celiac disease and the nickel patch test for food-induced nickel allergy, but the following will focus on IgE-mediated food allergies.

While total IgE may be an indicator of general atopy, it is rarely, if ever, helpful in discriminating persons with or without food allergy [11]. Likewise, acute measurements during challenge, such as plasma histamine or tryptase measurements, have not been documented to be of great clinical value [12]. This emphasizes that the diagnosis of food hypersensitivity is a clinical rather than a laboratory-based diagnosis.

A number of conditions, such as eosinophilic esophagitis or gastroenteritis IgE-mediated food allergy, may play a role in worsening of symptoms as well as in driving the pathology. The reader is referred to the specialty literature, but in terms of diagnosis, it is important to establish whether a specific food actually plays a role in patients with these diseases.

Which Is the Culprit Food?

Having focused suspicion on food allergy, the next step is to identify the culprit food that has elicited reactions in the past. Here, it is important to distinguish between meals, foods, and allergens. *Meals* are what most people ingest, and these may consist of a vast array of food ingredients, some of which may not even be directly recognizable by either taste or vision. By a *food*, we herein mean a biological source coming from a single species, such as celery or chicken. A single species may, however, give rise to different foods, e.g. celery roots vs. celery stalk or chicken meat vs. egg white vs. egg yolk, and it is important to identify (or exclude) not only the species of the food but also its precise form or fraction. Moreover, food items may have been *processed* in different ways, either processed during the preparation of a specific meal or used as raw materials as ingredients in the meal. In general, it not believed that processing increases the allergenicity of a food, but there are some important examples suggesting that this may actually be the case.

One process is fractionation of a food, which may concentrate certain proteins that may turn out to be allergens, as described for a soy protein isolate containing high amounts of the allergen Gly m 4 (which cross-reacts with the major allergen Bet v 1 of birch pollen) [13], which is otherwise not very abundant in soy beans. Studies of peanut processing have suggested that the roasting process may lead to intramolecular arrangements that stabilize the tertiary protein structure, enhancing the allergenicity of roasted vs. raw peanuts [14], as reviewed in [15].

Thus, one important aim of the diagnostic process should be the incrimination (or exclusion) of a food species, including definition of the form or fraction in which it has elicited reactions in the patient. This sets high demands on the quality of the diagnostic tools in order to be representative of the food in question (containing the right allergenic molecules). When performing challenges or prick-to-prick skin tests, it is possible to control the source materials (which may even be obtained from the patient to ascertain the eliciting food), but this is far more difficult when relying on commercial food allergen extracts for skin prick tests or when using in vitro analyses such as IgE tests or basophil histamine release or activation tests.

Which Allergens Are Involved?

With the advent of large numbers of purified or even cloned allergen molecules from foods [16] and both individual and multiplex analyses [17] for specific IgE against these, we have come one step closer to molecular-based diagnosis of food allergy. A word of caution might be warranted, however. Besides using sufficient quantities of pure and correctly folded variants of the proteins (see [18] and the following chapters for further discussion of analytical criteria for IgE tests), it may also be worth considering what an allergen actually is. By its immunologically based definition, an allergen is an antigen that will bind IgE, but this does not necessarily indicate clinical relevance. For practical reasons, a food allergen is normally considered to be an IgE-binding antigen from a food to which at least one patient has been demonstrated to have hypersensitivity, i.e. most often by a double-blind, placebo-controlled food challenge. By this definition, all IgE responses of a challenge-positive patient will be considered clinically relevant, but since completely pure allergen molecules rarely, if ever, have been used in challenge studies, there may be no formal proof of clinically relevant allergenicity. There are several examples of IgE binding to both carbohy-

drate [19–21] and protein epitopes [22] that have little clinical relevance, and results from both extract-based and molecular diagnostics should be evaluated with this in mind.

However, as described in detail in later chapters, knowledge of IgE reactivities on the molecular level gives rise to a higher likelihood of selecting the right foods for challenge [23], suggesting a milder or more severe disease prognosis [24], or points to which other foods should be considered for possible cross-reactions. While many new tests are available for research use, they should generally only be used routinely when there is an important clinical implication to be drawn from the test result.

How Much Is Too Much?

Patients' reactivities to the ingestion of allergenic foods experienced in the community are extremely difficult to describe [25], but it is generally assumed that the threshold dosages that can be determined in clinical settings are the most reasonable approximations, even though many real-life cofactors (infections, allergic co-morbidities, exercise, the matrix in which the food is given, alcohol, and drugs) may alter a patient's reactivity to challenges. Several groups have worked on defining dose ranges [26, 27], and it is clear that between individual patients, thresholds may vary by 4–5 decades in terms of dosage. Since the practical implications of living with a food allergy can differ widely, it is of great importance for patients and caretakers to know whether reactions may be expected to take place when administering gram quantities, which are often visible in foods and meals, or milligram quantities, which may be invisible. In the latter case, even small amounts of polluting allergenic foods not intended to go into a meal will present a significant problem.

For these reasons, to give both the patient and the doctor an estimate of the clinical sensitivity, it is of clear value to perform the challenge procedure in a titrated form to establish a no-effect level for each individual patient.

Prerequisites for Diagnosis

While each patient is unique, it is important to be aware of the characteristics of the patient population that visits a certain clinic. Overall climatic and geographical factors play a role in determining the inhalation allergies in a region, and some of these may cause cross-reactions with foods. The most frequent food allergy cross-reactivity is probably birch pollen among patients in the temperate areas of Northern and Central Europe, many of whom display symptoms upon exposure to hazelnuts and apples and to many other fruits, vegetables, and nuts. These reactions are well described and, in most cases, diagnosis of the underlying pollen allergy will be sufficient to advise the patient regarding food cross-reactions, with specific IgE tests and oral food challenges being of relatively small added value.

Typical eating habits, the main food variants, and weaning practices in a region may also be important background knowledge.

Finally, the age groups of the patients and whether there is a bias toward, e.g. skin-related or inhalation symptoms, are important to be aware of since food allergies in infants are often to milk or egg or other 'classical' foods (fig. 1) and tend to be outgrown more easily than food allergies in older children and adults. Additionally, worsening of atopic eczema by foods is much more frequent in small children than in adults. Thus, knowledge of the natural history of allergies in general and of food allergies in particular may provide good support for discerning the patterns seen in the clinic. Epidemiological studies have suggested that food allergy seems to change over time in a nonuniform matter in different areas of the world. The reasons for these changing patterns may be related to changes in food consumption patterns, but at present, it is unknown whether this is the sole or even the most important explanation. Accordingly, ongoing research and active monitoring of the scientific literature are crucial to maintain an optimal level of knowledge.

The Diagnostic Process

The individual elements of the diagnostic process are described in detail in later chapters, but basically, the process may be divided into the following steps:
– Anamnesis and physical examination
– In vivo and in vitro tests
– Oral food challenges

Recently, several groups and professional societies in the scientific research community working on food allergy have been revising, producing, and releasing guidelines on food allergy, including how to diagnose food allergy [9, 11, 12], and there are still more to follow from the European Society of Allergy and Clinical Immunology. While there is no total agreement between these guidelines, there is a clear trend indicating that all diagnoses should be based on a thorough examination of the patient, including taking the patient's history to decide whether he or she has a food allergy and, if confirmed, which food might be the cause. In a structured literature review process combined with the views of an expert panel [11], this trend was also emphasized, but the evidence behind it was not impressive (table 1). One must remember, however, that not all studies in medicine can be evidence based, just like there have been no double-blind, placebo-controlled studies to confirm that parachutes are relatively helpful when leaving an airplane at a high altitude. Likewise, it would be neither easy nor ethical to perform a study in which patients were randomized to talk or not talk to a doctor before being submitted to a number of diagnostic tests and food challenges. Thus, the evidence behind taking the patient's history and performing

Table 1. Summary of National Institute of Allergy and Infectious Diseases guidelines related to the diagnosis of food allergy based on an independent, systematic literature review and an expert panel [11]

Question	Guideline	Quality of evidence	Contribution of EP
Diagnosis of IgE-mediated FA (Is it FA?)			
Medical history and physical examination	#2: The EP recommends using medical history and physical examination to aid in the diagnosis of FA. #3: The EP recommends that parent and patient reports of FA must be confirmed because multiple studies have demonstrated that 50–90% of presumed FAs are not allergies.	Low High	Significant Minimal
Methods to identify the causative food (Which is the culprit food?)			
SPT	#4: The EP recommends performing an SPT to assist in the identification of foods that may be provoking IgE-mediated food-induced allergic reactions, but an SPT alone cannot be considered diagnostic of FA.	Moderate	Significant
Intradermal tests	#5: The EP recommends that intradermal testing should not be used to make a diagnosis of FA.	Low	Significant
Total sIgE	#6: The EP recommends that the measurement of total sIgE should not be routinely used to make a diagnosis of FA.	Low	Significant
Allergen-specific sIgE	#7: The EP recommends sIgE tests for identifying foods that potentially provoke IgE-mediated food-induced allergic reactions, but alone, these tests are not diagnostic of FA.	Moderate	Significant
APT	#8: The EP suggests that an APT should not be used in the routine evaluation of noncontact FA.	Low	Significant
Use of SPTs, sIgE tests, and APTs in combination	#9: The EP suggests that the combination of SPTs, sIgE tests, and APTs should not be used for the routine diagnosis of FA.	Low	Significant
Food elimination diets	#10: The EP suggests that elimination of 1 or a few specific foods from the diet may be useful in the diagnosis of FA, and especially in identifying foods responsible for some non-IgE-mediated food-induced allergic disorders, such as FPIES, food protein-induced AP, and Heiner syndrome, and some mixed IgE- and non-IgE-mediated food-induced allergic disorders, such as EoE.	Low	Significant
Oral food challenges	#11: The EP recommends using oral food challenges for diagnosing FA. The DBPCFC is the gold standard. However, a single-blind or open-food challenge may be considered diagnostic under certain circumstances. If either of these challenges elicits no symptoms (i.e. the challenge is negative), then FA can be ruled out, but when either challenge elicits objective symptoms (i.e. the challenge is positive) and those objective symptoms correlate with the medical history and are supported by laboratory tests, a diagnosis of FA is supported.	High	Moderate

Question	Guideline	Quality of evidence	Contribution of EP
Nonstandardized and unproven procedures	#12: The EP recommends not using any of the following nonstandardized tests for the routine evaluation of IgE-mediated FA: – Basophil histamine release/activation – Lymphocyte stimulation – Facial thermography – Gastric juice analysis – Endoscopic allergen provocation – Hair analysis – Applied kinesiology – Provocation neutralization – Allergen-specific IgG4 testing – Cytotoxicity assays – Electrodermal test (Vega) – Mediator release assay (Lifestyle, Eating, and Performance diet)	Low	Significant

FA = Food allergy; EP = expert panel; SPT = skin prick test; sIgE = serum IgE; APT = atopy patch test; EoE = eosinophilic esophagitis; FPIES = food protein-induced enterocolitis syndrome; AP = allergic proctocolitis; DBPCFC = double-blind, placebo-controlled food challenge.

a physical examination is likely to be based on expert opinions, rather than randomized clinical trials.

Based on such opinions, the anamnesis and physical examination should include a description of symptoms and their temporal relationship with food ingestion, and it is from the symptom description that the suspicion of an IgE-mediated reaction may arise. Food allergy often produces symptoms in more than one organ, and since the patient is often seen by the allergist some time after the reaction, when the patient is in an asymptomatic state, it is important to perform thorough questioning. While the dose may influence the reaction, symptoms are often stereotypic, meaning that if the patient has tolerated a food or a meal on one occasion, he or she is unlikely to react at another time. Thus, in particular, a food to which the patient has not recently been exposed should be sought. Symptoms often have an acute onset and occur within one hour of ingestion, one ex-

ception being reactions to the so-called alpha Gal epitope in meat, which is mainly described as causing symptoms initiating 3–4 hours after ingestion. Late reactions – even after total recovery from the acute symptoms – may occur but are rarely isolated. In regard to knowledge of the ingredients of different meals and raw materials for food preparation, an interview by a trained allergy dietician is often a valuable supplement to the doctor's investigations.

Since food allergy is closely linked to other allergies and may indeed elicit or worsen allergic symptoms in the skin or in the airways, it is important to have an overall picture of all of the patient's allergies, including a possible familial atopic disposition.

The anamnesis and the physical examination rarely yield a diagnosis without further investigation, but this may be the case in well-documented pollen allergies with known cross-reactivities to foods giving rise to oral allergy syndrome [28]. In most other cases, a further diagnostic work-up will include tests and oral food challenges.

The mainstay of diagnosis is the confirmation of clinical reactivity by oral challenge with the incriminated food as well as by a number of paraclinical tests, which were also evaluated in the above-mentioned investigation [11]. A summary of the results and the concluding guidelines are given in table 1, but the reader is referred to the original paper for a deeper discussion and the proper references. Here, it suffices to say that skin prick tests and specific IgE tests are the main diagnostic tests that – besides the case history – may be helpful in shaping the picture leading to the final diagnosis.

of a food allergy, and if the patient will have to be referred to another center that can perform oral food challenges anyway, it might be better to refer them right away. Moreover, if more tests than the doctor expected turn out positive, the doctor may end up in a situation in which the patient expects more clinical investigations than the doctor is prepared or able to deliver. Additionally, a much larger number of patients suspect that they have food allergy than can be proven by proper diagnostic measures. In this respect, the initial anamnesis and physical examination, including a thorough consideration of differential diagnoses, may be an important gatekeeper for the remaining diagnostic process.

Who Should Perform the Diagnosis?

In order to not waste the patient's time and the resources of the health care system, it is important to think ahead before entering the diagnostic process. If it is perceived that the patient will have to undergo an oral food challenge and the clinic does not have the facilities to perform this, it might be better to refer the patient at an early stage, rather than in the middle of the process. This particularly applies to the use of skin prick tests and IgE measurements. Such tests, when negative, are rarely sufficient to eliminate the risk

Conclusions

The diagnosis of food allergy requires responses to two important questions: Does the patient have a food allergy? If so, which foods will elicit allergic symptoms? The first question will most often have to be answered based on a physical examination and an interview with the patient and/ or caretakers. To respond to the next question, the anamnesis is highly important in selecting which tests and, ultimately, oral food challenges the patient should undergo to reach the final diagnosis.

References

1 Demoncheaux JP, Michel R, Mazenot C, Duflos G, Iacini C, de Laval F, Saware EM, Renard JC: A large outbreak of scombroid fish poisoning associated with eating yellowfin tuna (Thunnus albacares) at a military mass catering in Dakar, Senegal. Epidemiol Infect 2012; 140:1008–1012.

2 Jarvela I, Torniainen S, Kolho KL: Molecular genetics of human lactase deficiencies. Ann Med 2009;41:568–575.

3 Negri R, Morini G, Greco L: From the tongue to the gut. J Pediatr Gastroenterol Nutr 2011;53:601–605.

4 Spector AC, Glendinning JI: Linking peripheral taste processes to behavior. Curr Opin Neurobiol 2009;19:370–377.

5 Iwatsuki K, Uneyama H: Sense of taste in the gastrointestinal tract. J Pharmacol Sci 2012;118:123–128.

6 Ortolani C, Bruijnzeel-Koomen C, Bengtsson U, Bindslev-Jensen C, Bjorksten B, Host A, Ispano M, Jarisch R, Madsen C, Nekam K, Paganelli R, Poulsen LK, Wüthrich B: Controversial aspects of adverse reactions to food. European Academy of Allergology and Clinical Immunology (EAACI) Reactions to Food Subcommittee. Allergy 1999;54:27–45.

7 Bindslev-Jensen C, Stahl Skov P, Madsen F, Poulsen LK: Food allergy and food intolerance – what is the difference? Ann Allergy 1994;72:317–320.

8 Johansson SG, Hourihane JO, Bousquet J, Bruijnzeel-Koomen C, Dreborg S, Haahtela T, Kowalski ML, Mygind N, Ring J, Van CP, Van Hage-Hamsten M, Wuthrich B: A revised nomenclature for allergy. An EAACI position statement from the EAACI nomenclature task force. Allergy 2001;56:813–824.

9 Burks AW, Tang M, Sicherer S, Muraro A, Eigenmann PA, Ebisawa M, Fiocchi A, Chiang W, Beyer K, Wood R, Hourihane J, Jones SM, Lack G, Sampson HA: ICON: food allergy. J Allergy Clin Immunol 2012;129:906–920.

10 Menne T, Vejen N, Sjplin K-E, Maibach HI: Systemic contact dermatitis. Am J Cont Derm 1994;5:1–12.

11 Boyce JA, Assa'ad A, Burks AW, Jones SM, Sampson HA, Wood RA, Plaut M, Cooper SF, Fenton MJ, Arshad SH, Bahna SL, Beck LA, Byrd-Bredbenner C, Camargo CA Jr, Eichenfield L, Furuta GT, Hanifin JM, Jones C, Kraft M, Levy BD, Lieberman P, Luccioli S, McCall KM, Schneider LC, Simon RA, Simons FE, Teach SJ, Yawn BP, Schwaninger JM: Guidelines for the diagnosis and management of food allergy in the United States: report of the NIAID-sponsored expert panel. J Allergy Clin Immunol 2010;126:S1–S58.

12 Sampson HA, Gerth van WR, Bindslev-Jensen C, Sicherer S, Teuber SS, Burks AW, Dubois AE, Beyer K, Eigenmann PA, Spergel JM, Werfel T, Chinchilli VM: Standardizing double-blind, placebo-controlled oral food challenges: American Academy of Allergy, Asthma & Immunology-European Academy of Allergy and Clinical Immunology PRACTALL consensus report. J Allergy Clin Immunol 2012;130:1260–1274.

13 Mittag D, Vieths S, Vogel L, Becker WM, Rihs HP, Helbling A, Wuthrich B, Ballmer-Weber BK: Soybean allergy in patients allergic to birch pollen: clinical investigation and molecular characterization of allergens. J Allergy Clin Immunol 2004;113:148–154.

14 Maleki SJ, Chung SY, Champagne ET, Raufman JP: The effects of roasting on the allergenic properties of peanut proteins. J Allergy Clin Immunol 2000;106:763–768.

15 Maleki SJ: Food processing: effects on allergenicity. Curr Opin Allergy Clin Immunol 2004;4:241–245.

16 Sancho AI, Hoffmann-Sommergruber K, Alessandri S, Conti A, Giuffrida MG, Shewry P, Jensen BM, Skov P, Vieths S: Authentication of food allergen quality by physicochemical and immunological methods. Clin Exp Allergy 2010;40:973–986.

17 Hiller R, Laffer S, Harwanegg C, Huber M, Schmidt WM, Twardosz A, Barletta B, Becker WM, Blaser K, Breiteneder H, Chapman M, Crameri R, Duchene M, Ferreira F, Fiebig H, Hoffmann-Sommergruber K, King TP, Kleber-Janke T, Kurup VP, Lehrer SB, Lidholm J, Muller U, Pini C, Reese G, Scheiner O, Scheynius A, Shen HD, Spitzauer S, Suck R, Swoboda I, Thomas W, Tinghino R, Van Hage-Hamsten M, Virtanen T, Kraft D, Muller MW, Valenta R: Microarrayed allergen molecules: diagnostic gatekeepers for allergy treatment. FASEB J 2002;16:414–416.

18 Holzhauser T, Ree R, Poulsen LK, Bannon GA: Analytical criteria for performance characteristics of IgE binding methods for evaluating safety of biotech food products. Food Chem Toxicol 2008;46(suppl 10)S15–S19.

19 van Ree R, Aalberse RC: Specific IgE without clinical allergy. J Allergy Clin Immunol 1999;103:1000–1001.

20 Sten E, Stahl SP, Andersen SB, Torp AM, Olesen A, Bindslev-Jensen U, Poulsen LK, Bindslev-Jensen C: Allergenic components of a novel food, Micronesian nut Nangai (Canarium indicum), shows IgE cross-reactivity in pollen allergic patients. Allergy 2002;57:398–404.

21 Mari A, Ooievaar-de HP, Scala E, Giani M, Pirrotta L, Zuidmeer L, Bethell D, van Ree R: Evaluation by double-blind placebo-controlled oral challenge of the clinical relevance of IgE antibodies against plant glycans. Allergy 2008;63:891–896.

22 Martens M, Schnoor HJ, Malling H-J, Poulsen LK: Sensitization to cereals and peanut evidenced by skin prick test and specific IgE in food-tolerant, grass pollen allergic patients. Clin Transl Allergy 2011;1:15.

23 Eller E, Bindslev-Jensen C: Clinical value of component-resolved diagnostics in peanut-allergic patients. Allergy 2013;68:190–194.

24 Skamstrup Hansen K, Poulsen LK: Component resolved testing for allergic sensitization. Curr Allergy Asthma Rep 2010;10:340–348.

25 Hourihane JO, Grimshaw KE, Lewis SA, Briggs RA, Trewin JB, King RM, Kilburn SA, Warner JO: Does severity of low-dose, double-blind, placebo-controlled food challenges reflect severity of allergic reactions to peanut in the community? Clin Exp Allergy 2005;35:1227–1233.

26 Taylor SL, Hefle SL, Bindslev-Jensen C, Bock SA, Burks AW Jr, Christie L, Hill DJ, Host A, Hourihane JO, Lack G, Metcalfe DD, Moneret-Vautrin DA, Vadas PA, Rance F, Skrypec DJ, Trautman TA, Yman IM, Zeiger RS: Factors affecting the determination of threshold doses for allergenic foods: how much is too much? J Allergy Clin Immunol 2002;109:24–30.

27 Bindslev-Jensen C, Briggs D, Osterballe M: Can we determine a threshold level for allergenic foods by statistical analysis of published data in the literature? Allergy 2002;57:741–746.

28 Bindslev-Jensen C, Ballmer-Weber B, Bengtsson U, Blanco C, Ebner C, Hourihane JO, Knulst AC, Moneret-Vautrin D, Nekam K, Niggemann B, Osterballe M, Ortolani C, Ring J, Schnopp C, Werfel T: Standardization of food challenges in patients with immediate reactions to foods – position paper from the European Academy of Allergology and Clinical Immunology. Allergy 2004;59:690–697.

Lars K. Poulsen
Laboratory of Medical Allergology, Allergy Clinic
Copenhagen University Hospital at Gentofte, Department 22
Kildgaardsvej 28, DK–2900 Hellerup (Denmark)
E-Mail lkpallgy@mail.dk

Ebisawa M, Ballmer-Weber BK, Vieths S, Wood RA (eds): Food Allergy: Molecular Basis and Clinical Practice.
Chem Immunol Allergy. Basel, Karger, 2015, vol 101, pp 68–78 (DOI: 10.1159/000371675)

IgE-Related Examination in Food Allergy with Focus on Allergen Components

Magnus P. Borres[a, b] · Sakura Sato[c] · Motohiro Ebisawa[c]

[a]Department of Women's and Children's Health, Uppsala University, and [b]Thermo Fisher Scientific, Uppsala, Sweden; [c]Department of Allergy, Clinical Research Center for Allergology and Rheumatology, Sagamihara National Hospital, Sagamihara, Kanagawa, Japan

Abstract

Molecular allergology is a breakthrough science that enables the quantification of IgE antibodies against individual allergen protein components at the molecular level. The diagnosis of IgE-mediated allergic disorders is based on the clinical history and on sensitization demonstrated through an allergy test. Identifying whether the sensitization is primary (species specific) or due to cross-reactivity with proteins with similar protein structures helps the clinician to judge the risk of allergic reaction. This is possible today because allergen component tests for food allergy are now available for clinicians to use in everyday practice. © 2015 S. Karger AG, Basel

How IgE-Mediated Food Allergy Is Diagnosed

It is complicated to interpret food allergy symptoms in children because of the dynamic nature of the allergic response, which changes over time: acquisition of food tolerance and amelioration of symptoms have been reported in patients with all types of food allergy [1].

The various diagnostic errors and pitfalls in the management of food allergy suggest that utilizing all available tests more fully is in the best interests of the patient.

The diagnosis of IgE-mediated food allergic disorders is based on the clinical history and on sensitization demonstrated through an allergy test. Allergen-specific IgE is detected by in vitro and/or in vivo testing. In some cases, food provocation tests are performed to confirm an allergy diagnosis.

Sampson and Ho were the first to publish studies on utilization of serum-specific IgE in order to predict which food-allergic patients were likely to fail an oral food challenge [2]. They suggested threshold values for egg, milk, and peanut, i.e. food-specific serum IgE concentrations at which approximately 95% of patients are predicted to have a clinical reaction [2]. These diagnostic values were helpful for the physicians in deciding if a food challenge was necessary or potentially harmful to the patients and also led to interest among other researchers in investigating these relationships.

However, other groups have reported different diagnostic values, and the differences have been explained by the fact that the study populations differed. One explanation for the differences is that there is a relationship between allergen-specific IgE levels in response to egg and milk and oral food challenge outcomes and that this relationship is influenced by age, as shown by Komata et al. [3]. This means that younger children react via low levels of IgE antibody specific to egg and milk compared with older children.

Another explanation could be the difficulty of standardizing the allergens used as substrates. Extracts may differ in terms of their allergenic content due to the natural variability of the allergen source, such as peanut, wheat, or soy.

Furthermore, traditional tests used today are not capable of differentiating between primary sensitization and immunological cross-reactivity, which, in some cases, entails a significant risk of serious symptoms. This, together with the increased prevalence of childhood food allergy [1], causes difficulties for clinicians in their day-to-day work of interpreting the results of allergy tests.

Component-Resolved Diagnostics

The limitations described above have led to the initiation of intensive research activity in molecular allergology. The term 'component-resolved diagnostics' was introduced by Valenta et al. in 1999 [4]. However, the isolation and characterization of allergen components began far earlier. One of the first food allergen components to be described, Gad c 1 from cod, had already been purified by Kjell Aas and El Sayed in the late 1960s in Norway. Allergen components are named after their Latin family name: 'Gad c 1' stands for 'allergen 1 from *Gadus callarias*' (Baltic cod).

It is important to understand some basics of molecular allergology in order to understand how tests can be used clinically. Almost anything containing proteins can be an allergen source. Each source contains many different proteins, some of which can cause allergy. Knowledge of the proteins' structures, families, and stability during heating and digestion enables the use of allergen components in the clinic to be optimized.

Development of a Test for Allergen Components

The development of allergen components in pure form has made it possible to resolve many of these problems. In terms of production techniques, allergen components can be either produced biotechnologically in recombinant form or purified from their original sources. In other words, the main area of application of purified natural or recombinant allergen components is in the precise identification of the proteins that cause the disease [5]. Many allergen sources have not yet been fully characterized, and for the foreseeable future, allergen extracts will be needed for the diagnosis of unusual allergies and in cases of unusual sensitization patterns for common allergen sources. The different methods must complement each other.

Allergen components are available to clinicians (table 1) and are used in accordance with the same techniques and blood sampling as for usual ImmunoCAP® tests.

Allergen components are also available on an ImmunoCAP® Immuno Solid-phase allergen chip (ISAC) (see below).

Heat Stability in Proteins

The differences in stability mentioned above explain why some food allergens may be tolerated when raw, while others require cooking. An example of this is cow's milk, which is the most frequent food causing allergy among infants and young children, with a prevalence of 2–3%. Half of the cases of this condition are estimated to be IgE mediated and responsible for up to 13% of fatal food-induced anaphylaxis. The most important allergens in cow's milk are alpha-lactalbumin

Table 1. Commercially available in vitro IgE assays for allergen components

Molecule	Source	Protein family/function
Food allergens		
Gal d 1	Egg white	Ovomucoid
Gal d 2	Egg white	Ovalbumin
Gal d 3	Egg white	Conalbumin/ovotransferrin
Gal d 4	Egg	Lysozyme
Gal d 5	Egg yolk/chicken	Livetin/serum albumin
Bos d 4	Cow's milk	Alpha-lactalbumin
Bos d 5	Cow's milk	Beta-lactoglobulin
Bos d 6	Cow's milk and meat	Serum albumin
Bos d 8	Cow's milk	Casein
Bos d lactoferrin	Cow's milk	Transferrin
Cyp c 1	Carp	Parvalbumin
Gad c 1	Cod	Parvalbumin
Pen a 1	Shrimp	Tropomyosin
Pen m 1	Shrimp	Tropomyosin
Pen m 2	Shrimp	Arginine kinase
Pen m 4	Shrimp	Sarcoplasmic calcium-binding protein
Ana o 2	Cashew nut	Storage protein, 11S globulin
Ana o 3	Cashew nut	Storage protein, 2S albumin
Ber e 1	Brazil nut	Storage protein, 2S albumin
Cor a 1.0401	Hazelnut	PR-10
Cor a 8	Hazelnut	LTP
Cor a 9	Hazelnut	Storage protein, 11S globulin
Cor a 14	Hazelnut	Storage protein, 2S albumin
Jug r 1	Walnut	Storage protein, 2S albumin
Jug r 2	Walnut	Storage protein, 7S globulin
Jug r 3	Walnut	LTP
Ses i 1	Sesame	Storage protein, 2S albumin
Ara h 1	Peanut	Storage protein, 7S globulin
Ara h 2	Peanut	Storage protein, 2S albumin
Ara h 3	Peanut	Storage protein, 11S globulin
Ara h 6	Peanut	Storage protein, 2S albumin
Ara h 8	Peanut	PR-10
Ara h 9	Peanut	LTP
Gly m 4	Soybean	PR-10
Gly m 5	Soybean	Storage protein, beta-conglycinin
Gly m 6	Soybean	Storage protein, glycinin
Fag e 2	Buckwheat	Storage protein, 2S albumin
Tri a 14	Wheat	LTP
Tri a 19	Wheat	Omega-5 gliadin
Tri a gliadin	Wheat	Gliadin
Tri a aA_TI	Wheat	Alpha-amylase/trypsin inhibitor
Act d 1	Kiwi	Cysteine protease
Act d 2	Kiwi	Thaumatin-like protein
Act d 5	Kiwi	Kiwellin
Act d 8	Kiwi	PR-10
Dau c 1	Carrot	PR-10
Api g 1	Celery	PR-10
Mal d 1	Apple	PR-10

Molecule	Source	Protein family/function
Mal d 3	Apple	LTP
Mal d 4	Apple	Profilin
Pru av 1	Cherry	PR-10
Pru av 3	Cherry	LTP
Pru av 4	Cherry	Profilin
Pru p 1	Peach	PR-10
Pru p 3	Peach	LTP
Pru p 4	Peach	Profilin
Others allergens close to foods		
Ani s 1	Anisakis	Serine protease inhibitor
Ani s 3	Anisakis	Tropomyosin
MUXF3	Bromelain	CCD marker
Galactose-alpha-1, 3-galactose	Bovine	Alpha-Gal, thyroglobulin

LTP = Lipid transfer protein; CCD = cross-reactive carbohydrate domain.

(Bos d 4), beta-lactoglobulin (Bos d 5), and casein (Bos d 8). Beta-lactoglobulin, the most abundant protein in whey, is not present in human milk. Therefore, it was originally considered to be the major allergen in cow's milk. However, all milk proteins appear to be potential allergens, and patients are often sensitized to several of them. Casein has been shown to be both the most antigenic and the most allergenic of these three, indicating its role as an important milk allergen due to its heat stability [6].

It has now been shown that the level of casein-specific IgE measurements has significantly greater accuracy in predicting reactivity to baked milk compared with measurements of specific IgE to milk and beta-lactoglobulin [7]. The positive decision point for reactivity to baked milk is 20.2 kU for casein-specific IgE. In contrast, a concentration of less than approximately 0.94 kU (negative decision point) indicates a very low risk of reacting to baked milk, even though the patient might very well react to regular milk.

Most children recover spontaneously from their cow's milk allergy and develop tolerance. It was recently reported that the majority (75%) of children with cow's milk allergy tolerate baked milk products (e.g. muffins, waffles, cakes, and breads) [8]. The addition of baked milk to the diets of children tolerating such foods appears to accelerate the development of tolerance to regular milk compared with strict dietary avoidance. Identification of patients tolerating baked milk is therefore essential but challenging.

Combined with the clinical history and the expertise of the physician, cutoff decision points for casein-specific IgE levels could be used to identify the optimal candidates for open food challenges with baked milk and to improve the management of these children.

Species-Specific and Cross-Reactive Proteins

Some allergens cause clinical reactions ranging from mild to moderate and severe, whereas all allergens can induce sensitization without any clinical reaction. Identifying whether the sensitization is primary (species specific) or due to cross-reactivity with proteins with similar protein structures helps the clinician to judge the risk of allergic reaction. Some cross-reactions can cause severe reactions, e.g. cross-reactions with lipid-transfer protein and Gly m 4.

The value of identifying these species-specific allergen components lies in being able to narrow down the primary sensitizer that causes certain reactions to just one specific source, e.g. peanut.

In patients with suspected peanut allergy, measurement of IgE to peanut is a sensitive test but is not specific. Five peanut components are clinically relevant and available to clinicians. To date, 13 peanut allergens have been detected. The peanut seed storage proteins Ara h 1, Ara h 2, and Ara h 3 are all major allergens and are associated with primary sensitization to peanut in susceptible individuals [9, 10]. Among these seed storage proteins, Ara h 2 in particular is considered to be a marker for clinical reactions. In individuals sensitized to peanut, with a cutoff point of 0.35 kU/l, Ara h 2 was used to correctly classify 97.5% of the patients [9]. Importantly, all children with peanut allergy were correctly classified. Codreanu et al. showed that a cutoff of Ara h 2 >0.23 kU/l would be optimal to separate peanut-allergic patients from those who are tolerant [11]. Eller and Bindslev-Jensen found that a cutoff of Ara h 2 >1.63 kU/l yielded a specificity of 1.00, with a corresponding sensitivity of 0.70, which would have reduced the number of challenges performed from 205 to 92 [12]. The severity of symptoms elicited during challenge correlated significantly with the levels of Ara h 2 and with increasing age, but not with challenge thresholds, in this study. Sensitization to multiple allergens is a stronger indication of more severe reactions than sensitization to only one of the peanut components is [13]. Ara h 8 is a PR-10 protein and a Bet v 1 homolog and is thus a marker for secondary sensitization after primary sensitization to pollen from birch and alder.

Ebisawa et al. found that in Japanese children, the Ara h 2 test had a sensitivity and specificity of 88 and 84%, respectively. The combination of Ara h 1, Ara h 2, and Ara h 3 resulted in a higher specificity, or 94% [12].

Lieberman and coworkers showed that measurement of IgE to Ara h 2 was a more specific test for challenge-proven peanut allergy than IgE to peanut was, with specificity ranging from 85 to 95%, depending on whether the cohort examined was in the US or Sweden [14]. The increased specificity of IgE to Ara h 2 compared with IgE to peanut leads to a decrease in sensitivity. This is to be expected, however, because examining only one component of the total peanut extract could miss sensitivity to other relevant proteins.

New Allergen Component Test: An Emerging Field of Interest

Interest in allergen components is increasing because their usage opens up new possibilities for a more refined and precise diagnostic workup in allergy [5]. Currently, there are commercially available tests for more than one hundred allergen components, and the number is growing steadily, as several new ones are introduced each year. However, it is important that allergen component tests be clinically relevant; in other words, the test results must have clinical implications for patient management. A recent example of the importance of clinical documentation of allergen components in comparison with food challenges is related to the soy component Gly m 2S albumin.

Several soybean proteins have been suggested to have IgE reactivity, but only six of them have so far been recognized by the World Health Organization/International Union of Immunological Societies Allergen Nomenclature Subcommittee. Gly m 4, a pollen-related allergen, and the storage proteins Gly m 5 and Gly m 6 have been found to be associated with food allergy [15–17]. The storage protein 2S albumin has not yet been widely recognized as an important allergen in soybean (Gly m 2S albumin), and its association with clinical symptoms is not clearly established. We have recently shown that Gly m 2S albumin was found to be a major allergen in a group of soybean-allergic Japanese children and had a higher diagnostic value than soybean Gly m 5 and Gly m 6 did [18].

Temporal Development of Allergen Components

The characteristics of allergy are modified during an individual's lifetime. Symptoms related to the skin as well as to the gastroenteric tract, usually associated with food allergy, are more frequent in early infancy, while respiratory allergies (rhinitis/asthma) arising from inhalant allergens tend to appear later, in children older than 5 up to adolescence. This phenomenon, called the allergic march, has been partially explained by the evolution of the immune system during the first 3 years of life, in association with dietary changes and exposure to airborne allergens.

Despite numerous studies having monitored children during their first years of life, little is known about modifications of the capacity for recognizing allergen components during childhood and puberty.

It is conceivable that knowledge of the evolution of IgE sensitization over time could allow identification of unique characteristics and therefore could imply novel strategies for diagnosis, therapy, and follow-up protocols for pediatric and adolescent patients.

Melioli et al. have studied IgE to allergen components in serum samples from 901 allergic patients stratified into six groups according to age [19]. The authors found a clear time-related modification in the IgE repertoire at the component level. The percentage of positive components during the first period of life (from birth to the end of the second year) was relatively small (20–30% of the 103 ISAC molecules). This percentage increased during the subsequent periods. Three out of four ISAC components were recognized by children aged 3–6, and 88% were recognized by children aged 6–10. After 10 years of age, the percentage of

components remained stable. The presence of IgE specific to either milk or egg components in patients with IgE specific to Der f 2 indicates that simultaneous food and inhalant sensitization is possible during the second and third periods of life.

Onell et al. have also studied the temporal development of childhood IgE profiles specific to allergen components in a smaller cohort followed until 18 years of age [20]. IgE profiles were unique to each child and showed broad agreement with the results of skin prick tests (SPTs) and doctors' diagnoses. In young children, the most prevalent cross-reacting allergen was serum albumin. Conversely, PR-10 proteins were the most prevalent cross-reacting allergens among the older children, while PR-10 sensitization was absent in 6- to 9-month-old children. No detectable IgE antibodies to lipid transfer proteins or cross-reactive carbohydrate determinants were found. Anti-profilin antibodies were detected only in 18-year-old subjects. Anti-tropomyosin antibodies were detected in two children at 1.5 years of age, one of whom remained sensitized at 6 years of age, but not at 18 years of age. A number of offending allergens with IgE antibody responses prior to any reported clinical reactions to that allergen were identified (fig. 1). We could also document an increasing number of sensitizing components (fig. 2), which is known as molecular spreading.

It is well known that many food allergies (e.g. egg, milk, and wheat) are outgrown during childhood. Children with food allergy are often on elimination diets for long periods of time and are therefore at risk of nutritional deficiencies. They have lower weight-for-age and height-for-age, especially if they have multiple food allergies. Oral food challenges are often not performed, leading to overdiagnosis of food allergy and an unnecessary burden of allergen avoidance. In a recent large Canadian study of over three hundred children with an unclear history of peanut allergy recruited from specialized allergy clinics, only 6% were challenged, which is far from the actual need for these patients.

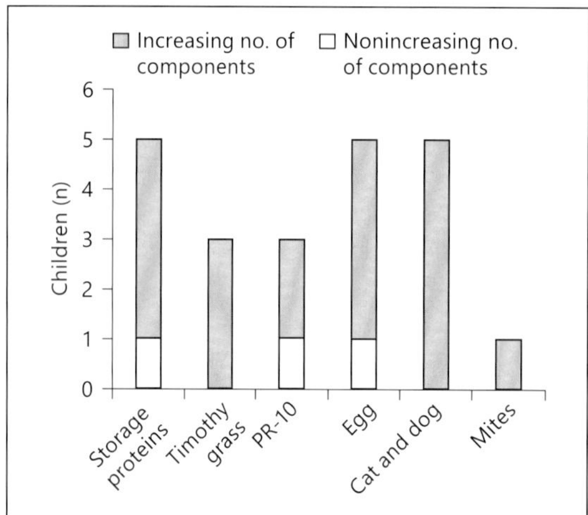

Fig. 1. Number of children sensitized to different allergens. The white bars represent children with IgE antibodies observed at the same time as the reporting of symptoms. The grey bars represent children with IgE antibodies observed at least one episode prior to the reporting of any symptoms to the given allergen [20].

Fig. 2. Number of children with increasing (grey, n = 19) and nonincreasing (white, n = 3) IgE-eliciting components in the initial phase of the IgE development process [20].

Monitoring of food-related serum IgE antibodies over time has been shown to be useful, demonstrating a relationship between the degree of the decrease in IgE antibody concentrations over time and the likelihood of developing tolerance. An interesting question is if it could be an advantage to monitor the development of tolerance to allergen components. Shibata et al. have studied the usefulness of measuring IgE antibod-

ies to the wheat component ω-5 gliadin in a follow-up of Japanese children with wheat allergy [21]. This group found that measuring IgE antibodies to ω-5 gliadin is even more useful than measuring IgE to wheat when monitoring wheat-allergic patients to assess whether their allergy has been outgrown or is persistent.

To summarize, modification of the IgE repertoire at the component level, from birth to adolescence, seems to accurately reflect the clinical characteristics of the allergic march.

Singleplex versus Multiplex Testing

IgE against allergen components may be measured using singleplex (one assay per sample) or multiplex (multiple assays per sample) testing. The newly introduced multiplex ISAC contains 112 allergen components from 51 allergen sources. Not all allergens derived from one source are presently available on the chip, and some important foods are underrepresented. It is advisable to start investigating a suspicion of food allergy by measuring IgE specific to an extract and, if positive, to continue with component testing in order to decide if food challenge is advisable or not. One of the most important implications of multiplex assays is their ability to distinguish specific sensitization from sensitization due to cross-reactivity.

Risk assessment of allergic individuals is one of the potential applications of molecular allergy diagnostics. The sensitization profile may differ among patients according to disease expression and severity. Therefore, detecting low-risk versus high-risk biomarkers is an area of major interest that may result in minimized risk of food challenge tests and improved recommendations (e.g. exposure reduction). This has been shown with the use of allergen components in food, venom, respiratory, and latex allergy. Lieberman et al. showed that relying on IgE to peanut alone would lead to 81 oral food challenges being conducted to identify 46 peanut-tolerant persons [14]. By simply adding IgE levels to Ara h 2 as a second diagnostic step for all patients positive for IgE to peanut and by only challenging patients who had undetectable levels of IgE to Ara h 2, they could have decreased the number of challenges to 56 and still have identified 44 tolerant patients.

Future Perspectives

In single-nut-allergic children, the question of whether avoidance should be generalized to all nuts or limited to the culprit nut is under discussion [22]. The general recommendation for peanut- or single-nut-allergic children used to be to avoid all nuts, given the clinical cross-reactivity between peanut and tree nuts and among tree nuts, to reduce the risk of contamination leading to inadvertent exposure. However, current clinical practice tends to change as the number of experienced clinicians increases, supporting the introduction of selected nuts while still avoiding the culprit nut. Advantages of this new approach are more accurate diagnosis and reductions in risk-taking behavior and in the psychosocial impact of allergen avoidance.

There are hopes and expectations that IgE to cashew and walnut components could reduce the number of positive oral food challenges, and hopefully, some of these clinically relevant and important components will be available in the near future.

Skin Prick Test

Since 1865, the SPT has been used to confirm sensitization to a specific allergen. This test is a useful tool because it possesses a number of advantages: simplicity; rapidity of results; good performance; low cost; and, finally, high sensitivity.

Various studies have examined the correlation between SPT results and the diagnosis of food allergy. In 1998, Eigenmann et al. reported that the size of the wheal and/or the positivity of the test (>3-mm mean diameter) was related to the diagnosis of food allergy [23]. In egg, milk, peanut, and wheat allergy, wheal sizes were significantly larger than in patients who were tolerant. Hill et al. showed SPT wheal diameters that were '100% diagnostic' of allergy to cow's milk (≥8 mm), egg (≥7 mm), and peanut (≥8 mm), with the SPT being more sensitive than specific IgE levels in diagnosing allergy to egg and peanut [24]. Moreover, Ogata et al. reported that 39 of 72 egg-allergic infants negative for egg-white-specific IgE showed positive SPT results [25]. By contrast, reactivity to soy could not be predicted based on SPT results [23]. SPT results should be interpreted according to populations as well as to antigens, and the diagnostic accuracy of the SPT in food allergy remains controversial.

Basophil Activation Test

Mechanisms of Basophil Activation
The mechanisms of IgE-receptor-mediated basophil activation and the subsequent transmission of signals lead to the release of histamine, the production of leukotrienes and cytokines [26, 27], and the expression of CD63 and CD203c on the cell membrane [28].

Histamine Release Test

In the 1960s, the histamine release test (HRT) was developed [29], and since then, a number of researchers have examined the relationship between HRT results and food allergy [30–33]. Lau et al. examined the utility of the HRT in the diagnosis of egg allergy, suggesting that the HRT was not effective in predicting the outcome of oral food challenges [32]. By contrast, Norgaard et al. reported that the sensitivity of the HRT in diagnosing egg and cow's milk allergy was 89% and showed that the HRT can be useful in food allergy diagnosis [33, 34]. They also suggested that the diagnostic ability of the HRT appears to be strongly influenced by the allergen quality.

In recent years, a novel HRT method that is more convenient and that requires a smaller volume of blood has been developed in Japan [35]. We examined whether the novel HRT kit could be useful in the diagnosis of food allergy [36]. Receiver operating characteristic analysis showed that the threshold of histamine release, which was defined as 'the minimum concentration of food antigen to induce a 10% net histamine release', was useful in the diagnosis of heated or raw egg, cow's milk, and wheat allergy. We were able to determine the cutoff value for the threshold of histamine release in relation to the outcome of oral food challenges. The cutoff values were 6 ng/ml for egg-white antigen in heated or raw egg allergy, 40 ng/ml for milk antigen in cow's milk allergy, and 500 ng/ml for wheat antigen in wheat allergy, with efficiencies of 70.3, 78.0, 77.6, and 70.7%, respectively. Therefore, the use of the HRT with food antigens seems to be useful in determining when oral food challenges should be performed. Multicenter studies are needed in the future.

Expression of the Basophil Activation Markers CD63 and CD203c

Recently, the flow cytometric basophil activation test (BAT), including testing for the expression of CD63 and CD203c, has attracted increasing attention. Food allergy will probably become one area of allergy diagnosis in which the BAT will prove to be a useful tool. In cow's milk allergy, Wanich et al. reported that patients able to tolerate heated cow's milk have suppressed basophil expression of milk-induced CD63 [37]. Ocmant et al. reported that the performance of an ovalbumin-induced BAT applied to egg allergy diagnosis was 62.5% for sensitivity and 96.4% for specificity, and therefore, the BAT may be helpful in diagnosing food allergy [38].

In 2010, we evaluated whether CD203c expression on basophils would be a useful predictor of symptoms associated with oral food challenge in children with hen's egg and milk allergy. In a receiver operating curve analysis, the CD203c stimulation index, which was the allergen-induced CD203c expression level divided by the baseline expression level, was as useful for diagnosing food allergy as antigen-specific IgE was. Additionally, the positive predictive value of the threshold of CD203c expression (the minimum concentration of antigen required to induce a CD203c stimulation index of 2 or greater) was 94.7% for egg white, 100% for ovomucoid, 85.7% for milk, and 75.0% for casein (fig. 3). Therefore, measurement of food antigen-induced CD63 and CD203c expression on basophils seems to be related to whether patients will outgrow food allergy. Unfortunately, there are few reports of BAT use in food allergy patients. Further studies are needed.

Correlation of the Skin Prick Test and the Basophil Activation Test with Oral Immunotherapy

Recently, oral immunotherapy (OIT) has been examined as a novel therapeutic approach for food allergy. SPT reactivity was found to decrease beginning after several months of OIT and remained decreased throughout a 3-year follow-up

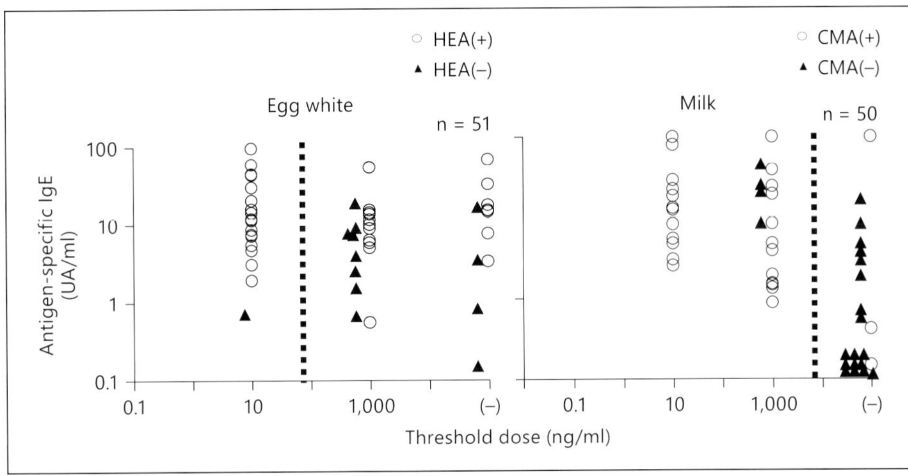

Fig. 3. The threshold of CD203c expression is related to hen's egg and cow's milk allergy. HEA = Heated egg allergy; CMA = cow's milk allergy.

[39]. In addition, allergen-induced CD63 expression on basophils was reduced. Although the mechanisms of OIT are not clear, suppression of effector cells is the predominant mechanism through which OIT might function.

In summary, molecular allergy diagnostics have found their way into routine diagnostics due to their ability to improve risk assessment, above all in food allergy. The stability of a component and the clinical history help the clinician to evaluate the risk of a systemic reaction versus local reactions. Labile components are linked to local reactions (typically oral symptoms), and cooked food is often tolerated.

Simplex allergen component tests decrease the need for provocation testing and support recommendation of allergen avoidance, which so far has been shown for peanut allergy. Multiplex component testing is especially suitable for patients with complex symptomatology.

References

1 Prescott S, Allen KJ: Food allergy: riding the second wave of the allergy epidemic. Pediatr Allergy Immunol 2011;22:155–160.

2 Sampson HA, Ho DG: Relationship between food-specific IgE concentrations and the risk of positive food challenges in children and adolescents. J Allergy Clin Immunol 1997;100:444–451.

3 Komata T, Soderstrom L, Borres MP, et al: The predictive relationship of food-specific serum IgE concentrations to challenge outcomes for egg and milk varies by patient age. J Allergy Clin Immunol 2007;119:1272–1274.

4 Valenta R, Lidholm J, Niederberger V, et al: The recombinant allergen-based concept of component-resolved diagnostics and immunotherapy (CRD and CRIT). Clin Exp Allergy 1999;29:896–904.

5 Borres MP, Ebisawa M, Eigenmann PA: Use of allergen components begins a new era in pediatric allergology. Pediatr Allergy Immunol 2011;22:454–461.

6 Ito K, Futamura M, Moverare R, et al: The usefulness of casein-specific IgE and IgG4 antibodies in cow's milk allergic children. Clin Mol Allergy 2012;10:1.

7 Caubet JC, Nowak-Wegrzyn A, Moshier E, et al: Utility of casein-specific IgE levels in predicting reactivity to baked milk. J Allergy Clin Immunol 2013;131:222–224.e1–e4.

8 Kim JS, Nowak-Wegrzyn A, Sicherer SH, et al: Dietary baked milk accelerates the resolution of cow's milk allergy in children. J Allergy Clin Immunol 2011;128:125–131.e2.

9 Nicolaou N, Poorafshar M, Murray C, et al: Allergy or tolerance in children sensitized to peanut: prevalence and differentiation using component-resolved diagnostics. J Allergy Clin Immunol 2010;125:191–197.e1–e13.

10 Ebisawa M, Moverare R, Sato S, et al: Measurement of Ara h 1-, 2-, and 3-specific IgE antibodies is useful in diagnosis of peanut allergy in Japanese children. Pediatr Allergy Immunol 2012;23:573–581.

11 Codreanu F, Collignon O, Roitel, et al: A novel immunoassay using recombinant allergens simplifies peanut allergy diagnosis. Int Arch Allergy Immunol 2011; 154:216–226.

12 Eller E, Bindslev-Jensen C: Clinical value of component-resolved diagnostics in peanut-allergic patients. Allergy 2013; 68:190–194.

13 Astier C, Morisset M, Roitel O, et al: Predictive value of skin prick tests using recombinant allergens for diagnosis of peanut allergy. J Allergy Clin Immunol 2006;118:250–256.

14 Lieberman JA, Glaumann S, Batelsson S, et al: The utility of peanut components in the diagnosis of IgE-mediated peanut allergy among distinct populations. J Allergy Clin Immunol Pract 2013;1:75–82.

15 Kosma P, Sjolander S, Landgren E, et al: Severe reactions after the intake of soy drink in birch pollen-allergic children sensitized to Gly m 4. Acta Paediatrica 2011;100:305–306.

16 Ito K, Sjolander S, Sato S, et al: IgE to Gly m 5 and Gly m 6 is associated with severe allergic reactions to soybean in Japanese children. J Allergy Clin Immunol 2011;128:673–675.

17 Holzhauser T, Wackermann O, Ballmer-Weber BK, et al: Soybean (Glycine max) allergy in Europe: Gly m 5 (beta-conglycinin) and Gly m 6 (glycinin) are potential diagnostic markers for severe allergic reactions to soy. J Allergy Clin Immunol 2009;123:452–458.

18 Ebisawa M, Brostedt P, Sjölander S, et al: Gly m 2S albumin is a major allergen with a high diagnostic value in soybean allergic children. J Allergy Clin Immunol 2013;132:976–978.e1–e5.

19 Melioli G, Marcomini L, Agazzi A, et al: The IgE repertoire in children and adolescents resolved at component level: a cross-sectional study. Pediatr Allergy Immunol 2012;23:433–440.

20 Onell A, Hjalle L, Borres MP: Exploring the temporal development of childhood IgE profiles to allergen components. Clin Transl Allergy 2012;2:24.

21 Shibata R, Nishima S, Tanaka A, et al: Usefulness of specific IgE antibodies to omega-5 gliadin in the diagnosis and follow-up of Japanese children with wheat allergy. Ann Allergy Asthma Immunol 2011;107:337–343.

22 Santos AF, Lack G: Food allergy and anaphylaxis in pediatrics: update 2010–2012. Pediatr Allergy Immunol 2012;23: 698–706.

23 Eigenmann PA, Sampson HA: Interpreting skin prick tests in the evaluation of food allergy in children. Pediatr Allergy Immunol 1998;9:186–191.

24 Hill DJ, Heine RG, Hosking CS: The diagnostic value of skin prick testing in children with food allergy. Pediatr Allergy Immunol 2004;15:435–441.

25 Ogata M, Sukuya A, Sugizaki C, et al: [Usefulness of skin prick test using bifurcated needle for the diagnosis of food allergy in infantile atopic dermatitis – 1st report. Case of egg allergy]. Arerugi 2008;57:843–852.

26 MacGlashan DW Jr, Peters SP, Warner J, et al: Characteristics of human basophil sulfidopeptide leukotriene release: releasability defined as the ability of the basophil to respond to dimeric cross-links. J Immunol 1986;136:2231–2239.

27 Schroeder JT, MacGlashan DW Jr, Kagey-Sobotka A, et al: IgE-dependent IL-4 secretion by human basophils. The relationship between cytokine production and histamine release in mixed leukocyte cultures. J Immunol 1994;153:1808–1817.

28 Buhring HJ, Simmons PJ, Pudney M, et al: The monoclonal antibody 97A6 defines a novel surface antigen expressed on human basophils and their multipotent and unipotent progenitors. Blood 1999;94:2343–2356.

29 Lichtenstein LM, Norman PS, Connell JT: Comparison between skin-sensitizing antibody titers and leukocyte sensitivity measurements as an index of the severity of ragweed hay fever. J Allergy 1967;40:160–167.

30 Norgaard A, Bindslev-Jensen C: Egg and milk allergy in adults. Diagnosis and characterization. Allergy 1992;47:503–509.

31 Kleine-Tebbe J, Galleani M, Jeep S, et al: Basophil histamine release in patients with birch pollen hypersensitivity with and without allergic symptoms to fruits. Allergy 1992;47:618–623.

32 Lau S, Thiemeier M, Urbanek R, et al: Immediate hypersensitivity to ovalbumin in children with hen's egg white allergy. Eur J Pediatr 1988;147:606–608.

33 Norgaard A, Skov PS, Bindslev-Jensen C: Egg and milk allergy in adults: comparison between fresh foods and commercial allergen extracts in skin prick test and histamine release from basophils. Clin Exp Allergy 1992;22:940–947.

34 Kleine-Tebbe J, Werfel S, Roedsgaard D, et al: Comparison of fiberglass-based histamine assay with a conventional automated fluorometric histamine assay, case history, skin prick test, and specific serum IgE in patients with milk and egg allergic reactions. Allergy 1993;48:49–53.

35 Nishi H, Nishimura S, Higashiura M, et al: A new method for histamine release from purified peripheral blood basophils using monoclonal antibody-coated magnetic beads. J Immunol Methods 2000;240:39–46.

36 Sato S, Tachimoto H, Shukuya A, et al: Utility of the peripheral blood basophil histamine release test in the diagnosis of hen's egg, cow's milk, and wheat allergy in children. Int Arch Allergy Immunol 2011;155(suppl 1):96–103.

37 Wanich N, Nowak-Wegrzyn A, Sampson HA, et al: Allergen-specific basophil suppression associated with clinical tolerance in patients with milk allergy. J Allergy Clin Immunol 2009;123:789–794.e20.

38 Ocmant A, Mulier S, Hanssens L, et al: Basophil activation tests for the diagnosis of food allergy in children. Clin Exp Allergy 2009;39:1234–1245.

39 Jones SM, Pons L, Roberts JL, et al: Clinical efficacy and immune regulation with peanut oral immunotherapy. J Allergy Clin Immunol 2009;124:292–300. e1–e97.

Motohiro Ebisawa, MD, PhD
Department of Allergy, Clinical Research Center for Allergology and Rheumatology
Sagamihara National Hospital, 18–1, Sakuradai, Minami-ku
Sagamihara, Kanagawa 228–8522 (Japan)
E-Mail m-ebisawa@sagamihara-hosp.gr.jp

Ebisawa M, Ballmer-Weber BK, Vieths S, Wood RA (eds): Food Allergy: Molecular Basis and Clinical Practice.
Chem Immunol Allergy. Basel, Karger, 2015, vol 101, pp 79–86 (DOI: 10.1159/000371676)

Non-IgE-Related Diagnostic Methods (LST, Patch Test)

Kenji Matsumoto

Department of Allergy and Immunology, National Research Institute for Child Health and Development,
Tokyo, Japan

Abstract

Although most food allergy patients have immediate-type reactions, some have delayed-type reactions. Unlike for the detection of food-specific IgE antibody in immediate-type (IgE-mediated) food allergies, only a few tests are currently available to aid in the diagnosis of delayed-type (non-IgE-mediated) food allergies. This chapter summarizes our current understanding of one in vitro test and one in vivo test for non-IgE-mediated food allergies: the lymphocyte stimulation test (LST) and the atopy patch test (APT). Although the LST is not yet standardized, a food protein-specific LST might be a useful tool for diagnosing delayed-type food allergies, and especially those manifesting with gastrointestinal symptoms but not skin symptoms. Various remaining issues – including basophil contamination of the peripheral blood mononuclear cell fraction and lipopolysaccharide contamination of food antigen preparations – are also discussed. The APT uses an epicutaneous patch technique to occlusively apply food antigens to the skin to induce inflammatory reactions at the patch application site. Because the APT shows modest sensitivity and specificity, the clinical benefit of the APT in the diagnosis of food allergies in patients with atopic dermatitis is limited. A position paper on the APT issued by the European Academy of Allergy and Clinical Immunology/Global Allergy and Asthma European Network in 2006 is briefly summarized, and several recent APT-related topics, including APT use for the diagnosis of food protein-induced enterocolitis syndrome, are discussed. © 2015 S. Karger AG, Basel

Introduction

Although most food allergy patients have immediate-type reactions, approximately 10 and 1% of food allergy patients with and without atopic dermatitis, respectively, have delayed-type reactions. Food-specific serum IgE antibody titers, skin prick tests, and basophil activation tests are regularly used for the diagnosis of immediate-type (IgE-mediated) food allergies. However, only a few tests are currently available to aid in the diagnosis of delayed-type (non-IgE-mediated) food

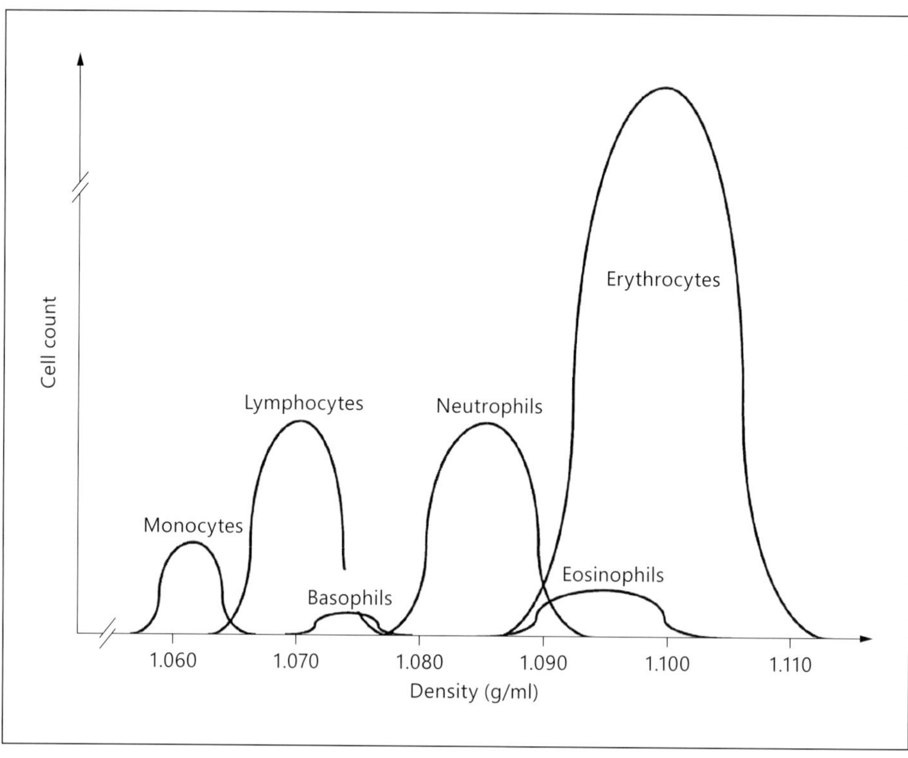

Fig. 1. Density distribution of human blood cells. Peripheral blood mononuclear cells isolated using conventional lymphocyte separation media (d = 1.077 g/ml) include monocytes and basophils.

allergies. This chapter summarizes our current understanding of an in vitro test and an in vivo test for non-IgE-mediated food allergies: the lymphocyte stimulation test (LST) and the atopy patch test (APT).

Lymphocyte Stimulation Test

The LST, also called the lymphoproliferation test or the lymphocyte transformation test, was introduced in the early 1960s, using several mitogens or lectins, such as phytohemagglutinin and pokeweed mitogen, in order to test for non-specific lymphocyte activation. Later, antigen-specific responses were determined using antigens such as drugs to stimulate autologous/ allogenic lymphocytes. These examinations mainly aimed to determine Th1-type immune responses, such as contact hypersensitivity and metal allergies. Lymphocyte responses to food antigens in patients with atopic dermatitis were first reported in 1990 [1]. However, use of the LST method for food antigens has not yet been standardized.

Peripheral Blood Mononuclear Cells
The peripheral blood mononuclear cell (PBMC) fraction is usually purified by density gradient centrifugation using separation reagents (Percoll, Ficoll-Paque, Lymphocyte Separation Medium, LymphoPrep, etc.). However, this fraction also contains monocytes and basophils (fig. 1). Therefore, if the patient has IgE antibody specific

to the test antigen in the LST, the antigen activates not only T cells but also contaminating basophils. This leads to the release of various mediators, including histamine and IL-4, both of which are known to suppress Th1-type immune responses [2]. The cytokine profiles in the supernatants can be affected by these basophil-derived mediators.

Antigens

Several commercially available food protein preparations, including ovalbumin, β-lactoglobulin, and caseins, reportedly contain lipopolysaccharides (LPS) at levels high enough to activate mainly monocytes in the PBMC fraction and to cause antigen-nonspecific immune responses [3–5]. PBMCs from younger children show more pronounced lymphoproliferation in response to LPS [5], and depletion of LPS in food protein antigen preparations prior to use is thus strongly recommended. In addition, some plant proteins can act as an adjuvant, partly through their lectin activity, inducing lymphoproliferative responses [6]. PBMCs from age matched healthy subjects should be used as a control. The possible effects of food processing on lymphocyte responses remain to be determined [7]. The optimal antigen concentration varies with the antigen and with the patient [1, 5], and thus, several concentrations should be used.

Culture System

PBMCs are suspended at a concentration of $1–2 \times 10^6$/ml in culture medium such as RPMI 1640. Autologous serum or pooled human serum, but not fetal bovine serum, should be added to a final concentration of 5–15%. The lymphoproliferative response usually reaches a plateau within 3–5 days of culture [1, 5].

Measurements

For the LST, measurement of ^{3}H-thymidine incorporation is the most sensitive method and has the widest dynamic range. Other methods, such as enzymatic assays that evaluate the turnover of mitochondrial dehydrogenases (3-(4,5-dimethylthiazol-2-yl)-2,5-diphenyltetrazolium bromide test) and lysosomal hexosaminidase (N-acetyl-beta-D-glucosaminidase test), are reportedly less sensitive [8]. Measurement either of incorporation of the nucleotide analog 5-bromo-2'-deoxyuridine or of the DNA content using propidium iodide or 4'6'-diamidino-2-phenylindole was shown to be a practicable, nonradioactive alternative [8, 9]. Cell proliferation can also be assessed by measuring the fluorescence of carboxyfluorescein diacetate succinimidyl ester by flow cytometry [10].

Some studies have measured cytokine concentrations in the supernatants of cultured PBMCs. Lymphoproliferation correlated best with IL-2 production [5, 11, 12].

Interpretation

Definitive cut-off points (stimulation index) in the LST for food antigens have not yet been determined. The proliferative responses may vary depending on the patient, antigen, and culture system. Use of appropriate age-matched control subjects may help in defining cut-off points, but this could be very difficult, especially if the patients are children.

An appropriately designed LST provides information about the presence/absence of antigen-specific T-cell clones in the peripheral blood, regardless of the cytokine production profile. In fact, the LST is reportedly useful for the detection delayed-type sensitization to nonprotein antigens such as metals (nickel, mercury, gold, beryllium, palladium, cobalt, chromium), drugs, and haptens. With respect to food allergies, the LST has been used mainly to evaluate the involvement of food antigens in the pathogenesis (especially delayed-type) of atopic dermatitis [1, 13]. However, lymphocyte responses decrease significantly as a result of avoidance of offending foods, regardless of acquisition of immune tolerance, suggesting that the LST is not suitable for diagnosing immune tolerance [14].

In delayed-type food allergies of the gastrointestinal (GI) tract (GI allergy) [15], such as food protein-induced enterocolitis syndrome (FPIES), food protein-induced proctocolitis, and food protein-induced enteropathy, a food protein-specific LST might be a useful tool for diagnosis [16, 17], especially when LPS is depleted from the antigens [5]. Patients with GI allergy show more pronounced proliferation in the LST compared with patients with IgE-mediated food allergy [5]. Interestingly, the cytokine secretion profiles of milk antigen-stimulated PBMCs from GI allergy patients not only include several proinflammatory cytokines (TNF-α and IL-6) but are also skewed toward Th2.

Future Perspectives
Unlike measurement of antigen-specific IgE titers, the LST requires both sterile technique in cell culture facilities and fresh blood. In addition, depletion of LPS from food antigen preparations is essential for the LST, especially if the patient is a young child, but this depletion is expensive. However, the LST is probably the only in vitro test for delayed-type allergic disorders, and we sincerely hope that standardization of the method, as well as affordable commercially available services and cost-effectiveness, will be achieved soon. Ethical issues regarding recruiting age-matched healthy controls need to be resolved by academic societies including allergy specialists.

Recent short-term clinical studies have revealed that dietary food antigens are involved in the pathogenesis of eosinophilic GI diseases (EGIDs), including eosinophilic esophagitis and eosinophilic gastroenteritis [18–20]. In addition, local expression of antigen-presenting molecules (MHC class II and co-stimulatory molecules) strongly points to involvement of food antigen-specific lymphocytes in EGIDs [21]. For these reasons, the LST may prove diagnostically useful in patients with EGIDs.

Patch Test/Atopy Patch Test

The patch test was originally designed to investigate delayed-type immune reactions to antigens, and especially metals, drugs, and haptens, among others. The APT involves the same procedure using protein antigens and is performed in patients with atopic dermatitis. In 2000, Niggemann et al. studied the APT using food antigens in patients with atopic dermatitis and found it to be a useful tool for diagnosing food allergies in children with atopic dermatitis [22]. Since then, a number of studies have been published, and a position paper on the APT was issued by the Section on Dermatology and the Section on Pediatrics of the European Academy of Allergy and Clinical Immunology and the Global Allergy and Asthma European Network [23]. Although the APT using food antigens has not been standardized for use in clinical practice, the position paper describes several practical issues, including the indication for testing, the APT technique, practical methods, the APT readout, and side effects.

This section briefly summarizes the European Academy of Allergy and Clinical Immunology/ Global Allergy and Asthma European Network position paper (2006) and discusses several APT-related topics that have arisen since the paper's release.

Indication for Testing
Performance of the APT using food antigens may increase the identification of food allergies in patients with atopic dermatitis in the following situations:
- suspicion of food allergy in children without specific IgE above published predictive levels or a positive skin prick test;
- severe and/or persistent atopic dermatitis with unknown trigger factors;
- multiple IgE sensitizations without proven clinical relevance in patients with atopic dermatitis.

In addition, the APT may help in diagnosing delayed-type food allergies, and especially those manifesting with GI symptoms but not skin symptoms (non-IgE-dependent food allergies of the GI tract). However, appropriately controlled and prospective studies are lacking.

Atopy Patch Test Methods
The APT is recommended to be performed using a 12-mm-diameter Finn Chamber (Epitest Ltd.) mounted on Scanpor tape and applied for 48 h to skin of the upper back that is not irritated, abraded, or tape stripped. The test reaction is evaluated after 48 and 72 h. However, recently, a commercially available APT kit using milk was introduced in France (Diallertest®), and it showed good sensitivity and specificity, without any side effects [24]. More such products, using various food antigens, may be the way of the future.

Food Antigens
Since the first study of the use of food antigens in the APT by Niggemann et al. [22], fresh foods have generally been used, but this has not yet been standardized. The diagnostic accuracy of the APT in children with food allergy-related GI symptoms was compared between using fresh foods and using commercially available freeze-dried food extracts [25]. The diagnostic accuracy was higher with the fresh foods than with the freeze-dried food extracts, even though both contained similar protein components (as determined by SDS-PAGE) [26], suggesting that the protein conformation, and especially disulfide bond-related structures, may be important for the responses in the APT. The actual effects of food processing on the APT need to be determined.

Reading of Atopy Patch Test Results
APT results were originally assessed in accordance with a report by the International Contact Dermatitis Research Group [27], and the reading key was updated for both aeroallergens

and food allergens in 2004 [28] and 2006 [29]. Recently, the co-presence of erythema and papules was demonstrated to have high specificity and a high positive predictive value [30]. Further study on how to best read APT results is needed.

Atopy Patch Test for Non-IgE-Mediated Gastrointestinal Allergy
The APT was originally used to diagnose non-IgE-mediated food allergy in patients with atopic dermatitis. In 2004, the APT's diagnostic accuracy for non-IgE-mediated food allergy in children without atopic dermatitis was investigated [31]. That initial trial failed to find any clinical usefulness for the APT, but subsequent studies enrolling children with FPIES [32, 33] or eosinophilic esophagitis [18] found the APT to be helpful for identifying causative food proteins. Canani et al. investigated the diagnostic accuracy of the APT in children with allergy-related GI symptoms and found very high sensitivity and specificity when fresh foods were used [25]. Recently, the APT also showed high diagnostic accuracy in detecting offending foods among exclusively breast-fed infants with allergic proctocolitis refractory to a maternal hypoallergenic diet [34]. However, the APT was poor in predicting the development of tolerance in patients with FPIES [33].

Epicutaneous IgE Sensitization and Antigen Absorption via the Skin
The results of recent epidemiological studies strongly suggest that ingestion of food promotes immune tolerance to food antigens, especially in young children, whereas exposure to food antigens through the skin leads to IgE sensitization. A 'dual-allergen-exposure hypothesis' was proposed to explain those findings [35]. However, recurrent exposure to food proteins via normal skin can reportedly induce antigen-specific tolerance and reduce allergic symptoms in food allergy patients (epicutaneous immunotherapy) [36], suggesting that not only epicutaneous

exposure but also some other factors may be involved in the induction of IgE sensitization via the skin. We have proposed that exposure to food antigens, especially via eczematous skin, is critical for the onset of allergic diseases [37], and that hypothesis was supported by the results of both a basic study [38] and an epidemiological study [39]. Protein antigens applied to the skin are engulfed by epidermis-dwelling Langerhans cells/dendritic cells, processed, and presented to T cells in the draining lymph nodes. However, the precise mechanisms of how food proteins – which are large molecules – cross the skin barrier remain unclear. Nagao et al. demonstrated that mechanical perturbation or inflammation of the hair follicles induces pre-Langerhans cell migration into the hair follicles through C-C chemokine receptor 6-dependent mechanisms [40]. Their study explains how penetration of antigenic proteins and epicutaneous sensitization occur in patients with skin inflammation

and partly explains why the APT does not induce sensitization when performed on normal skin [23].

Future Perspectives
Even though the direct application of protein antigens to the skin is an interesting approach, a comprehensive review [41] and a large-scale, well-designed clinical study [42] showed only limited additional clinical benefit of the APT in the diagnosis of food allergies in patients with atopic dermatitis.

The APT may potentially provide rare and valuable information regarding in vivo reactions to a food protein, with minimal risks. Because the precise mechanisms of non-IgE-mediated local reactions induced 48 and 72 h after antigen application are of particular interest, standardization of the methods and clarification of the suitable phenotype of patients should be further investigated.

References

1 Kondo N, Agata H, Fukutomi O, Motoyoshi F, Orii T: Lymphocyte responses to food antigens in patients with atopic dermatitis who are sensitive to foods. J Allergy Clin Immunol 1990;86:253–260.
2 Turjanmaa K, Rasanen L, Lehto M, Makinen-Kiljunen S, Reunala T: Basophil histamine release and lymphocyte proliferation tests in latex contact urticaria. In vitro tests in latex contact urticaria. Allergy 1989;44:181–186.
3 Brix S, Bovetto L, Fritsche R, Barkholt V, Frokiaer H: Immunostimulatory potential of beta-lactoglobulin preparations: effects caused by endotoxin contamination. J Allergy Clin Immunol 2003;112:1216–1222.
4 Watanabe J, Miyazaki Y, Zimmerman GA, Albertine KH, McIntyre TM: Endotoxin contamination of ovalbumin suppresses murine immunologic responses and development of airway hyper-reactivity. J Biol Chem 2003;278:42361–42368.
5 Morita H, Nomura I, Orihara K, Yoshida K, Akasawa A, Tachimoto H, Ohtsuka Y, Namai Y, Futamura M, Shoda T, Matsuda A, Kamemura N, Kido H, Takahashi T, Ohya Y, Saito H, Matsumoto K: Antigen-specific T-cell responses in patients with non-IgE-mediated gastrointestinal food allergy are predominantly skewed to T(H)2. J Allergy Clin Immunol 2013;131:590–592.
6 Shreffler WG, Castro RR, Kucuk ZY, Charlop-Powers Z, Grishina G, Yoo S, Burks AW, Sampson HA: The major glycoprotein allergen from Arachis hypogaea, Ara h 1, is a ligand of dendritic cell-specific ICAM-grabbing nonintegrin and acts as a Th2 adjuvant in vitro. J Immunol 2006;177:3677–3685.
7 Nishida T, Kondo N, Agata H, Fukutomi O, Shinoda S, Suzuki Y, Shimozawa N, Tomatsu S, Orii T: Proliferative responses towards native, heat-denatured and pepsin-treated ovalbumin by peripheral blood mononuclear cells from patients with hen's egg-sensitive atopic dermatitis. Biotherapy 1994;8:33–40.
8 Wemme H, Pfeifer S, Heck R, Muller-Quernheim J: Measurement of lymphocyte proliferation: critical analysis of radioactive and photometric methods. Immunobiology 1992;185:78–89.
9 Farris GM, Newman LS, Frome EL, Shou Y, Barker E, Habbersett RC, Maier L, Smith HN, Marrone BL: Detection of beryllium sensitivity using a flow cytometric lymphocyte proliferation test: the Immuno-Be-LPT. Toxicology 2000;143:125–140.
10 Milovanova TN: Comparative analysis between CFSE flow cytometric and tritiated thymidine incorporation tests for beryllium sensitivity. Cytometry B Clin Cytom 2007;72:265–275.

11 Agata H, Kondo N, Fukutomi O, Shino-
    da S, Orii T: Interleukin-2 production of
    lymphocytes in food sensitive atopic
    dermatitis. Arch Dis Child 1992;67:280–
    284.
12 Spiewak R, Moed H, von Blomberg BM,
    Bruynzeel DP, Scheper RJ, Gibbs S, Rus-
    temeyer T: Allergic contact dermatitis to
    nickel: modified in vitro test protocols
    for better detection of allergen-specific
    response. Contact Dermatitis 2007;56:
    63–69.
13 Werfel T, Ahlers G, Schmidt P, Boeker
    M, Kapp A: Detection of a kappa-casein-
    specific lymphocyte response in milk-
    responsive atopic dermatitis. Clin Exp
    Allergy 1996;26:1380–1386.
14 Fujimura M, Masuda K, Hayashiya M,
    Okayama T: Flow cytometric analysis
    of lymphocyte proliferative responses
    to food allergens in dogs with food al-
    lergy. J Vet Med Sci 2011;73:1309–
    1317.
15 Nomura I, Morita H, Hosokawa S,
    Hoshina H, Fukuie T, Watanabe M, Oht-
    suka Y, Shoda T, Terada A, Takamasu T,
    Arai K, Ito Y, Ohya Y, Saito H, Matsu-
    moto K: Four distinct subtypes of non-
    IgE-mediated gastrointestinal food aller-
    gies in neonates and infants,
    distinguished by their initial symptoms.
    J Allergy Clin Immunol 2011;127:685–
    688.
16 Giavi S, Megremis S, Papadopoulos NG:
    Lymphocyte stimulation test for the
    diagnosis of non-IgE-mediated cow's
    milk allergy: a step closer to a noninva-
    sive diagnostic tool? Int Arch Allergy
    Immunol 2012;157:1–2.
17 Kimura M, Oh S, Narabayashi S, Tagu-
    chi T: Usefulness of lymphocyte stimu-
    lation test for the diagnosis of intestinal
    cow's milk allergy in infants. Int Arch
    Allergy Immunol 2012;157:58–64.
18 Spergel JM: Eosinophilic esophagitis in
    adults and children: evidence for a food
    allergy component in many patients.
    Curr Opin Allergy Clin Immunol 2007;7:
    274–278.
19 Henderson CJ, Abonia JP, King EC, Put-
    nam PE, Collins MH, Franciosi JP,
    Rothenberg ME: Comparative dietary
    therapy effectiveness in remission of pe-
    diatric eosinophilic esophagitis. J Allergy
    Clin Immunol 2012;129:1570–1578.

20 Lucendo AJ, Arias A, Gonzalez-Cervera
    J, Yague-Compadre JL, Guagnozzi D,
    Angueira T, Jimenez-Contreras S, Gon-
    zalez-Castillo S, Rodriguez-Dominguez B,
    De Rezende LC, Tenias JM: Empiric
    6-food elimination diet induced and
    maintained prolonged remission in pa-
    tients with adult eosinophilic esophagi-
    tis: a prospective study on the food
    cause of the disease. J Allergy Clin Im-
    munol 2013;131:797–804.
21 Mulder DJ, Pooni A, Mak N, Hurlbut DJ,
    Basta S, Justinich CJ: Antigen presenta-
    tion and MHC class II expression by
    human esophageal epithelial cells: role
    in eosinophilic esophagitis. Am J Pathol
    2011;178:744–753.
22 Niggemann B, Reibel S, Wahn U: The
    atopy patch test (APT) – a useful tool
    for the diagnosis of food allergy in chil-
    dren with atopic dermatitis. Allergy
    2000;55:281–285.
23 Turjanmaa K, Darsow U, Niggemann B,
    Rance F, Vanto T, Werfel T: EAACI/
    GA2LEN position paper: present status
    of the atopy patch test. Allergy 2006;61:
    1377–1384.
24 Kalach N, Soulaines P, de Boissieu D,
    Dupont C: A pilot study of the useful-
    ness and safety of a ready-to-use atopy
    patch test (Diallertest) versus a compar-
    ator (Finn Chamber) during cow's milk
    allergy in children. J Allergy Clin Immu-
    nol 2005;116:1321–1326.
25 Canani RB, Ruotolo S, Auricchio L, Cal-
    dore M, Porcaro F, Manguso F, Terrin
    G, Troncone R: Diagnostic accuracy of
    the atopy patch test in children with
    food allergy-related gastrointestinal
    symptoms. Allergy 2007;62:738–743.
26 Ballabio C, Fiocchi A, Martelli A, Pecora
    S, Burastero SE, Restani P: A method for
    the analysis of milk and egg allergens for
    the atopy patch test. Exp Dermatol 2009;
    18:886–888.
27 Darsow U, Vieluf D, Ring J: Evaluating
    the relevance of aeroallergen sensitiza-
    tion in atopic eczema with the atopy
    patch test: a randomized, double-blind
    multicenter study. Atopy Patch Test
    Study Group. J Am Acad Dermatol 1999;
    40:187–193.

28 Darsow U, Laifaoui J, Kerschenlohr K,
    Wollenberg A, Przybilla B, Wuthrich B,
    Borelli S Jr, Giusti F, Seidenari S, Drzi-
    malla K, Simon D, Disch R, Borelli S,
    Devillers AC, Oranje AP, De Raeve L,
    Hachem JP, Dangoisse C, Blondeel A,
    Song M, Breuer K, Wulf A, Werfel T,
    Roul S, Taieb A, Bolhaar S, Bruijnzeel-
    Koomen C, Bronnimann M, Braathen
    LR, Didierlaurent A, Andre C, Ring J:
    The prevalence of positive reactions in
    the atopy patch test with aeroallergens
    and food allergens in subjects with atop-
    ic eczema: a European multicenter
    study. Allergy 2004;59:1318–1325.
29 Heine RG, Verstege A, Mehl A, Staden
    U, Rolinck-Werninghaus C, Niggemann
    B: Proposal for a standardized interpre-
    tation of the atopy patch test in children
    with atopic dermatitis and suspected
    food allergy. Pediatr Allergy Immunol
    2006;17:213–217.
30 Canani RB, Buongiovanni A, Nocerino
    R, Cosenza L, Troncone R: Toward a
    standardized reading of the atopy patch
    test in children with suspected cow's
    milk allergy-related gastrointestinal
    symptoms. Allergy 2011;66:1499–1500.
31 Osterballe M, Andersen KE, Bindslev-
    Jensen C: The diagnostic accuracy of the
    atopy patch test in diagnosing hypersen-
    sitivity to cow's milk and hen's egg in
    unselected children with and without
    atopic dermatitis. J Am Acad Dermatol
    2004;51:556–562.
32 Zapatero Remon L, Alonso Lebrero E,
    Martin Fernandez E, Martinez Molero
    MI: Food-protein-induced enterocolitis
    syndrome caused by fish. Allergol Im-
    munopathol (Madr) 2005;33:312–316.
33 Fogg MI, Brown-Whitehorn TA, Paw-
    lowski NA, Spergel JM: Atopy patch test
    for the diagnosis of food protein-in-
    duced enterocolitis syndrome. Pediatr
    Allergy Immunol 2006;17:351–355.
34 Lucarelli S, Di Nardo G, Lastrucci G,
    D'Alfonso Y, Marcheggiano A, Federici
    T, Frediani S, Frediani T, Cucchiara S:
    Allergic proctocolitis refractory to ma-
    ternal hypoallergenic diet in exclusively
    breast-fed infants: a clinical observation.
    BMC Gastroenterol 2011;11:82.
35 Lack G: Epidemiologic risks for food
    allergy. J Allergy Clin Immunol 2008;
    121:1331–1336.
36 Moingeon P, Mascarell L: Novel routes
    for allergen immunotherapy: safety,
    efficacy and mode of action. Immuno-
    therapy 2012;4:201–212.

37 Matsumoto K, Saito H: Epicutaneous immunity and onset of allergic diseases – per-'eczema'tous sensitization drives the allergy march. Allergol Int 2013;62:291–296.

38 Newell L, Polak ME, Perera J, Owen C, Boyd P, Pickard C, Howarth PH, Healy E, Holloway JW, Friedmann PS, Ardern-Jones MR: Sensitization via healthy skin programs Th2 responses in individuals with atopic dermatitis. J Invest Dermatol 2013;133:2372–2380.

39 Flohr C, Perkin M, Logan K, Marrs T, Radulovic S, Campbell LE, Maccallum SF, Irwin McLean WH, Lack G: Atopic dermatitis and disease severity are the main risk factors for food sensitization in exclusively breastfed infants. J Invest Dermatol 2014;134:345–350.

40 Nagao K, Kobayashi T, Moro K, Ohyama M, Adachi T, Kitashima DY, Ueha S, Horiuchi K, Tanizaki H, Kabashima K, Kubo A, Cho YH, Clausen BE, Matsushima K, Suematsu M, Furtado GC, Lira SA, Farber JM, Udey MC, Amagai M: Stress-induced production of chemokines by hair follicles regulates the trafficking of dendritic cells in skin. Nat Immunol 2012;13:744–752.

41 Niggemann B, Rolinck-Werninghaus C, Mehl A, Binder C, Ziegert M, Beyer K: Controlled oral food challenges in children – when indicated, when superfluous? Allegy 2005;60:865–870.

42 Mehl A, Rolinck-Werninghaus C, Staden U, Verstege A, Wahn U, Beyer K, Niggemann B: The atopy patch test in the diagnostic workup of suspected food-related symptoms in children. J Allergy Clin Immunol 2006;118:923–929.

Kenji Matsumoto, MD, PhD
Department of Allergy and Immunology
National Research Institute for Child Health and Development
2–10–1, Okura, Setagaya-ku, Tokyo 157–8535 (Japan)
E-Mail matsumoto-k@ncchd.go.jp

Ebisawa M, Ballmer-Weber BK, Vieths S, Wood RA (eds): Food Allergy: Molecular Basis and Clinical Practice.
Chem Immunol Allergy. Basel, Karger, 2015, vol 101, pp 87–95 (DOI: 10.1159/000371680)

Diagnostic Elimination Diets and Oral Food Provocation

Robert A. Wood

Division of Pediatric Allergy and Immunology, Johns Hopkins University School of Medicine, and
Department of International Health, Johns Hopkins Bloomberg School of Public Health, Baltimore, Md., USA

Abstract

Accurately diagnosing patients with suspected food allergy is obviously critically important. The patient's health may be compromised if problem foods are left in the diet, while nutrition and quality of life may be negatively affected if foods are unnecessarily removed from the diet. In some patients, the diagnosis is very straightforward, such as with anaphylaxis with the first known exposure to peanut, but in many cases, the diagnosis will not be clear based on the history, skin tests, and serologic tests, especially because these tests often yield falsely positive results. In these instances, further testing will be needed, typically including diagnostic elimination diets and/or oral food challenges, which are the gold standard for the diagnosis of food allergy.   © 2015 S. Karger AG, Basel

Introduction

Although diagnostic testing methods for food hypersensitivity have improved over time, both in vivo and in vitro methods are sufficiently limited to allow elimination diets and oral food challenges (OFCs) to remain essential tools in the diagnosis and management of food allergy. In fact, the double-blind, placebo-controlled food challenge (DBPCFC) remains the gold standard for the diagnosis of food allergy [1–3]. In this chapter, the rational use of elimination diets and the indications for and methodologies and risks of OFCs will be reviewed in detail.

Elimination Diets

Elimination diets may be used diagnostically to determine if symptoms, usually chronic in nature, resolve after the suspect food(s) are removed from the diet. Overall, three general types of elimination diets are used in the care of patients with suspected food allergy: (1) elimination of one or several foods suspected to be causing symptoms, usually based on the history or preliminary test results; (2) elimination of most foods, just allowing the patient to eat a defined group of allowed foods (often referred to as an oligoantigenic diet); and (3) an elemental diet consisting of a hydrolyzed formula or an amino acid-based formula.

The type of elimination diet chosen depends on the age of the patient, the clinical history, and the results of other allergy tests. In patients with a clinical history consistent with an acute IgE-mediated allergy, it may be appropriate to recommend avoidance of several potential causal foods if a reaction occurred but a single causal food allergen could not be identified based on testing or history. Elimination diets are far more likely to be needed, however, in patients with chronic illness with a suspected allergic etiology. In this case, elimination of multiple foods (using an oligoantigenic or elemental diet) may be indicated. This will most often be indicated for patients with atopic dermatitis or allergic gastrointestinal disease, in which history is rarely helpful in identifying the culprit food(s) and the reactions are usually non-IgE mediated or mixed IgE and non-IgE mediated [4–6]. In these cases, and especially in the case of an infant or young child with significant gastrointestinal symptoms or poor growth, elimination of multiple foods may be needed to determine if the disorder is food responsive.

Adherence to these diets is difficult, especially in older children, adolescents, and adults. Thus, while an elimination diet may be quite easy in an infant on formula and eating a limited number of solid foods, it may be extraordinarily difficult for older patients. Needless to say, such limited diets may also pose nutritional risk. It is therefore important to choose elimination diets carefully to exclude the fewest foods possible and to have a planned endpoint for the reintroduction of foods into the diet. While food allergy is likely if there is significant clinical improvement, as documented based on history, symptoms, physical examination, or biopsy results, reintroduction of the suspect foods will still often be needed to confirm the diagnosis. This is accomplished either through careful introduction in the home setting or as an OFC, which would be needed for most suspected IgE-mediated reactions. However, it is also important to recognize that some patients who previously only had chronic symptoms may have acute reactivity to the same food after a period of avoidance [7].

Oral Challenge Testing

There are a number of reasons that oral challenge testing should be considered, both for clinical and for research purposes [1–3]. In the clinical setting, challenges are typically done for three major reasons. First, OFCs are used to establish an accurate diagnosis when the diagnosis is still not clear after performing other standard diagnostic tests, including history taking, skin testing, measurement of specific IgE levels, and/or elimination diets. Therefore, if a patient recently experienced an acute, severe reaction to his or her first peanut exposure and has a strongly positive skin test or markedly elevated peanut-specific IgE levels, an OFC with peanut would not be necessary or appropriate. Second, if a patient has a chronic allergic condition, such as atopic dermatitis or allergic gastrointestinal disease, skin tests or specific IgE levels that are not in the diagnostic range, and an unclear response to an elimination diet, one or more challenge tests may be very appropriate.

Third, OFCs are frequently used to determine if a patient with a known food allergy has developed tolerance to that food. For example, in a patient with a known allergy to egg or peanut who has remained reaction free over a period of time, usually considered as a minimum of 1 year, and whose test results suggest that the allergy may have been outgrown, a challenge should be considered to determine the degree of tolerance. While complete tolerance is certainly the goal, if a reaction occurs during the challenge, that information can still be used to guide the patient and the patient's family regarding the approach to the diet, such as the need for strict avoidance of the problem food or possibly some liberalization of the diet.

In the clinical setting, in addition to the potential for risk and the chances of success, decision-making about challenges is largely based on the preferences of the patient and the patient's family and the importance of the food to the diet. Clinicians would typically be much quicker to do an

OFC with a major food item, such as milk, egg, or wheat, even if the chances of success are less, because it would be so advantageous to be able to reintroduce that food into the diet. It is also very important to recognize that a food that might be unimportant to one family might be extremely important to another. For example, one family may not care if lentils are ever introduced into the diet, while for another practicing a vegetarian diet, this might be an extremely important food.

In the research setting, food challenges have been used with great success for numerous indications. First, they have been used to assess the accuracy of other diagnostic methods, including skin tests, patch tests, and measurement of allergen-specific IgE levels [8–15]. Second, they have been used to assess threshold doses for different allergenic foods, providing essential data for the establishment of guidelines for the food industry and revealing the potential risks of low-level allergen exposure [16–18]. Third, they have been used to determine the effects of food processing on the allergenicity of different foods [19, 20].

Methodology

The general concepts underlying all oral challenge procedures are the same. The food in question is introduced in gradually increasing doses under observation in a controlled setting until a specific goal dose is reached. The major differences among the various methods that are employed include the use of blinding and variations in dosing strategy.

Open Challenges

An open challenge refers to an OFC in which the suspect food is administered without blinding or use of a placebo. The limitations of open challenges relate to the chance of bias on the part of both the patient and the observer. This bias will most often result in falsely positive challenge results, with some suggesting up to 30% false-positive results [2]. This is especially common when the patient has significant anxiety about the challenge or when the patient's prior symptoms have been more subjective in nature. When a patient has only subjective complaints during a challenge, such as abdominal pain or pruritus, with no objective signs of reaction, the interpretation of the challenge outcome can be difficult. However, this difficulty can be markedly reduced when experienced observers conduct challenges.

Even with these potential limitations, open challenges do still have significant utility in the clinical setting for several reasons. First, an open challenge may be the first approach when the probability of a negative outcome is estimated to be high (for example, while studying an adverse reaction believed to be IgE mediated when a food skin test and in vitro determination of specific IgE are completely negative). Second, when an open challenge is negative, it is likely to be very accurate and may obviate the need for a DBPCFC. Third, in infants and young children, in whom the impact of anxiety and other psychological factors is likely to be minimal, the risk of bias is significantly reduced, and open challenges may be appropriate as a first-line challenge procedure. Lastly, for practical reasons, open challenges are significantly easier to perform since food preparation will be far simpler than with a blinded challenge and since the entire challenge can be performed with a single visit. This can make a huge difference for busy practitioners limited in the number of challenges that they are capable of performing.

Single-Blind Challenges

In a single-blind challenge, the patient is blinded to the challenge material, while the observer is not. Single-blind challenges still have the potential limitation of observer bias, and, in reality, the only advantage that they provide is a minor reduction in the personnel needed for food preparation since the same individual can both prepare the challenge foods and act as an observer of the

Table 1. Examples of foods and vehicles for double-blind, placebo-controlled food challenges

Food	Challenge material	Placebo	Vehicle
Egg	Dried egg white	Corn starch, oat flour, rice flour	Applesauce, oatmeal, pudding, mashed potato
Milk	Dried milk, milk	Soy milk or formula, corn starch, wheat or rice flour	Formula (soy, hydrolyzed, or elemental), soy or rice milk (chocolate), applesauce, pudding
Peanut	Peanut flour, peanut butter, crushed peanuts	Oat or wheat flour, soy butter	Hamburger, other meat patties, chili, oatmeal, pudding, cookies, candy
Soy	Soy flour, soy milk or formula	Flour (wheat, oat, rice, corn), safe formula	Formula (hydrolyzed or elemental), rice milk (chocolate), applesauce, oatmeal, pudding
Wheat	Wheat flour	Oat, rice, or corn flour	Applesauce, oatmeal, pudding
Tree nuts	Crushed nuts, nut butter	Oat or wheat flour, soy or peanut butter	Applesauce, oatmeal, pudding

challenge. Therefore, there is little or no role for single-blind challenges in either the clinical or the research setting.

Double-Blind, Placebo-Controlled Challenges
The DBPCFC remains the gold standard for the diagnosis of food allergy since both patient and observer biases are minimized. It is the preferred method for all scientific research protocols and for the clinical evaluation of patients who present with a history of delayed reactions, chronic symptoms, or primarily subjective symptoms, such as abdominal pain, pruritus, chronic fatigue, multiple chemical sensitivities, or headache. The limitations of DBPCFCs are entirely practical, including considerable time requirements for staff in the preparation of adequately blinded challenge materials and the requirement for two visits to accomplish both segments of the blinded challenge. Suggestions of foods, placebos, and vehicles for DBPCFCs to several common food allergens are presented in table 1.

Although it is the best available test to diagnose food allergy, even the DBPCFC is not perfect, and false-positive and false-negative rates have been estimated to be between 1 and 3% [21]. The use of an open challenge after a blinded challenge will help to reduce or eliminate false-negative challenges, but all challenges need to be interpreted with care. Increasing the number of challenges, with multiple active and placebo challenges, will improve accuracy but is usually not practical and may increase risk by providing more doses of the active substance. It has also been suggested that a final challenge be conducted on a subsequent day, as one study demonstrated that over 10% of negative challenges will prove positive when the entire provocative dose is given as a single challenge on a separate day [22]. The likely explanation for this phenomenon is that there may be an element of desensitization during a graded challenge, leading to falsely negative results.

Challenge Settings and Procedures

In some instances, food introduction can be conducted at home, without physician supervision. This should be the case only when the physician determines that there is no risk of a severe reaction.

This approach might be appropriate for patients who present with complaints that are usually not associated with food allergy and when skin or in vitro testing has been negative. It may also be appropriate to do a home reintroduction of a food that has been temporarily discontinued as part of an elimination diet but that had been present in the diet previously. However, the caveat here is that if there has been prolonged avoidance, or avoidance for more than a few weeks to a few months, the pattern of reactivity may have changed, so a home introduction may no longer be safe [7]. Thus, if a child with atopic dermatitis and a positive skin test for egg undergoes a 3-week trial off egg, reintroducing egg at home would be safe for most patients, although no challenge may be needed at that time if there was a dramatic improvement in the atopic dermatitis on the avoidance diet. However, if it is felt that the family may have difficulty interpreting the results of the home introduction or if the avoidance has been more prolonged, then the reintroduction should be done as a formal challenge under observation. Additionally, in all cases in which there is even a remote chance of a severe or anaphylactic reaction, challenges should only be conducted with physician supervision.

OFCs should be performed in an environment that maximizes comfort and safety. The risks and benefits of the challenge should be discussed in detail; in most settings, informed consent should be obtained. The personnel involved in challenge procedures must be specially trained in the management of acute allergic reactions, and these trained personnel should continuously monitor patients undergoing challenge. Medications and equipment for resuscitation must be readily available. At a minimum, this should include injectable epinephrine, intravenous fluids, oral and parenteral antihistamines, oral and parenteral corticosteroids, inhaled or nebulized beta-agonists, oxygen, and resuscitation equipment. In cases in which a severe reaction is suspected, the challenge should be performed in an inpatient setting or intensive care unit. Ideally, challenges should be conducted in a setting where patients and their families can be comfortable and relaxed. Particularly for anxious children, activities that help to provide distraction are of great benefit.

Before proceeding with a challenge, patients should have a stable baseline examination, without significant symptoms of atopic dermatitis, rhino-conjunctivitis, urticaria, or other symptoms evaluated during food challenges. They should have no wheezing or repetitive cough prior to the challenge, and they should not have been treated for a significant asthma exacerbation within a minimum of 1 week prior to undergoing the challenge. They must have no current illness (e.g., fever, vomiting, diarrhea) at the time of the challenge. Prior to challenges, patients should discontinue antihistamines and bronchodilators for appropriate periods, based on their elimination half-lives and duration of action. The challenge food should be provided gradually, at 15–30 min intervals or longer, beginning with a dose unlikely to trigger a reaction and progressing stepwise with escalating doses, with an option to repeat doses or delay doses longer if symptoms may be developing (e.g., subjective signs of a reaction). Vital signs (heart rate, blood pressure, respiratory rate) should be monitored at the start and end of the challenge, with a brief examination focusing on the oral mucosa, skin, and respiratory system prior to each dose. Pulse oximetry, spirometry, or assessment of peak expiratory flow may also be used for individual patients when deemed appropriate. Challenges should be stopped and medications administered in the event of any significant objective symptoms (e.g., a challenge might be continued if there are just one or two hives, especially where the food may have touched the skin). Challenges may also be stopped for subjective symptoms, such as significant abdominal pain, at the discretion of the supervising personnel. All challenge procedures, including the baseline exam, doses administered, vital signs, subjective complaints, objective signs, medications given, discharge examination, and discharge instructions, should be fully documented in the patient's medical record.

In addition, patients with a diagnosis of food protein-induced enterocolitis syndrome deserve special consideration [23]. Reactions in this syndrome are often very severe, frequently including hypotension. All such challenges should be done with intravenous access established since the primary treatment for such reactions is fluid resuscitation. Some may also benefit from intravenous corticosteroids. Reactions are typically delayed by at least 1 h after ingestion and more commonly by 2–3 h, so observation times must be adjusted accordingly.

Upon discharge from all challenges, patients should be given detailed instructions on how the food should or should not be introduced into the diet as well as information on the signs and symptoms that might indicate a problem with that food in the future. As a general rule, foods can be introduced in unlimited quantities after a successful challenge, although for most patients, it is recommended that they eat no more than one serving per day for the first several days. For those with failed challenges, specific post-challenge dietary instruction should also be provided, which might range from continued strict avoidance in those with significant reactions after small doses to the introduction of small amounts of the food into the diet, such as milk or egg in baked products, in patients with lesser reactions after larger doses. In some specific instances, such as in patients with resolved peanut allergy, it may also be important both to maintain the food in the diet on a regular basis to lower the risk of a recurrence of the allergy and to continue to keep self-injectable epinephrine on hand until tolerance has been documented over a minimum of 6 months.

Dosing Strategies

Although the general approach to dosing is similar from one protocol to another, there is no consensus about a single best strategy [1–3, 24–26]. In all challenges, the food is given in gradually increasing amounts. For most IgE-medicated reactions, typical total doses administered are 8–10 g for dry food and 100 ml for wet food, doubling the amounts for meat or fish, or an approximate full serving for fruits and vegetables. Doses are typically given every 15–30 min over 1–2 h, although the dosing interval can be lengthened if clinically indicated. For example, if a patient has had prior severe reactions to a food, a 30 min or even 40–60 min interval might be selected between doses. It is also reasonable to delay individual doses or to repeat prior doses if a reaction is suspected but not yet confirmed.

One common dosing scheme is to divide the total challenge into seven incremental doses: 1, 4, 10, 15, 20, 25, and 25% (table 2). For patients deemed to be at higher risk of a severe reaction, it may be prudent to begin with one or more smaller doses, such as 0.1 and/or 0.5%. This may be particularly appropriate when doing challenges in the research setting, such as for a treatment study, where more highly sensitive patients may be undergoing challenges compared with in the clinical setting, where challenges are most often being done in less sensitive patients. Some centers

Table 2. Suggested challenge dosing regimen (for a liquid challenge totaling 100 ml)

Dose #	Time, min	Percentage	Volume, ml
1	0	1	1
2	15	4	4
3	30	10	10
4	45	15	15
5	60	20	20
6	75	25	25
7	90	25	25

The dosing is shown here as a percentage of the total and can be calculated as a weight or volume, depending on the substance being used. For example, if the total weight of a final challenge is 20 g, then 1% = 200 mg.

Table 3. Steps to minimize challenge risks

Table 3. Steps to minimize challenge risks

Adjust the starting dose and challenge protocol for individual patients who might be at higher risk of a severe reaction.

Utilize experienced observers who have been trained to do food challenges and who are present throughout the challenge, continually interacting with and reexamining the patient at regular intervals.

Stop the challenge as soon as one or more observers are convinced that a reaction is occurring.

Prepare all medications that might be needed before the challenge so that they can be administered without delay.

Perform challenges only in settings where all measures that might be needed to treat a severe reaction are readily available.

also begin with a labial challenge, placing a small amount of the challenge material on the lower lip for 1–2 min and observing for localized (or systemic) signs of a reaction.

Risk and Treatment of Oral Food Challenges

Several studies have focused on the types of reactions that occur as well as on the types of treatment needed after positive (failed) OFCs [27 30]. The expected reactions are those seen with food-induced reactions in general, involving some combination of cutaneous, gastrointestinal, respiratory, and cardiovascular reactions. Skin and gastrointestinal reactions are most common, and severe or life-threatening reactions are rare. Many patients describe localized pruritus in the mouth, throat, or ears as their first symptom, sometimes with visible urticaria in or around the mouth. While these symptoms do indicate a localized allergic response, they do not automatically mean that the challenge must stop, as they are often transient and may occur during challenges that are otherwise successful. Distinct behavioral changes are also very common, especially in young children. It is common to see children change suddenly from happy and playful to quiet and frightened with the onset of a reaction. These signs should always be taken seriously, as they likely herald the onset of a reaction.

The risk of challenges can be minimized by following several guidelines (table 3). First, as discussed above, the starting dose and challenge protocol should be adjusted for individual patients who might be at higher risk of a severe reaction. Second, experienced observers who are present throughout the challenge, continually interacting with and reexamining the patient at regular intervals, can dramatically reduce risk. Third, the challenge should be stopped as soon as one or more observers are convinced that a reaction is occurring. While there is a risk that stopping too early will result in a false-positive challenge, the risk of waiting too long or giving an extra dose is much more significant. Fourth, all medications that might be needed should be prepared in appropriate doses before starting the challenge so that they can be administered without delay. Finally, the challenge should be performed in a setting where all measures that might be needed to treat a severe reaction are readily available.

Challenges should be terminated whenever the observer is reasonably convinced that a reaction is occurring, and treatment should be administered as indicated. Some challenges may have only minor, localized signs and symptoms, in which case treatment may not be necessary. In the vast majority of instances, however, treatment with at least an antihistamine is warranted. Other therapies, including intramuscular epinephrine, oral or parenteral corticosteroids, inhaled or nebulized beta-agonists, an H_2 antagonist, oxygen, or intravenous fluids, should be administered at the discretion of the treating physician. While there may be a greater role for cautious observation than there would be after accidental ingestions, it is still critical that reactions be treated as aggressively as necessary to prevent possible progression to something more severe or dangerous.

Although all OFCs carry risk, they remain an essential tool in the management of patients with suspected food allergy. Given the enormous nutritional and social benefits that can result from a negative challenge, these risks are reasonable when the risk-to-benefit ratio is carefully considered for each patient and challenges are performed under the guidance of an experienced practitioner in a properly equipped setting.

Summary

Elimination diets and OFCs are essential tools in the diagnosis of food allergy. The OFC remains the single most accurate test for the diagnosis of food allergy. The basic methodology underlying all OFCs relies on the administration of the suspect food in gradually increasing doses under close observation in a medical setting. Variations in challenge methodology include the inclusion of placebo controls, blinding, and different dosing strategies. Challenges should be terminated and treatment administered at the first sign that a reaction is occurring. OFCs carry the potential for significant risk, but this risk can be minimized by appropriate dosing and by performing challenges in an appropriate setting with experienced personnel.

References

1 Bindslev-Jensen C, Ballmer-Weber BK, Bengtsson U, et al: Standardization of food challenges in patients with immediate reactions to foods – position paper from the European Academy of Allergology and Clinical Immunology. Allergy 2004;59:690–697.

2 Nowak-Wegrzyn A, Assa'ad AH, Bahna SL, et al: Work Group report: oral food challenge testing. J Allergy Clin Immunol 2009;123:S365–S383.

3 Sampson HA, Gerth van Wijk R, Bindslev-Jensen C, et al: Standardizing double-blind, placebo-controlled oral food challenges: American Academy of Allergy, Asthma & Immunology-European Academy of Allergy and Clinical Immunology PRACTALL consensus report. J Allergy Clin Immunol 2012;130:1260.

4 Eigenmann PA, Sicherer SH, Borkowski TA, et al: Prevalence of IgE-mediated food allergy among children with atopic dermatitis. Pediatrics 1998;101:E8.

5 Sicherer SH, Sampson HA: Food hypersensitivity and atopic dermatitis: pathophysiology, epidemiology, diagnosis, and management. J Allergy Clin Immunol 1999;104:S114.

6 Liacouras CA, Spergel JM, Ruchelli E, et al: Eosinophilic esophagitis: a 10-year experience in 381 children. Clin Gastroenterol Hepatol 2005;3:1198.

7 Barbi E, Gerarduzzi T, Longo G, et al: Fatal allergy as a possible consequence of long-term elimination diet. Allergy 2004;59:668–669.

8 Niggemann B, Reibel S, Wahn U: The atopy patch test (APT) – a useful tool for the diagnosis of food allergy in children with atopic dermatitis. Allergy 2000;55:281–285.

9 Sampson HA, Ho DG: Relationship between food-specific IgE concentrations and the risk of positive food challenges in children and adolescents. J Allergy Clin Immunol 1997;100:444–451.

10 Sampson HA: Utility of food-specific IgE concentrations in predicting symptomatic food allergy. J Allergy Clin Immunol 2001;107:891–896.

11 Boyano MT, Garcia-Ara C, Diaz-Pena JM, et al: Validity of specific IgE antibodies in children with egg allergy. Clin Exp Allergy 2001;31:1464–1469.

12 DunnGalvin A, Daly D, Cullinane C, et al: Highly accurate prediction of food challenge outcome using routinely available clinical data. J Allergy Clin Immunol 2011;127:633–639.

13 Perry TT, Matsui EC, Conover-Walker MK, et al: The relationship of allergen-specific IgE levels and oral food challenge outcome. J Allergy Clin Immunol 2004;114:144–149.

14 Wood RA: The likelihood of remission of food allergy in children: when is the optimal time for challenge? Curr Allergy Asthma Rep 2012;12:42–47.

15 Rance F, Juchet A, Bremont F, et al: Correlations between skin prick tests using commercial extracts and fresh foods, specific IgE, and food challenges. Allergy 1997;52:1031–1035.

16 Taylor SL, Hefle SL, Bindslev-Jensen C, et al: Factors affecting the determination of threshold doses for allergenic foods: how much is too much? J Allergy Clin Immunol 2002;109:24–30.

17 Taylor SL, Hefle SL, Bindslev-Jensen C, et al: A consensus protocol for the determination of the threshold doses for allergenic foods: how much is too much? Clin Exp Allergy 2004;34:689–695.

18 Taylor SL, Moneret-Vautrin DA, Crevel RW, et al: Threshold dose for peanut: risk characterization based upon diagnostic oral challenge of a series of 286 peanut-allergic individuals. Food Chem Toxicol 2010;48:814.

19 Ballmer-Weber BK, Hoffmann A, Wuthrich B, et al: Influence of food processing on the allergenicity of celery: DBPCFC with celery spice and cooked celery in patients with celery allergy. Allergy 2002;57:228–235.

20 Nowak-Wegrzyn A, Bloom KA, Sicherer SH, et al: Tolerance to extensively heated milk in children with cow's milk allergy. J Allergy Clin Immunol 2008;122:342–347.

21 Caffarelli C, Petroccione T: False negative food challenges in children with suspected food allergy. Lancet 2001;358:1871–1872.

22 Niggemann B, Lange L, Finger A, et al: Accurate oral food challenge requires a cumulative dose on a subsequent day. J Allergy Clin Immunol 2012;130:261–263.

23 Sicherer S: Food protein-induced enterocolitis syndrome: case presentations and management lessons. J Allergy Clin Immunol 2005;115:149–156.

24 Bindslev-Jensen C: Standardization of double-blind, placebo-controlled food challenges. Allergy 2001;56(suppl 67):75–77.

25 Järvinen KM, Sicherer SH: Diagnostic oral food challenges: procedures and biomarkers. J Immunol Methods 2012;383:30–38.

26 Rancé F, Deschildre A, Villard-Truc F, et al: Oral food challenge in children: an expert review. Eur Ann Allergy Clin Immunol 2009;41:35–49.

27 Reibel S, Rohr C, Ziegert M, et al: What safety measures need to be taken in oral food challenges in children? Allergy 2000;55:940–944.

28 Perry TT, Matsui EC, Conover-Walker MK, et al: The risk of oral food challenges. J Allergy Clin Immunol 2004;114:1164–1168.

29 Järvinen KM, Amalanayagam S, Shreffler WG, et al: Epinephrine treatment is infrequent and biphasic reactions are rare in food-induced reactions during oral food challenges in children. J Allergy Clin Immunol 2009;124:1267–1272.

30 Rolinck-Werninghaus C, Niggemann B, Grabenhenrich L, et al: Outcome of oral food challenges in children in relation to symptom-eliciting allergen dose and allergen-specific IgE. Allergy 2012;67:951–957.

Robert A. Wood, MD
Division of Pediatric Allergy and Immunology
Johns Hopkins University School of Medicine, CMSC 1102
600 N. Wolfe Street, Baltimore, MD 21287 (USA)
E-Mail rwood@jhmi.edu

Ebisawa M, Ballmer-Weber BK, Vieths S, Wood RA (eds): Food Allergy: Molecular Basis and Clinical Practice.
Chem Immunol Allergy. Basel, Karger, 2015, vol 101, pp 96–105 (DOI: 10.1159/000374080)

Pharmacological Management of Acute Food-Allergic Reactions

Stephanie Richards[a] · Mimi Tang[a–c]

[a]Department of Allergy and Immunology, The Royal Children's Hospital Melbourne, Melbourne, Vic.,
[b]Allergy and Immune Disorders Research, Murdoch Childrens Research Institute, Melbourne, Vic., and
[c]Department of Paediatrics, The University of Melbourne, Melbourne, Vic., Australia

Abstract

There is currently no well-established disease-modifying treatment for food allergy, so management relies upon strict avoidance of food allergen(s), implementation of risk minimisation strategies to avoid inadvertent exposure and allergic reactions, and prompt management of acute allergic reactions, should they occur. The pharmacological management of acute food-induced allergic reactions is dependent on the underlying pathophysiology of the allergic reaction and the severity of clinical symptoms and signs. Mild to moderate symptoms of an immunoglobulin E-mediated acute allergic reaction may be treated effectively with an oral anti-histamine. In patients exhibiting the clinical features of anaphylaxis, adrenaline is the only first-line therapy recommended by expert consensus. Adjunctive therapies, including anti-histamines, beta-agonists and glucocorticoids, may be used in the subsequent management of immunoglobulin E-mediated anaphylaxis. Here, we present the current recommendations for the pharmacological management of acute food-induced allergic reactions, together with a summary of the evidence supporting these recommendations.

© 2015 S. Karger AG, Basel

Introduction

As discussed by Kim and Burks (pp. 8–17), food allergy can be classified by its underlying pathophysiological mechanism into immunoglobulin E (IgE)-mediated, mixed IgE/non-IgE mediated, and non-IgE-mediated food allergy [1]. IgE-mediated food allergy reactions are characterised by acute onset of symptoms within 1–2 hours of exposure to food allergen. IgE-mediated food allergy occurs as a result of the production of food-specific IgE. This circulating, food-specific IgE binds to the surface of tissue mast cells and circulating

Table 1. Symptoms of acute food-induced allergic reactions (modified from [3])

Target organ	Immediate symptoms
Cutaneous	Erythema Pruritis Urticaria Angioedema
Ocular	Pruritis Conjunctival erythema Tearing Periorbital oedema
Upper respiratory	Nasal congestion Pruritis Rhinorrhoea Sneezing Laryngeal oedema Hoarseness Dry staccato cough
Lower respiratory	Persistent cough Chest tightness Dyspnea Wheezing Intercostal retractions Accessory muscle use
Gastrointestinal (oral)	Angioedema of the lips, tongue or palate Oral pruritis Tongue swelling
Gastrointestinal (lower)	Nausea Colicky abdominal pain Reflux Vomiting Diarrhoea
Cardiovascular	Pallor and drowsiness (in infants and young children) Tachycardia (occasionally bradycardia in anaphylaxis) Hypotension Dizziness Collapse Loss of consciousness

basophils. Upon re-exposure to the food, the food allergen cross-links cell surface-bound, allergen-specific IgE and initiates mast cell degranulation and the rapid release of vasoactive and inflammatory mediators, including histamine, tryptase and leukotrienes [1, 2], which are responsible for the clinical manifestations of immediate food-induced allergic reactions, as outlined in table 1 [3]. In contrast to IgE-mediated food allergy, the non-IgE-mediated and mixed IgE/non-IgE-mediated food allergy syndromes typically present with delayed onset of symptoms hours after allergen exposure and involve cell-mediated immune mechanisms (see Kim and Burks, pp. 8–17).

There is currently no well-established disease-modifying treatment or cure for food allergy, so management relies upon strict avoidance of the specific food allergen(s), together with implementation of risk minimisation strategies to avoid future inadvertent food allergen exposure and to promote early recognition and treatment of allergic reactions [1]. However, allergen avoidance is difficult to achieve, and individuals with food allergy will commonly have accidental exposure to food allergens, resulting in acute allergic reactions. Hence, a sound understanding of the management of acute reactions is important not only for the physician but also for the patient (and their family, if the patient is a child). This chapter will discuss the pharmacological management of acute allergic reactions to food and its supporting evidence base, with focus on acute IgE-mediated allergic reactions.

Pharmacological Management of IgE-Mediated, Food-Induced Acute Allergic Reactions

Mild to Moderate Reactions
Histamine is one of the principal pre-formed mediators that are released by mast cells and basophils during an IgE-mediated allergic reaction. Histamine induces many of the clinical features of IgE-mediated food-allergic reactions through activation of H1 and/or H2 receptors in the skin, intestine, airway and cardiovascular tissues [4]. Symptoms in the skin include cutaneous erythema, angio-oedema, urticaria and pruritus, while intestinal symptoms include abdominal pain, vomiting and diarrhoea. Accordingly, histamine antagonists or anti-histamine medications are widely used in the management of IgE-mediated, food-induced acute allergic reactions.

Anti-histamines may selectively target H1 and/or H2 receptors and preferentially bind to the inactive receptor, thereby inhibiting receptor signalling in the presence of endogenously released histamine and promoting the inactive state [4, 5]. The clinical utility of this class of medications is in the management of mild to moderate symptoms of an IgE-mediated, food-induced allergic reaction, particularly in the management of cutaneous symptoms such as urticaria, pruritus, erythema and angio-oedema as well as localised upper respiratory symptoms such as rhinorrhoea and sneezing [6].

Importantly, there is no high-quality evidence to support the use of anti-histamines in the initial management of anaphylaxis, as they do not prevent or relieve airway obstruction or hypotensive shock [6, 7]. Expert guidelines continue to recommend the administration of anti-histamine in the event of clinical symptoms and/or signs of an IgE-mediated allergic reaction, but this should never delay the administration of adrenaline in the management of anaphylaxis [8] (see Pesek and Jones, pp. 191–198).

The choice of anti-histamine is dependent upon multiple patient factors, and prescribing practices vary internationally [9]. As a general rule, first-generation sedating H1 anti-histamines should be avoided, with a preference for newer generation, less-sedating anti-histamines that are available in liquid form for ease of administration and rapidity of onset [8]. Generally, the onset of action following a single oral dose of H1 anti-histamine is within 1–3 hours, and the duration of action is at least 24 hours [5]. First-generation H1 anti-histamines (e.g. chlorpheniramine and promethazine) have a number of side effects that limit their usefulness in the management of acute, IgE-mediated allergic reactions. In particular, these first-generation H1 anti-histamines characteristically induce central nervous system effects, such as drowsiness, psychomotor retardation and confusion due to interference with neurotransmitters in the central nervous system [5]. In contrast, second-generation H1 anti-histamines are more specific for H1 receptors and, due to their lipophobicity, are less able to penetrate the central

Anaphylaxis is highly likely when any one of the following 3 criteria are fulfilled:

1. Acute onset of an illness (minutes to several hours), with involvement of the skin, mucosal tissue, or both (e.g. generalised hives, pruritis or flushing, swollen lips-tongue-uvula) and at least one of the following:
   a. Respiratory compromise (e.g. dyspnoea, wheeze-bronchospasm, stridor, reduced peak expiratory flow, hypoxemia).
   b. Reduced blood pressure (BP) or associated symptoms of end-organ dysfunction (e.g. hypotonia, syncope, incontinence).

2. Two or more of the following that occur rapidly after exposure to a likely allergen for that patient (minutes to several hours):
   a. Involvement of the skin-mucosal tissue (e.g. generalised hives, itch-flush, swollen lips-tongue-uvula).
   b. Respiratory compromise (e.g. dyspnoea, wheeze-bronchospasm, stridor, reduced peak expiratory flow hypoxemia).
   c. Reduced BP or associated symptoms of end-organ dysfunction (e.g. hypotonia, syncope, incontinence).
   d. Persistent gastrointestinal symptoms (e.g. crampy abdominal pain, vomiting).

3. Reduced BP after exposure to known allergen for that patient (minutes to several hours):
   a. Infants and children: low systolic BP (age-specific) or greater than 30% decrease in systolic BP.
   b. Adults: systolic BP of less than 90 mm Hg or greater than 30% decrease from baseline.

nervous system. Given this, second-generation H1 anti-histamines are less frequently associated with neurological side effects [5]. This is especially relevant in the management of IgE-mediated allergic reactions in younger children, since circulatory system compromise in this age group may present as pallor and drowsiness (pale and floppy infant or child) rather than hypotension, and the use of a first-generation (sedating) anti-histamine can cause drowsiness that may mask the signs of progressive circulatory system compromise. Other relevant side effects of first-generation H1 anti-histamines to be aware of include reflex tachycardia and QT interval prolongation (predominantly associated with first-generation H1 anti-histamines). These side effects are less often reported for second-generation H1 anti-histamines [5].

Less data are available for the use of H2 anti-histamines in the management of IgE-mediated allergic reactions. Two randomised control trials have demonstrated improved efficacy for the treatment of urticaria using a combination of H1 and H2 anti-histamines when compared to using H1 anti-histamines in isolation. However, a similar effect was not evident for the management of other common symptoms and signs of an acute IgE mediated allergic reaction, including itch, angio-oedema and cutaneous erythema [4, 10].

Anaphylaxis
Adrenaline
The most severe form of an acute IgE-mediated allergic reaction is anaphylaxis, which is life-threatening. Anaphylaxis is clinically defined as a severe, systemic allergic reaction characterised by involvement of the respiratory or cardiovascular systems or both [8]. Reactions can be further classified as uniphasic (single episode), biphasic (second reaction after the initial therapy) or protracted (no initial recovery period) [11]. Expert consensus criteria for the diagnosis of anaphylaxis can be found in table 2 [12] (and are discussed by Pesek and Jones, pp. 191–198).

As involvement or compromise of the airway and/or circulation can be life-threatening, anaphylaxis represents a medical emergency, and prompt assessment and initiation of management is essential. Initial management requires rapid assessment of the patient's airway, breathing, circulation, and removal of further allergen exposure (if possible) [6]. Adrenaline should be administered immediately once a diagnosis of anaphylaxis is established. The patient should be placed in a supine position (unless contraindicated by respiratory difficulty or vomiting), ideally with the lower limbs elevated to ensure adequate venous return, as a change to an upright posture may have contributed to fatality in some cases of anaphylaxis [1, 13]; the patient should not be asked to ambulate to a different location.

Adrenaline is the first-line pharmacological treatment for anaphylaxis, and delay in its administration has been associated with increased morbidity and mortality [3, 14, 15]. The evidence base for the use of adrenaline in anaphylaxis is derived from observational, epidemiologic and *in vitro* studies as well as animal models [3]. Although there are no randomised control trials examining adrenaline use in anaphylaxis, expert consensus is that adrenaline is the only first-line treatment for anaphylaxis, and all other pharmacologic treatments represent adjunctive therapies [3, 15].

Importantly, there is no high-quality evidence to support the use of anti-histamines in the initial management of anaphylaxis, as this class of therapeutic agents does not prevent or reverse the life-threatening features of airway obstruction or hypotension [6, 7]. Administration of adrenaline should never be delayed or replaced by treatment with anti-histamine in the setting of anaphylaxis [8].

The therapeutic and life-saving effects of adrenaline in the management of anaphylaxis are due to several mechanisms of action. First, adrenaline acts as an agonist of α1-adrenergic receptors, resulting in vasoconstriction, increased peripheral vascular resistance and decreased mucosal oedema. Adrenaline also has β1- and β2-adrenergic agonist properties, resulting in an increased rate and force of cardiac contractions, reduced inflammatory mediator release and bronchodilation [3, 6, 8]. These combined actions result in resolution or improvement of respiratory and circulatory compromise in anaphylaxis. Although the onset of action of adrenaline occurs within minutes of administration, it is also readily metabolised. Consequently, the effects may be short-lived, and repeated doses may be required in up to 20% of patients whose symptoms do not improve or resolve with a single dose [3, 14]. Repeat doses of adrenaline can be administered every 5–15 minutes, as required.

Intramuscular (IM) injection of adrenaline into the upper anterolateral thigh is the recommended route of administration. The recommended dose of IM adrenaline is 0.01 mg/kg of a 1:1,000 solution, up to a maximum dose of 0.5 mg. The efficacy of IM adrenaline administration has been compared to the subcutaneous route in several studies, all of which have demonstrated a higher and more rapid peak in plasma and tissue concentrations of adrenaline following IM administration [15]. Adrenaline may also be administered through the intraosseous and endotracheal routes.

Intravenous (IV) adrenaline is not recommended for use in the initial management of anaphylaxis, but it may be required for patients who do not respond to IM adrenaline or are profoundly hypotensive [4, 6]. In this setting, a more dilute (1:10,000) solution should be administered by slow infusion, and the dose should be titrated according to the response. In the event of cardiac arrest, a bolus of IV adrenaline (rather than slow infusion) is indicated. Additionally, if IV adrenaline is required, invasive cardiac monitoring is recommended [6, 15], as IV adrenaline infusion may be associated with an increased risk of adverse cardiovascular effects, especially in the elderly and adults with cardiovascular disease [3, 6]. It is advisable that IV adrenaline be administered by emergency or intensive care physicians who have experience with this route of administration.

Alternative routes of adrenaline administration have been explored in the literature, including oral, inhaled and, more recently, sublingual therapy. Oral adrenaline administration is ineffective in the management of anaphylaxis due to its rapid inactivation by enzymes in the gastrointestinal tract [16]. Inhalation of adrenaline via a metered-dose inhaler results in high concentrations of adrenaline in the upper and lower airways. Potential benefits of this include local effects at the site of airway obstruction during anaphylaxis as well as providing a large surface area for systemic absorption [16]. One of the significant disadvantages of this route of administration is that a large number of inhalations (10–20 inhalations in children and 20–30 inhalations in adults) are required over a short period of time to provide adequate plasma concentrations necessary for treatment of the systemic effects of anaphylaxis [15, 16]. Currently, inhaled or nebulised adrenaline is only recommended as an adjunct to IM therapy to assist with the management of oral mucosal swelling or oedema [8]. Recently, a preclinical study evaluating the utility of sublingual adrenaline tablets was published and demonstrated a rapid absorption of adrenaline via this route with similar bioavailability to IM adrenaline [17]. Clinical trials are now required to further investigate this route as a possible alternative to the currently recommended IM administration of adrenaline.

Given the cardiac, respiratory and vascular effects of adrenaline, several side effects of adrenaline administration can be noted. Common, but transient side effects of adrenaline administration include tremor, pallor, restlessness, palpitations, dizziness and headache. Major side effects are rare but include ventricular arrhythmias, acute coronary syndrome, hypertension and pulmonary oedema [6, 15, 18]. There are no absolute contraindications for the use of adrenaline, although careful monitoring and a reduced dose may be considered for patients with co-morbid cardiac conditions.

Adjunctive Therapies

Oxygen: Supplemental oxygen is recommended for patients with anaphylaxis, particularly those with a history of reactive airway disease, chronic respiratory disease or evidence of respiratory distress and/or hypoxemia. In addition to improving end-organ perfusion, provision of supplemental oxygen also facilitates bronchodilation [3, 6].

Anti-Histamines: The use of anti-histamines in the management of anaphylaxis is the most common reason for delayed or non-administration of adrenaline [14, 15]. As discussed previously, there is little evidence to support the use of histamine antagonists in the initial management of anaphylaxis, as they do not prevent or relieve airway obstruction or hypotension [6, 7, 15]. International guidelines for the management of anaphylaxis vary in their recommendations for anti-histamine use; however, it is agreed that anti-histamines may have a role in the treatment of the cutaneous manifestations such as urticaria, pruritus, flushing, angio-oedema and rhinorrhoea, which are commonly evident in anaphylaxis [6, 9]. Importantly, the use of anti-histamines should never delay the administration of adrenaline in the management of anaphylaxis [8].

Glucocorticoids: Glucocorticoids are commonly prescribed in anaphylaxis to prevent biphasic (late phase) and protracted reactions, although there is limited evidence to support their use in this setting [19]. The proposed mechanism of this effect is by altered transcription of pro-inflammatory genes and subsequent down-regulation of the late-phase inflammatory response [4, 19]. As the onset of action of glucocorticoids is between 4 and 6 hours, there is no role for their use in the initial emergency management of acute anaphylaxis [3, 19]. The choice of glucocorticoid is variable among international guidelines; however, oral prednisolone, IM hydrocortisone or IV methylprednisolone are among the more commonly used drugs [9]. In general, glucocorticoid is used for anaphylaxis as a single dose following the initial resuscitation, and in some cases, this may be followed by additional doses over the next 2–3 days [19]. Short-term administration of systemic glucocorticoids in this manner is not reported to be associated with known adverse effects, such as hypertension, skin thinning and altered bone and glucose metabolism [4, 6].

Beta-Agonists: Inhaled beta-2 adrenergic agonists, such as salbutamol, are used in the management of acute asthma and chronic obstructive pulmonary disease. Their mechanism of action is through direct relaxation of airway smooth muscle, facilitating bronchodilation [20]. Given the known benefits in relieving acute airway obstruction, inhaled or nebulised beta-2 agonists may be used as additional therapy in anaphylaxis management, particularly for refractory wheeze and shortness of breath that is not relieved by adrenaline [6]. Importantly, beta-2 agonists should not be used in place of adrenaline in the treatment of anaphylaxis, as they do not have the additional systemic beta-1 agonist effects of adrenaline and do not prevent or relieve airway angio-oedema, upper airway obstruction, hypotension or shock [3, 6].

Intravenous Fluids: Vascular permeability is increased in anaphylaxis, and this may result in large volumes of fluid moving from the patient's circulation into the interstitial tissue, resulting in intravascular depletion and subsequent hypotension [3, 6]. Aggressive fluid resuscitation is indicated in patients with cardiovascular compromise. The clinical response to fluid resuscitation should be monitored, and volume replacement should be titrated to reach the desired effect.

Vasopressors: Patients with persistent hypotension, despite appropriate doses of adrenaline and IV fluid resuscitation, may require additional inotropic support with medications such as dopamine, noradrenaline and vasopressin [3, 6]. Administration of these medications requires concomitant invasive monitoring and ideally should be provided in an intensive care environment.

Glucagon: Glucagon may be indicated in the management of patients with anaphylaxis if the patient is known to be taking a beta-adrenergic antagonist at the time of presentation. Beta-adrenergic antagonist medications impair the response to adrenaline, and glucagon is used to treat refractory hypotension and bradycardia in these patients [3, 6]. Glucagon acts via alternative pathways to provide similar inotropic and chronotropic effects as adrenaline. The recommended dosage for an adult is 1–5 mg administered intravenously over 5 minutes, and in children, a dose of 20–30 µg/kg up to a maximum of 1 mg may be used [3, 21].

Subsequent Management of IgE-Mediated Food-Induced Allergic Reactions

Observation

Biphasic anaphylaxis is known to occur in 1–20% of adults and in up to 11% of children with anaphylaxis [11, 22]. Several pathogenic mechanisms have been proposed to underlie the biphasic response, including inadequate initial therapy, bimodal synthesis of mediators from mast cells and activation of secondary inflammatory pathways during the initial event [11]. Identified risk factors for the development of a biphasic response include oral allergen exposure, delayed onset of initial symptoms after allergen exposure and delayed or inadequate administration of adrenaline during the initial episode [11]. In children, additional risk factors for developing a biphasic reaction include the requirement of >1 dose of adrenaline and fluid resuscitation during the primary anaphylaxis episode [22]. In the majority of patients, recurrence of symptoms occurs within 8 hours of the initial episode, and the symptoms may be less severe, similar to, or more severe than the initial event [11]. There is no consensus in the literature regarding the optimal period of observation of a patient following treatment for anaphylaxis. In the authors' experience, patients who respond well to an initial dose of adrenaline are observed

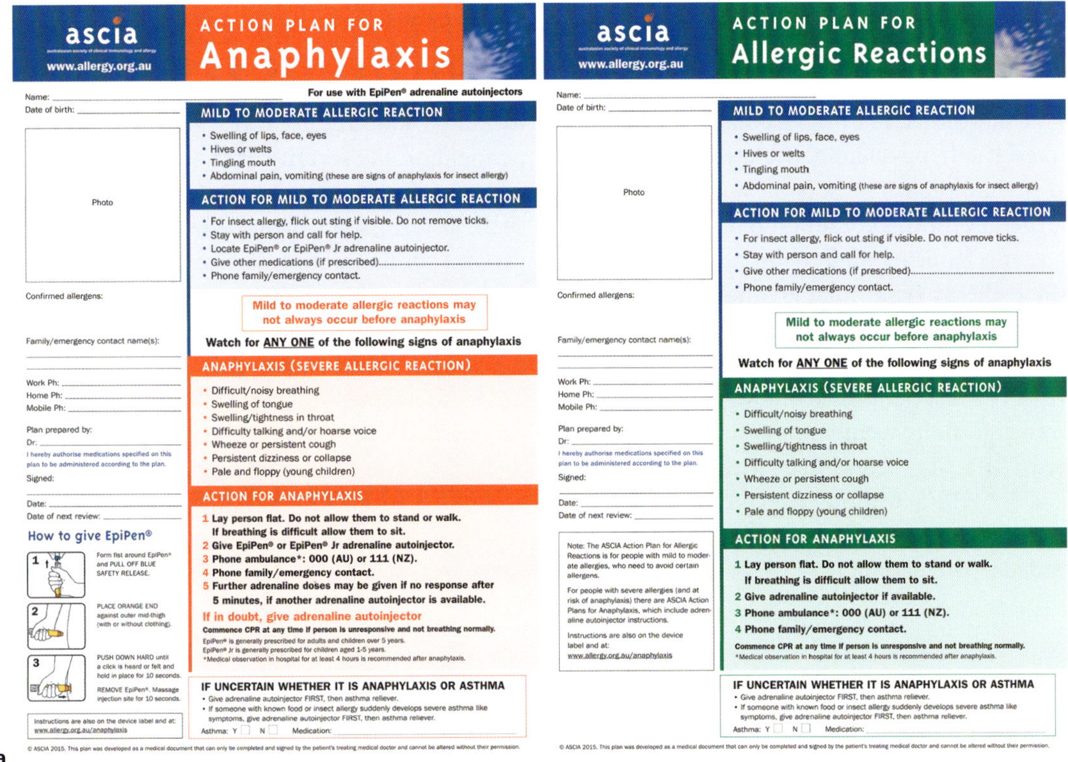

Fig. 1. Australasian Society of Clinical Immunology and Allergy (ASCIA) allergy action plans. **a** Anaphylaxis action plan, **b** allergy action plan. Reproduced with permission from the ASCIA website http://www.allergy.org.au.

for 4 hours before discharge. Patients who require multiple doses of adrenaline or have significant cardiovascular and/or respiratory compromise are typically admitted for overnight observation and discharged the following morning.

Risk Minimisation
Several studies have identified the value of emergency action plans in reducing the frequency and severity of subsequent reactions [8, 23, 24]. There is a lack of agreement on the required content of action plans and no universally accepted action plan, but proposed key areas to address include personal identification information, specific identification of the allergens to be avoided and well-defined, step-wise instructions for the management of symptoms, ranging from mild symp-

toms to anaphylaxis [8]. Two examples of the currently used allergy action plans provided by the peak professional body of clinical allergy and immunology in Australia and New Zealand are provided in figure 1.

Pharmacological Management of Non-IgE-Mediated Food-Induced Allergic Reactions

Infants and children with food protein-induced enterocolitis syndrome (FPIES), a non-IgE-mediated food allergy, may sometimes (in up to 15% of cases) present with intractable vomiting, hypotension and shock that develop 2–4 hours after ingestion of an allergen [1, 25]. This acute presentation can mimic anaphylaxis; however, management requires fluid resuscitation rather than adrenaline administration. The cardiovascular compromise in FPIES is considered to occur as a result of hypovolemic shock (rapid fluid loss), and so fluid replacement is the appropriate first-line therapy for this condition [25, 26]. As the immune mechanisms underlying non-IgE-mediated food allergy syndromes are thought to involve cell-mediated pathways, corticosteroids have also been recommended for the management of severe FPIES reactions involving hypotension [25]. Adrenaline alone would not be sufficient to treat a food reaction associated with hypovolemic shock in FPIES without concomitant fluid replacement therapy and so is generally not recommended in this setting [25].

Conclusions

The pharmacological management of acute IgE-mediated food-induced allergic reactions is dependent on the severity of the clinical symptoms and signs. For mild to moderate allergic reactions, such as urticaria, angio-oedema and pruritus, prompt administration of an anti-histamine is the current recommended treatment. In patients exhibiting symptoms and signs of anaphylaxis, namely respiratory or cardiovascular compromise, adrenaline is the only first-line therapy recommended by consensus guidelines. Adjunctive therapies, such as anti-histamines, beta-agonists and glucocorticoids, may be administered concurrently but should never replace or delay the administration of adrenaline.

References

1 Burks AW, Tang M, Sicherer S, Muraro A, Eigenmann PA, Ebisawa M, Fiocchi A, Chiang W, Beyer K, Wood R, Hourihane J, Jones SM, Lack G, Sampson HA: ICON: food allergy. J Allergy Clin Immunol 2012;129:906–920.

2 Eigenmann PA: Mechanisms of food allergy. Pediatr Allergy Immunol 2009; 20:5–11.

3 Boyce JA, Assa'ad A, Burks AW, Jones SM, Sampson HA, Wood RA, Plaut M, Cooper SF, Fenton MJ, Arshad SH, Bahna SL, Beck LA, Byrd-Bredbenner C, Camargo CA Jr, Eichenfield L, Furuta GT, Hanifin JM, Jones C, Kraft M, Levy BD, Lieberman P, Luccioli S, McCall KM, Schneider LC, Simon RA, Simons FE, Teach SJ, Yawn BP, Schwaninger JM: Guidelines for the diagnosis and management of food allergy in the United States: report of the NIAID-sponsored expert panel. J Allergy Clin Immunol 2010;126:S1–S58.

4 Keet C: Recognition and management of food-induced anaphylaxis. Pediatr Clin North Am 2011;58:377–388.

5 Simons FE: Advances in H1-antihistamines. N Engl J Med 2004;351:2203–2217.

6 Simons FE, Ardusso LR, Bilo MB, El-Gamal YM, Ledford DK, Ring J, Sanchez-Borges M, Senna GE, Sheikh A, Thong BY, World Allergy O: World Allergy Organization anaphylaxis guidelines: summary. J Allergy Clin Immunol 2011;127:587–593.e1–e22.

7 Sheikh A, ten Broek V, Brown SG, Simons FE: H1-antihistamines for the treatment of anaphylaxis with and without shock. Cochrane Database Syst Rev 2007;1:CD006160.

8 Muraro A, Roberts G, Clark A, Eigenmann PA, Halken S, Lack G, Moneret-Vautrin A, Niggemann B, Rance F, EAACI Task Force on Anaphylaxis in Children: The management of anaphylaxis in childhood: position paper of the European academy of allergology and clinical immunology. Allergy 2007;62:857–871.

9 Alrasbi M, Sheikh A: Comparison of international guidelines for the emergency medical management of anaphylaxis. Allergy 2007;62:838–841.

10 Lin RY, Curry A, Pesola GR, Knight RJ, Lee HS, Bakalchuk L, Tenenbaum C, Westfal RE: Improved outcomes in patients with acute allergic syndromes who are treated with combined H1 and H2 antagonists. Ann Emerg Med 2000; 36:462–468.

11 Tole JW, Lieberman P: Biphasic anaphylaxis: review of incidence, clinical predictors, and observation recommendations. Immunol Allergy Clin North Am 2007;27:309–326, viii.

12 Sampson HA, Munoz-Furlong A, Campbell RL, Adkinson NF Jr, Bock SA, Branum A, Brown SG, Camargo CA Jr, Cydulka R, Galli SJ, Gidudu J, Gruchalla RS, Harlor AD Jr, Hepner DL, Lewis LM, Lieberman PL, Metcalfe DD, O'Connor R, Muraro A, Rudman A, Schmitt C, Scherrer D, Simons FE, Thomas S, Wood JP, Decker WW: Second symposium on the definition and management of anaphylaxis: summary report – Second National Institute of Allergy and Infectious Disease/Food Allergy and Anaphylaxis Network symposium. J Allergy Clin Immunol 2006;117:391–397.

13 Pumphrey RS: Fatal posture in anaphylactic shock. J Allergy Clin Immunol 2003;112:451–452.

14 Chipps BE: Update in pediatric anaphylaxis: a systematic review. Clin Pediatr (Phila) 2013;52:451–461.

15 Sheikh A, Shehata YA, Brown SG, Simons FE: Adrenaline (epinephrine) for the treatment of anaphylaxis with and without shock. Cochrane Database Syst Rev 2008;4:CD006312.

16 Simons FE, Gu X, Johnston LM, Simons KJ: Can epinephrine inhalations be substituted for epinephrine injection in children at risk for systemic anaphylaxis? Pediatrics 2000;106:1040–1044.

17 Rachid O, Rawas-Qalaji MM, Simons FE, Simons KJ: Epinephrine (adrenaline) absorption from new-generation, taste-masked sublingual tablets: a preclinical study. J Allergy Clin Immunol 2013;131:236–238.

18 Simons FE: First-aid treatment of anaphylaxis to food: focus on epinephrine. J Allergy Clin Immunol 2004;113:837–844.

19 Choo KJ, Simons FE, Sheikh A: Glucocorticoids for the treatment of anaphylaxis. Cochrane Database Syst Rev 2012; 4:CD007596.

20 Cazzola M, Page CP, Calzetta L, Matera MG: Pharmacology and therapeutics of bronchodilators. Pharmacol Rev 2012; 64:450–504.

21 Ellender TJ, Skinner JC: The use of vasopressors and inotropes in the emergency medical treatment of shock. Emerg Med Clin North Am 2008;26:759–786, ix.

22 Mehr S, Liew WK, Tey D, Tang ML: Clinical predictors for biphasic reactions in children presenting with anaphylaxis. Clin Exp Allergy 2009;39:1390–1396.

23 Nurmatov U, Worth A, Sheikh A: Anaphylaxis management plans for the acute and long-term management of anaphylaxis: a systematic review. J Allergy Clin Immunol 2008;122:353–361. e1–e3.

24 Ewan PW, Clark AT: Efficacy of a management plan based on severity assessment in longitudinal and case-controlled studies of 747 children with nut allergy: proposal for good practice. Clin Exp Allergy 2005;35:751–756.

25 Sicherer SH: Food protein-induced enterocolitis syndrome: case presentations and management lessons. J Allergy Clin Immunol 2005;115:149–156.

26 Sampson HA. Update on food allergy. J Allergy Clin Immunol 2004;113:805–819.

Prof. Mimi Tang
Department of Allergy and Immunology
The Royal Children's Hospital Melbourne
50 Flemington Road
Parkville, VIC 3052 (Australia)
E-Mail mimi.tang@rch.org.au

Ebisawa M, Ballmer-Weber BK, Vieths S, Wood RA (eds): Food Allergy: Molecular Basis and Clinical Practice.
Chem Immunol Allergy. Basel, Karger, 2015, vol 101, pp 106–113 (DOI: 10.1159/000371697)

Oral Immunotherapy and Potential Treatment

Sakura Sato · Noriyuki Yanagida · Motohiro Ebisawa

Department of Allergy, Clinical Research Center for Allergology and Rheumatology, Sagamihara National Hospital, Sagamihara, Kanagawa, Japan

Abstract

The standardized therapeutic approach for food allergy is based on avoidance of allergens in foods. Oral immunotherapy (OIT) is a significant focus of food allergy research and appears to be effective in inducing desensitization. However, most patients receiving OIT have mild to moderate symptoms during the therapy, and it has not been clearly established whether OIT is effective in inducing permanent tolerance. Recently, novel therapeutic approaches for food allergy, or sublingual immunotherapy and epicutaneous immunotherapy using an anti-IgE monoclonal antibody (omalizumab), have been examined in some studies. These studies showed that the frequency of adverse reactions is lower than with OIT and that patients can increase their food tolerance. Other novel approaches, including the use of omalizumab in combination with OIT, may be useful in food allergy treatment. There is some evidence that a combination of OIT with omalizumab increases threshold doses of food without causing symptoms. OIT offers a new approach for treating food allergy, although further study is needed to demonstrate long-term safety and benefits in larger numbers of patients. © 2015 S. Karger AG, Basel

Introduction

The standard therapeutic approach for food allergy is the identification of causative foods and allergen avoidance [1] along with nutritional counseling. Unfortunately, accidental exposures to causative foods are quite common [2], and rapid medical treatment for accidental exposure is necessary. Recently, oral immunotherapy (OIT) has been investigated as a novel therapeutic approach for food allergy [3–10], and it continues to be an active area of investigation in food allergy research. In this chapter, we will discuss progress in developing OIT and novel treatments to modulate the food allergy response.

Oral Immunotherapy for Food Allergy

Efficacy and Safety of Oral Immunotherapy
Recently, OIT has become the most actively and extensively utilized therapeutic approach for food allergy. The OIT method generally includes an initial rapid dose-escalation phase, followed by a slower

Table 1. Summary of OIT trials for food allergy

Allergen	Study (publication year)	Cases (n)	Adverse reactions (% of total OIT dose)	Symptoms during therapy	Use of adrenaline (n)	Efficacy (desensitization rate, %)
Peanut	Jones et al. [5] (2009)	OIT: 29	Initial day: 92% (of the subjects) At home: 3.7%	Mainly upper respiratory and mild to moderate skin symptoms	4	OIT: threshold dose ↑
	Blumchen et al. [7] (2010)	OIT: 23	Rush phase: 7.9% At home: 2.6%	Mild skin and gastrointestinal (GI) symptoms were most common	0	OIT: 52%
Milk	Longo et al. [9] (2008)	OIT: 30 Control: 30	Rush phase: 100% (of the subjects) At home: 57% (of the subjects)	Mainly skin, mucosal membrane and GI symptoms	4	OIT: 36% Control: 0%
	Skripak et al. [3] (2008)	OIT: 13 Control: 7	45.4%	Mostly local symptoms, then GI and respiratory symptoms	4	Control: no change
	Pajno et al. [12] (2010)	OIT: 15 Control: 15	80% (of the subjects)	Mostly mild skin symptoms, then GI and respiratory symptoms	2	OIT: 67% Control: 0%
Egg	Burks et al. [11] (2012)	OIT: 40 Placebo: 15	Initial day: 27.4% At home: 24.2%	Mild to moderate symptoms only	0	OIT: 75% OIT: 28%[#] Placebo: 0%

[#] Tolerance rate.

build-up phase to reach the maintenance dose. Finally, treatment effectiveness is evaluated by an oral food challenge (OFC) following allergen avoidance for a certain period of time. Many studies have shown that OIT is effective, although allergic reactions, mainly mild to moderate, occur in the majority of patients receiving OIT [3, 4, 7, 9–11] (table 1).

There is a larger number of studies focusing on peanut OIT than on egg or milk OIT. In 2009, Jones et al. [5] reported a study of peanut OIT in 29 subjects with peanut allergy. The study was divided into 3 phases (initial escalation day, build-up phase, and maintenance phase). In a post-maintenance OFC, 27 of the 29 subjects (93%) were able to ingest 3.9 g of peanut protein, whereas the remaining 2 subjects stopped at doses lower than or equal to 2.1 g of peanut protein. Most subjects showed symptoms during the initial escalation day, and 3.7% of patients who received the total OIT dose showed symptoms at home. Most symptoms resolved spontaneously or with antihistamines; however, 2 subjects received an adrenaline injection at home.

Another study of peanut OIT was reported by Blumchen et al. [7]. The protocol was divided into 3 phases and was therefore similar to that of Jones et al. Of the 23 enrolled patients, 14 patients were fully desensitized, tolerating a peanut dose of 0.5–2 g, while 1 patient was partially desensitized. The remaining 8 patients dropped out of the study due to adverse reactions and compliance issues. In 2.6% of patients who received the total OIT dose, mild to moderate reactions that did not require injection of adrenaline were observed.

Several controlled studies of milk OIT found significant differences between those who underwent OIT and those who were on an elimination diet [3, 9, 12]. In 2008, Longo et al. [9] enrolled 60 severely milk-allergic subjects with milk-specific IgE levels above 85 kUA/l. The subjects were divided into 2 groups: one group underwent OIT for cow's milk, and the other group was kept on a milk-free diet (control group). After 1 year, 11 (36%) of the 30 children in the OIT group were successfully desensitized (daily intake of 150 ml or more), 16 (54%) were partially desensitized (daily intake of 5–150 ml), and 3 (10%) could not complete the protocol because of allergic side effects. None of the subjects in the control group could tolerate 5 ml of cow's milk. During the rush phase, all subjects showed some symptoms, and then around 60% of the subjects presented adverse reactions at home. Subsequently, 1 out of 4 subjects received treatment with an adrenaline injection at home. In other studies of milk OIT, therapies were proven to be effective regarding increases in the threshold for reactions to milk [3, 12]. Unfortunately, the frequency of symptoms caused by OIT was relatively high, and adrenaline injections were sometimes used to treat severe reactions.

More recently, results from a double-blind, randomized, placebo-controlled study of OIT in 55 children with egg allergy have been published [11]. After 10 months of therapy, none of the children who received a placebo and 55% of those who received OIT passed an OFC and were considered to be desensitized. At 22 months after the therapy, 75% of children in the OIT group were desensitized. Furthermore, after 2 months of complete egg avoidance, in the OIT group, 28% (11 of 40 children) passed an OFC at 24 months and were considered to have sustained unresponsiveness to the allergen. At 30 and 36 months, all children who had passed the OFC at 24 months were consuming egg without any problems [11].

Factors Affecting Safety of Oral Immunotherapy
The issue of patient safety is critical for successful OIT. The most common factors affecting adverse reactions are infection and exercise [3, 13]. In food allergy patients, infections with virus or bacteria are generally known to affect symptom severity, especially in cases of gastrointestinal infections. Complications from bronchial asthma, especially if poorly controlled, and pollen allergy [13] are important triggers of a lower-threshold reaction to OIT. Other factors may be associated with increased reactions to allergens, including nonsteroidal anti-inflammatory drugs, physical exertion after dosing, and dosing during menses [14]. Therefore, patients should be regularly monitored by an experienced allergist, even after successful tolerance induction.

Mechanisms of and Immunologic Responses to Oral Immunotherapy
OIT is a strategy that has been tested for its ability to induce desensitization, although the precise mechanisms of OIT remain unclear. The immunologic responses of antigen-specific immunoglobulins, mast cells, basophils, and T cells with OIT mirror those seen with allergen immunotherapy for inhalant allergens and seem to be similar to the natural development of tolerance to food allergens [15].

Jones et al. reported that antigen-specific IgE levels in children receiving OIT tended to increase early in the dose-escalation phase and to subsequently decrease compared with baseline values at 12 and 18 months. Then, for all subsequent time points, peanut-specific IgE levels tended to significantly decrease (fig. 1a) [5]. A significant increase in specific IgG levels started at 3 months of therapy, remained high until 24 months, and gradually returned to baseline by 33 months. In contrast, specific IgG4 levels increased initially, reaching statistical significance at 3 months, and remained elevated until the end of the study (fig. 1b, c). These changes in antigen-specific immunoglobulins were seen only in patients receiving OIT, so the effect of OIT on antigen-specific IgE levels seems to occur in an allergen-specific manner [16].

Suppression of effector cells is a predominant mechanism through which immunotherapy might function. Skin prick test reactivity shows a significant decrease beginning at several months and remains decreased throughout a 3-year follow-up [5]. Studies have identified basophils as a key cell type underlying clinical desensitization. Some early studies reported decreased allergen-induced CD63 expression in whole blood during OIT [5, 17], but not in washed suspensions

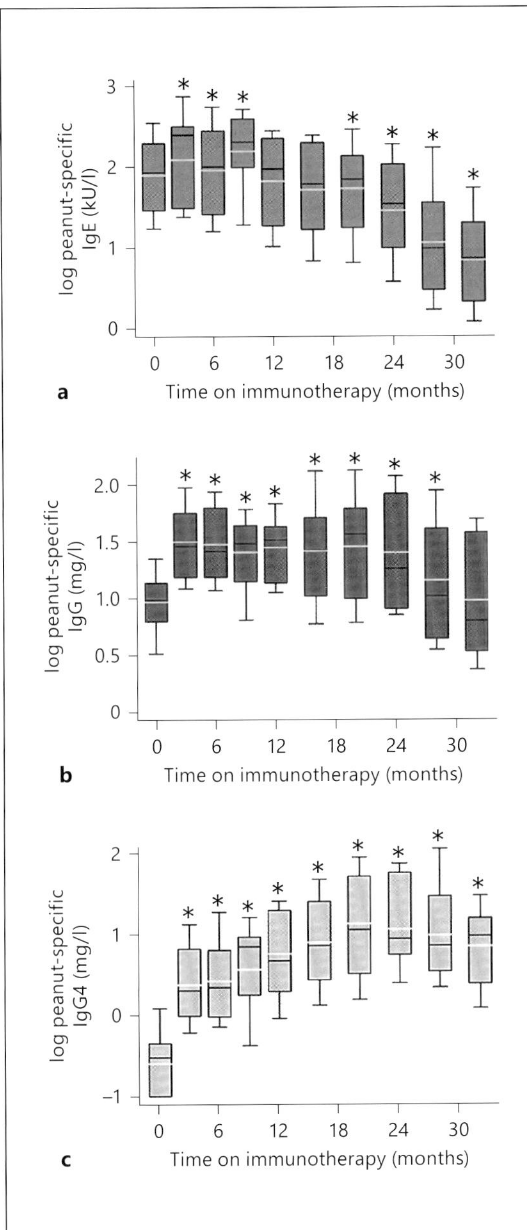

Fig. 1. Changes in peanut-specific immunoglobulin levels during peanut oral immunotherapy. Peanut-specific IgE (**a**), IgG (**b**), and IgG4 (**c**) were measured by using ImmunoCAP. The values are log transformed, and median and mean values are represented by the black and yellow horizontal lines, respectively. Mixed-model, repeated-measures analysis of variance was used to determine the statistical significance of differences between baseline and the treatment time points (* p < 0.0005) [5].

(serum free). This discrepancy may indicate that washing actually disrupted the binding of IgG or another serum inhibitory factor. This may indicate a state of reduced extrinsic basophil activation in vivo.

Jones et al. [5] and Varshney et al. [18] reported that forkhead box P3-expressing T regulatory (Treg) cells increased after OIT and returned to baseline levels by 20 months after peanut stimulation [5]. In contrast, placebo-treated subjects showed no change in Treg cells. The mechanisms of Treg cell-induced immunosuppression remain unclear, and further studies are needed.

Clinical Use of Oral Immunotherapy

The results of previous studies indicate that OIT for food allergy is effective in increasing the amount of food tolerated in 50% or more of treated patients [3, 5, 7, 9, 11, 12]. However, many other patients continue to be resistant to desensitization or achieve only partial desensitization. A goal of OIT is to develop a safe and effective protocol that can be performed in routine clinical practice, without too many allergic reactions, but an evidence base for the protocol has not yet been established.

Desensitization and Permanent Tolerance

In any discussion of OIT for food allergy, the concepts of desensitization and tolerance must be addressed. Desensitization is defined as 'a change in the threshold dose of an ingested food allergen necessary to cause allergic symptoms' and can be short term or prolonged, with ongoing therapy [19]. By contrast, tolerance should be defined as a permanent loss of reactivity correlated with the ability to ingest food without symptoms and without ongoing therapy [20]. However, whether desensitization will lead to tolerance to food is not yet clear. There are little data available on whether OIT for food allergy induces permanent tolerance or if the effects represent transient desensitization. Despite the relatively good results of OIT reported by Buchanan et al. [4] and Blumchen et al. [7], a lot of patients fail to be desensitized after stopping OIT. In a recent published study by Keet et al. [8], 6 of the 15 subjects who passed a full milk challenge after 60 weeks of maintenance lost desensitization within 6 weeks, and 2 patients required adrenaline for severe abdominal pain/vomiting and urticaria/erythema after 1 week off the therapy. Together, these results suggest that desensitization by OIT seemed to have failed after a short time. Therefore, it seems likely that the state of desensitization requires ongoing exposure to be maintained.

Optimal Dose and Duration of Oral Immunotherapy
Although previous studies of OIT for food allergy seem to be promising, critical questions, such as about the optimal dose and length of therapy, remain. How long would it take before a lack of continued allergen intake would result in loss of desensitization? Previous studies suggest that desensitization by OIT does not quickly lead to tolerance. Therefore, it is possible that a longer period of daily maintenance treatment may be required for most patients to develop tolerance, or at least a maintenance period similar to that for subcutaneous immunotherapy for inhaled allergens. Moreover, it is not yet clear whether even those who pass an OFC without receiving therapy can be considered to have permanent tolerance or, rather, transient desensitization.

Previous studies of OIT have used a variety of doses [3, 10, 12, 21] and heterogeneous protocols, making comparisons among them difficult. In 2012, Keet et al. [8] demonstrated that sublingual immunotherapy (SLIT) followed by OIT was much more effective for desensitization than SLIT alone was. They also examined two OIT maintenance doses (1,000 vs. 2,000 mg) and found no significant differences in either the overall rate of reaction or efficacy between these regimens. The results of this and other studies cited above point to the need for more studies with longer intervention periods and larger numbers of patients to resolve these issues.

Novel Treatment for Food Allergy

Current OIT protocols are associated with significant adverse reactions, a necessity of providing treatment for longer periods, and a failure of some patients to respond to the treatment. Therefore, additional approaches for food allergy treatment should be examined to assess whether the therapy can induce tolerance, the safety of the therapy, and if it is possible to identify who might most benefit or who has benefitted while receiving the therapy (table 2).

Sublingual Immunotherapy
In several previous studies, it was demonstrated that SLIT with hazelnut, milk, and peanut can increase the amount of the food tolerated during OFC, and adverse reactions were mostly mild enough to not require oral antihistamine administration [8, 22, 23]. However, an important issue with the use of SLIT is the limited maximum dose that can be used sublingually. Another study of SLIT for food allergy, by Keet et al., involved 30 randomized children with milk allergy receiving SLIT alone or SLIT followed by OIT. This protocol consisted of 3 phases: (1) initial SLIT escalation, (2) continued SLIT escalation or commencement of OIT at 2 maintenance doses, and (3) OFC after 12 and 60 weeks of maintenance. After therapy, only 1 in the SLIT group, 6 in the lower-dose OIT group, and 8 in the higher-dose OIT group passed an OFC with 8 g of milk. Systemic reactions were more common during OIT than during SLIT. These results showed SLIT followed by OIT is more effective than SLIT alone is in achieving desensitization. This combination therapy (SLIT and OIT) may benefit from the safety of SLIT and the potential for achieving higher doses of food with OIT.

Table 2. Novel treatments for food allergy

Treatment	Allergen	Efficacy	Study (publication year)
SLIT	Hazelnut	45% of the subjects reached 20 g after 8–12 weeks of therapy	Enrique et al. [22] (2005)
	Peanut	70% of 20 subjects were able to increase the threshold doses after 44 weeks of therapy	Fleischer et al. [23] (2013)
SLIT + OIT	Milk	70% of 20 subjects were able to pass the 8 g oral challenge after 80 weeks of therapy	Keet et al. [8] (2012)
Omalizumab	Peanut	89% of 9 subjects could tolerate higher doses than at the baseline oral challenge	Sampson et al. [24] (2011)
OIT + Omalizumab	Milk	9 of 11 subjects reached 2,000 mg and passed the oral challenge in week 24 of the study	Nadeau et al. [25] (2012)
Epicutaneous immunotherapy	Milk	90% of 10 subjects tended to have increased threshold doses during the follow-up oral challenge (day 90)	Dupont et al. [26] (2010)

Anti-IgE Monoclonal Antibodies (Omalizumab) for Food Allergy

The anti-IgE monoclonal antibody omalizumab is a recombinant humanized IgE-blocking monoclonal antibody. It works by decreasing or preventing the allergic response triggered by IgE molecules.

In 2011, a phase II, multicenter, randomized, double-blind, placebo-controlled, parallel-group trial using omalizumab for peanut allergy was reported by Sampson et al. [24]. This trial was designed to determine whether omalizumab could be effective in reducing allergic reactions to small amounts of peanut. Although the data were limited, the treatment using omalizumab resulted in an improved threshold of reactivity to peanut ingestion.

Nadeau et al. conducted a phase I pilot study by combining omalizumab treatment with milk OIT [25]. The study was divided into 3 phases, or 9 weeks of omalizumab pretreatment, 7–11 weeks of oral desensitization with omalizumab treatment, and 9 weeks of maintenance OIT without omalizumab, followed by a double-blind, placebo-controlled food challenge (DBPCFC) at week 24. One subject discontinued the study because of gastrointestinal symptoms during the desensitization phase; the other 9 of the 10 subjects achieved the target dose and passed the DBPCFC. Concerning the issue of safety, the frequency of adverse reactions was 1.6%, and most symptoms were defined as mild. Only 1 subject showed rhinitis and generalized urticaria and responded to adrenaline at the time of the DBPCFC. These results demonstrated that such a combination approach is safe and might allow for faster desensitization in children with food allergy and without too many adverse reactions.

Epicutaneous Immunotherapy

Epicutaneous immunotherapy may be a novel approach for food allergy. Dupont et al. examined this approach in 18 children with milk allergy [26]. Subjects in the active treatment group showed higher tolerated doses of milk during an OFC during follow-up visits when compared with subjects in the placebo group. Adverse reactions consisted mostly of local skin reactions at the site of application and repeated episodes of diarrhea in one child but did not include any severe systemic reactions. While this pilot study suggests that epicutaneous immunotherapy is safe and well tolerated, additional studies are required to assess the clinical efficacy and the maximum doses that can be applied epicutaneously and tolerated orally.

Conclusion

OIT appears to be effective in inducing desensitization without major morbidity or mortality and may reduce the risk of severe reaction upon accidental ingestion. However, the data on the side effects of long-term therapy are limited, and further studies are needed to demonstrate OIT's long-term safety and benefits in larger numbers of patients. Combination OIT therapy, particularly in conjunction with omalizumab, allows patients to increase their food tolerance without symptoms. As a novel approach for food allergy treatment, the efficacy has not yet been fully assessed, with data from only a few studies using small sample sizes.

OIT could offer a reasonable new therapy for food allergy, even without tolerance. The final protocol will need to have standardized entry criteria, treatment dosages, and maintenance dosages during an optimal follow-up period, and a stronger safety protocol will have to be developed before utilization in the community. For patients with severe reactions, the inclusion of anti-IgE monoclonal antibodies may be useful.

Acknowledgments

We are supported by the Health and Labor Sciences Research Grants (Research on Allergic Disease and Immunology) from the Ministry of Health, Labor and Welfare (Japan).

References

1 Sampson HA: Food allergy. Part 2: diagnosis and management. J Allergy Clin Immunol 1999;103:981–989.

2 Sicherer SH, Furlong TJ, Munoz-Furlong A, et al: A voluntary registry for peanut and tree nut allergy: characteristics of the first 5,149 registrants. J Allergy Clin Immunol 2001;108:128–132.

3 Skripak JM, Nash SD, Rowley H, et al: A randomized, double-blind, placebo-controlled study of milk oral immunotherapy for cow's milk allergy. J Allergy Clin Immunol 2008;122:1154–1160.

4 Buchanan AD, Green TD, Jones SM, et al: Egg oral immunotherapy in nonanaphylactic children with egg allergy. J Allergy Clin Immunol 2007;119:199–205.

5 Jones SM, Pons L, Roberts JL, et al: Clinical efficacy and immune regulation with peanut oral immunotherapy. J Allergy Clin Immunol 2009;124:292–300. e1–e97.

6 Meglio P, Bartone E, Plantamura M, et al: A protocol for oral desensitization in children with IgE-mediated cow's milk allergy. Allergy 2004;59:980–987.

7 Blumchen K, Ulbricht H, Staden U, et al: Oral peanut immunotherapy in children with peanut anaphylaxis. J Allergy Clin Immunol 2010;126:83–91.e1.

8 Keet CA, Frischmeyer-Guerrerio PA, Thyagarajan A, et al: The safety and efficacy of sublingual and oral immunotherapy for milk allergy. J Allergy Clin Immunol 2012;129:448–455.e1–e5.

9 Longo G, Barbi E, Berti I, et al: Specific oral tolerance induction in children with very severe cow's milk-induced reactions. J Allergy Clin Immunol 2008;121:343–347.

10 Staden U, Blumchen K, Blankenstein N, et al: Rush oral immunotherapy in children with persistent cow's milk allergy. J Allergy Clin Immunol 2008;122:418–419.

11 Burks AW, Jones SM, Wood RA, et al: Oral immunotherapy for treatment of egg allergy in children. New Engl J Med 2012;367:233–243.

12 Pajno GB, Caminiti L, Ruggeri P, et al: Oral immunotherapy for cow's milk allergy with a weekly up-dosing regimen: a randomized single-blind controlled study. Ann Allergy Asthma Immunol 2010;105:376–381.

13 Staden U, Rolinck-Werninghaus C, Brewe F, et al: Specific oral tolerance induction in food allergy in children: efficacy and clinical patterns of reaction. Allergy 2007;62:1261–1269.

14 Varshney P, Steele PH, Vickery BP, et al: Adverse reactions during peanut oral immunotherapy home dosing. J Allergy Clin Immunol 2009;124:1351–1352.

15 Akdis M, Akdis CA: Mechanisms of allergen-specific immunotherapy. J Allergy Clin Immunol 2007;119:780–791.

16 Vickery BP, Pons L, Kulis M, et al: Individualized IgE-based dosing of egg oral immunotherapy and the development of tolerance. Ann Allergy Asthma Immunol 2010;105:444–450.

17 Wanich N, Nowak-Wegrzyn A, Sampson HA, et al: Allergen-specific basophil suppression associated with clinical tolerance in patients with milk allergy. J Allergy Clin Immunol 2009;123:789–794.e20.

18 Varshney P, Jones SM, Scurlock AM, et al: A randomized controlled study of peanut oral immunotherapy: clinical desensitization and modulation of the allergic response. J Allergy Clin Immunol 2011;127:654–660.

19 Rolinck-Werninghaus C, Staden U, Mehl A, et al: Specific oral tolerance induction with food in children: transient or persistent effect on food allergy? Allergy 2005;60:1320–1322.

20 Scurlock AM, Vickery BP, Hourihane JO, et al: Pediatric food allergy and mucosal tolerance. Mucosal Immunol 2010;3:345–354.

21 Patriarca G, Nucera E, Pollastrini E, et al: Oral specific desensitization in food-allergic children. Dig Dis Sci 2007;52:1662–1672.

22 Enrique E, Pineda F, Malek T, et al: Sublingual immunotherapy for hazelnut food allergy: a randomized, double-blind, placebo-controlled study with a standardized hazelnut extract. J Allergy Clin Immunol 2005;116:1073–1079.

23 Fleischer DM, Burks AW, Vickery BP, et al: Sublingual immunotherapy for peanut allergy: a randomized, double-blind, placebo-controlled multicenter trial. J Allergy Clin Immunol 2013;131:119–127.e1–e7.

24 Sampson HA, Leung DY, Burks AW, et al: A phase II, randomized, doubleblind, parallelgroup, placebocontrolled oral food challenge trial of Xolair (omalizumab) in peanut allergy. J Allergy Clin Immunol 2011;127:1309–1310.e1.

25 Nadeau KC, Kohli A, Iyengar S, et al: Oral immunotherapy and anti-IgE antibody-adjunctive treatment for food allergy. Immunol Allergy Clin North Am 2012;32:111–133.

26 Dupont C, Kalach N, Soulaines P, et al: Cow's milk epicutaneous immunotherapy in children: a pilot trial of safety, acceptability, and impact on allergic reactivity. J Allergy Clin Immunol 2010;125:1165–1167.

Sakura Sato, MD
Department of Allergy, Clinical Research Center for Allergology and Rheumatology
Sagamihara National Hospital, 18–1, Sakuradai, Minami-ku
Sagamihara, Kanagawa 252–0392 (Japan)
E-Mail s-satou@sagamihara-hosp.gr.jp

Ebisawa M, Ballmer-Weber BK, Vieths S, Wood RA (eds): Food Allergy: Molecular Basis and Clinical Practice.
Chem Immunol Allergy. Basel, Karger, 2015, vol 101, pp 114–123 (DOI: 10.1159/000375415)

Cow's Milk Allergy in Children and Adults

Alessandro Fiocchi[a] · Lamia Dahdah[a] · Marco Albarini[b] ·
Alberto Martelli[c]

[a]Division of Allergy, Department of Pediatrics, Pediatric Hospital Bambino Gesù, Rome; [b]Melloni Paediatria,
Melloni University Hospital, Milan; [c]The Garbagnate, Bollate Santa Corona Hospital, Milan, Italy

Abstract

Cow's milk allergy is among the more frequent food allergies in infants and children. Because its suspicion stems from a plethora of symptoms, it is frequently reported. However, the development of a rigorous diagnostic pathway will reduce the diagnosed children to less than 50% of those reported. Cow's milk allergy is the only specific food allergy for which an EBM guideline exists. According to the guidelines (Diagnosis and Rationale for Action against Cow's Milk Allergy), a diagnostic process based on the pre-test probability of this condition is available. Treatments include avoidance, the substitution of cow's milk with an appropriate formula, and in some cases, oral immunotherapy. Treatment choice is also guided by these guidelines. © 2015 S. Karger AG, Basel

Introduction

According to the general definition of food allergy, cow's milk allergy (CMA) is an adverse health effect arising from a specific immune response that occurs reproducibly on exposure to a given food' [1]. This definition includes both IgE-mediated and non-IgE-mediated immune responses as well as a combination of both, and it is in agreement with international guidelines [2–4] and statements [5]. Thus, CMA is not a single clinical condition but includes a spectrum of IgE, non-IgE and mixed conditions affecting different organs and systems (table 1).

Epidemiology

The estimated prevalence of confirmed CMA varies from 0.25 to 4.9% and is higher in children than in adults. Adult CMA is not an unknown phenomenon, and cow's milk is the second most reported food offender in adults on food allergy surveys [6].

CMA can develop in exclusively or partially breast-fed infants when cow's milk protein is introduced into the feeding regime. The incidence of CMA is lower in exclusively breast-fed infants compared to formula-fed or mixed-fed infants, and clinical reactions in the breast-fed group are mostly mild to moderate. These findings might be related to the lower levels of CMP in breast milk compared to cow's milk. Immunomodulators in breast milk and differences in gut flora between breast-fed and formula-fed infants may also play roles.

Table 1. The spectrum of conditions associated with IgE-mediated reactions to cow's milk [1]

I	Systemic IgE-mediated reactions (anaphylaxis) A Immediate-onset reactions B Late-onset reactions
II	IgE-mediated gastrointestinal reactions A Oral allergy syndrome B Immediate gastrointestinal allergy
III	IgE-mediated respiratory reactions A Asthma and rhinitis secondary to ingestion of milk B Asthma and rhinitis secondary to inhalation of milk (e.g. occupational asthma)

IV	IgE-mediated cutaneous reactions
	A Immediate-onset reactions
	    1. Acute urticaria or angioedema
	    2. Contact urticaria
	B Late-onset reactions
	    Atopic dermatitis

Pathogenesis

Milk can give rise to several food hypersensitivities, which are usually classified as milk allergy or milk intolerance [7]. The immunological basis of CMA distinguishes it from other adverse reactions to cow's milk protein, such as lactose intolerance, which is attributable to a beta-galactosidase (lactase) deficiency [8]. This chapter does not address lactase deficiency or other cow's milk-induced hypersensitivities that are not mediated by immune mechanisms. Other classes of immunoglobulins, immune complexes, or cell-mediated reactions are involved in allergies that are not mediated by IgE. IgE and non-IgE-mediated mechanisms may play roles in the pathogeneses of atopic dermatitis (AD) and eosinophilic gastrointestinal disorders (EGIDs). In IgE-mediated allergy, circulating antibodies recognize specific molecular regions on the antigen surface *(epitopes)*, which are classified according to their specific amino acid sequences *(linear epitopes)* or the folding and conformation of their protein chains *(conformational epitopes)*.

Allergens

Cow's milk contains several proteins, some of which are considered to be major allergens (i.e. IgE prevalence ≥50%), while some are minor allergens, and other milk proteins have hardly or never been associated with clinical reactions. The proteins in the casein and whey fractions of cow's milk are listed in table 2. Each of these two fractions contains five major components [9–11]. The casein fraction contains 80% of the total proteins in cow's milk, while alpha$_{s1}$ and beta-casein comprise 70% of this fraction. Whey proteins are less abundant, and beta-lactoglobulin accounts for 50% of this fraction. Because beta-lactoglobulin is not present in human milk, this protein has been previously considered to be the most important cow's milk allergen, but it has since been shown that other proteins, such as casein, are also dominantly involved in the etiology of the disease.

By convention in the international nomenclature, allergens are designated by an abbreviation formed by the genus (capitalized, with the first three letters abbreviated) and species (reduced to one letter) names of the Linnaean taxonomical system in italics, followed by an Arabic numeral reflecting the chronological order in which the allergen was identified and characterized (e.g. *Bos d* [omesticus] 4) [11] (see: http://www.allergen.org/). In CMA, the determination of an IgE-mediated response to sequenced and characterized allergens may be more useful in predicting the presence and severity of clinical allergy than the currently used skin test or serological tests performed with whole allergen extracts [12].

Clinical Manifestations

The clinical manifestations of CMA depend to a great extent on the type of immunological reaction involved.

Table 2. The proteins in cow's milk

Fraction/protein	Allergen [1]	g/l	% Total protein	MW (kDa)	AA	PI
		~30	80			
Caseins						
Alpha$_{s1}$-casein		12–15	29	23.6	199	4.9–5.0
Alpha$_{s2}$-casein		3–4	8	25.2	207	5.2–5.4
Beta-casein		9–11	27	24.0	209	5.1–5.4
Gamma$_1$-casein	*Bos d 8*			20.6	180	5.5
Gamma$_2$-casein		1–2	6	11.8	104	6.4
Gamma$_3$-casein				11.6	102	5.8
Kappa-casein		3–4	10	19.0	169	5.4–5.6
		~5.0	20			
Whey proteins						
Alpha-lactalbumin	*Bos d 4*	1–1.5	5	14.2	123	4.8
Beta-lactoglobulin	*Bos d 5*	3–4	10	18.3	162	5.3
Immunoglobulin	*Bos d 7*	0.6–1.0	3	160.0	–	–
BSA	*Bos d 6*	0.1–0.4	1	67.0	583	4.9–5.1
Lactoferrin	–	0.09	traces	800.0	703	8.7

AA = Amino acids; BSA = bovine serum albumin.

Immediate Reactions

These reactions occur at <2 hours after ingestion. The most frequent manifestations are IgE-mediated cutaneous (urticaria, angioedema, or an acute flare-up of atopic eczema) and gastrointestinal (GI) (vomiting, diarrhea, or colic) reactions. Cow's milk protein-induced enterocolitis syndrome is an immediate-onset, non-IgE-mediated condition. It is characterized by initial symptoms presenting during the first months of life as repeated vomiting episodes, sometimes leading to dehydration. Symptoms might be very severe and mimic sepsis. A characteristic feature of this syndrome is a symptom-free interval of up to several hours between the ingestion of milk, most often a cow's milk protein-based formula, and the first symptoms [13]. Milk-induced proctocolitis is mostly observed in young infants that are exclusively breast-fed [14]. Respiratory manifestations (asthma or allergic rhinitis) are infrequent, especially as isolated symptoms. There is a belief among some members of the lay public that the consumption of milk and dairy products increases the production of mucus in the respiratory tract; however, this view has not been confirmed by scientific evidence [15]. Anaphylaxis is the most severe manifestation of immediate-type CMA.

Delayed Reactions

These immunological, non-IgE-mediated reactions occur at several hours or days after milk consumption. AD is observed in approximately 10–15% of young children. It is primarily associated with dry skin and is linked to hereditary factors; however, approximately one third of patients with moderate to severe AD present with flares of eczema linked to a food allergy [16]. Cow's milk, hen's egg, and peanuts are the most frequently involved foods. GI disorders include food protein-induced enteropathy and proctocolitis [17]. CMA-enteropathy usually presents with diarrhea, mild to moderate steatorrhea (80% of cases) and poor weight gain. Rectal bleeding is the usual presenting feature of CMA-colitis, and the infant is otherwise well and thriving. The EGIDs include eosinophilic esophagitis, gastritis, gastroenteritis and colitis. While in children, the symptoms of eosinophilic esophagitis are similar to gastroesophageal reflux, in adults, dysphagia and food impaction are common. Symptoms of EGIDs are usually chronically relapsing, and the clinical presentation includes failure to thrive (due to chronic diarrhea, refusal of food and/or vomiting), iron deficiency anemia (due to occult or macroscopic blood loss), and hypoalbuminemia or recurrent abdominal pain. A rare milk reaction is milk-induced chronic pulmonary disease (Heiner's syndrome).

Diagnosis

Clinical Evaluation

A comprehensive history (including a family history of atopy) and careful physical examination form the basis of the diagnosis and management of CMA. Unfortunately, there is no one symptom that is pathognomonic for CMA. The timing and pattern of symptoms aid in its diagnosis. Symptoms of CMA occur often, but not always, within the first weeks after the introduction of cow's milk proteins. Many children with CMA develop symptoms in at least two of the following organ systems: GI (50–60%), skin (50%) and respiratory tract. A temporal relationship between milk ingestion and the onset of symptoms should also be assessed to distinguish immediate from non-IgE-mediated reactions.

Diagnostic Tests
IgE-Mediated CMA
Skin-prick testing (SPT) with fresh milk or commercial allergen products and serological tests for determining specific IgE (sIgE) against cow's milk proteins (e.g. ImmunoCAP™) are the currently available tests. The performance characteristics of these tests have been evaluated in different settings. The use of sensitization tests is dependent on the clinical setting and on the pre-test probability of disease. For this reason, this matter has been fully subjected to systematic review and meta-analysis in the preparation of the Diagnosis and Rationale for Action against Cow's Milk Allergy (DRACMA) guidelines. Including studies published up to September 2009, DRACMA has reviewed evidence summaries and has made recommendations on CMA diagnosis. According to these recommendations,

– Oral food challenge (OFC) with cow's milk remains the best diagnostic test;
– It should be performed under a physician's supervision regardless of the food-specific IgE levels;
– Outside of the research setting, sensitization tests may not be necessary if food challenge tests are positive;
– In settings where OFC is not considered to be a requirement for making a diagnosis of IgE-mediated CMA, a positive SPT and/or ImmunoCAP (cut-off: 0.35 kUI/l) can be used as diagnostic tests in the case of a high pre-test probability;
– In such settings, a negative SPT and/or ImmunoCAP (cut-off: 0.35 kUI/l) can be used as rule-out tests in the case of a low pre-test probability; and
– In any case of high uncertainty, challenges remain necessary.

Non-IgE-Mediated CMA
There are no reliable tests for the diagnosis of non-IgE mediated CMA. Initial diagnosis is based on a suggestive history and the absence of a positive SPT or ImmunoCAP-RAST. In these patients, diagnosis primarily relies on a successful milk-avoidance diet with clinical relapses after re-exposure to cow's milk proteins. In patients with AD in whom non-IgE-mediated CMA is suspected, atopy patch testing may be a

helpful diagnostic tool [18]; however, no sufficient data exists to evaluate its clinical utility [3].

Elimination-Challenge Testing
Unless a clear immediate anaphylactic reaction follows the ingestion of milk, food challenges are necessary and remain the definitive procedure for the diagnosis of CMA. If symptoms substantially improve or disappear after 2–4 weeks on an elimination diet, an open challenge with a formula based on whole cow's milk protein should be performed. Clinicians should be aware that the severity of a past reaction might not predict the severity of a challenge reaction, particularly after a period of avoidance. Previous mild reactions may be followed by anaphylactic reactions in some infants with CMA. For this reason, open challenges should ideally be performed in a setting where resuscitation facilities are available. In the case of cow's milk-induced anaphylaxis, a challenge is contraindicated unless SPTs and/or sIgE measurements show improvement. In these cases, the challenge should always be performed in a hospital setting.

Positive Challenge: CMA Confirmed. If symptoms of CMA re-appear, the suspected diagnosis of CMA is confirmed, and the infant should be maintained on an elimination diet using a milk substitute (discussed below) for at least 6 months. The challenge is then repeated. If it is possible to follow the infant with IgE-mediated allergy with SPTs and/or sIgE determination, the normalization or improvement of these tests would help in the timing of the challenge. Supplementary feeding should be introduced carefully to avoid the accidental intake of cow's milk protein.

Negative Challenge: No CMA. Children who do not develop symptoms after ingesting cow's milk formula during a challenge and for up to 1 week after follow-up can resume their normal diet, although they should still be carefully monitored. Clinicians should advise parents to be attentive for delayed reactions, which may evolve over several days following the challenge.

Natural History

Earlier studies have reported a good overall prognosis for CMA (developing tolerance to cow's milk protein), with most children outgrowing their allergy by 3 years of age. However, its prognosis appears to vary depending on whether the CMA is IgE-mediated or non-IgE-mediated, the titer of sIgE at the time of diagnosis and the age of onset of the CMA. The most important determining factor is the nature of the study. In birth cohorts, CMA has been estimated to run its course within 1 year [19]. Referral-based, prospective studies have indicated that in most cases (80%), tolerance is achieved within 3–4 years [20]. In a cohort of pediatric patients referred to a tertiary center in Italy for a double-blind placebo-controlled food challenge to cow's milk, the median duration of CMA was 23 months, while 23% of the children acquired tolerance at 13 months following diagnosis, and 75% were diagnosed after 43 months [21]. A longer duration has been found in retrospective referral studies. A study has reported that less than half of children diagnosed with IgE-mediated CMA during the first 9 years of life will outgrow it [22]. A retrospective study involving 807 patients with IgE-meditated CMA has reported the following resolution rates: 19% by the age of 4 years, 42% by 8 years, 64% by 12 years, and 79% by 16 years [23]. The same group has reported a shorter duration of the condition in a different caseload [24]. Children of all ages with very high levels of sIgE are likely to have a persistent milk allergy. Their decline is associated with tolerance [25]. The onset of CMA in infancy has the most favorable prognosis.

Treatment of Cow's Milk Allergy

Avoidance of Cow's Milk Protein
Patients with CMA must strictly avoid cow's milk and cow's milk protein-based products. Pa-

tients and their families must be instructed to read labels and to identify milk-containing products. Particularly in young children, a well-balanced diet with the sufficient intake of calcium and other essential nutriments is warranted. The input of a pediatric dietician is the most helpful for these patients. Mothers of breast-fed infants with CMA should continue breast-feeding but avoid causal foods. Recent studies have raised the possibility of monitoring incomplete milk avoidance in less severe cases of CMA. No acute milk-induced allergic reactions have been reported in children receiving limited amounts of extensively heated milk as a result of this diet, suggesting that a change from a milk-avoidance diet to one containing limited amounts of milk could provide substantial improvement to the quality of life of milk-allergic individuals [26, 27]. Moreover, baked milk-tolerant patients consuming baked products have been recently reported to be more likely to have unheated milk tolerance than subjects that do not consume such products [28]. This finding is in conflict with the observation that CMA children exposed to small doses of milk proteins in extensively hydrolyzed formula (eHF) may display a longer duration of CMA [29]. Thus, exposing such children to milk allergens remains an unwarranted practice [30].

Alternative Formulae (Milk Substitutes)
Partially hydrolyzed formulae are contra-indicated in the treatment of CMA because of their high residual allergen contents (only 12–26% of cow's milk protein is hydrolyzed in the currently available partially hydrolyzed formulae) and the definite risk of allergic reactions to these products. Goat, sheep, buffalo, and horse milk, unmodified soya and whole rice milk are also not recommended – these milks are not nutritionally adequate and often cross-react with proteins in cow's milk.

International guidelines [31, 32] recommend eHF or amino acid-based formulae (AAFs) as first-line alternatives for children with CMA (table 3). In general, eHFs are nutritionally adequate and well tolerated by children who are allergic to cow's milk and other foods, but their main drawbacks are their bitter taste, expense (2–3 times the cost of standard formulae) and potential to cause anaphylaxis. Rice hydrolyzed formulae (rHFs) are considered to be a second-line resource due to their nonuniversal availability [6]. Where available, rHF can be considered instead of eHF. AAFs are safe and palatable but are exorbitantly expensive (6–8 times the cost of eHFs) and are not widely available. Reimbursement for AAFs by the health care system or medical insurance is also a potential problem because they are not generally considered to be therapeutic agents.

Soy formula is well tolerated in up to 85% of infants with IgE-mediated CMA but only in 50% of those with non-IgE-mediated CMA. However, soya is not recommended in infants below 6 months of age because of concerns about its possible hormonal effects on the reproductive system (shown in animal studies), presumably due to phyto-estrogens in the form of isoflavones (genistein, daidzein and their glycosides) present in soya protein. To date, no studies have evaluated the safety of soya formula in humans, and such studies are greatly needed.

Oral Immunotherapy
Avoidance of cow's milk protein is difficult because it is ubiquitous, and accidental allergic reactions in children with CMA are common [11]. Oral immunotherapy (OIT) or desensitization is a promising treatment for IgE-mediated CMA. Randomized controlled trials have reported that about 35% of children become fully tolerant to cow's milk protein after OIT. A total of 15–20% of children may not complete the procedure because of severe adverse reactions, but no fatal events have been documented. Follow-up data on children who become tolerant to cow's milk protein are inadequate, and it is unclear whether

Table 3. Choosing the appropriate substitute formula in different presentations

Clinical presentation	1st choice	2nd choice	3rd choice
Anaphylaxis	AAF[+]	eHF[#, §]	SF
Immediate gastrointestinal allergy	eHF[§, b]	AAF[^]/SF[°]	
Food protein-induced enterocolitis syndrome	AAF	eHF[*]	
Asthma and rhinitis	eHF[§, b]	AAF[^]/SF[°]	
Acute urticaria or angioedema	eHF[§, b]	AAF[^]/SF[°]	
Atopic dermatitis	eHF[§, b]	AAF[^]/SF[°]	
Gastroesophageal reflux disease	eHF[b]	AAF	
Allergic eosinophilic esophagitis	AAF		
Cow's milk protein-induced enteropathy	eHF[§, b]	AAF	
Constipation	eHF[b]	AAF	Donkey milk[★]
Severe irritability (colic)	eHF[b]	AAF	
CM protein-induced gastroenteritis and proctocolitis	eHF[b]	AAF	
Milk-induced chronic pulmonary disease (Heiner's syndrome)[**]	AAF[^]	SF	eHF

[+] Recommendation 7.1.
[b] Recommendation 7.2.
[*] If AAF is refused.
[§] Subject to local availability; rHF can be considered instead of eHF (7.4).
[#] A negative SPT must be obtained with the specific formula (panel recommendation).
[^] AAF if a relatively high value on avoiding sensitization to soy formula (SF) and/or a low value on resource expenditure are placed.
[°] SF if a relatively low value on avoiding sensitization to SF and/or a high value on resource expenditure are placed. Given that more than 50% of such children are allergic to soy, a careful clinical evaluation is necessary (panel recommendation).
[**] This suggestion attributes a high value to avoiding exposure to even residual antigenic cow's milk proteins.
[★] Based on reports from 1 case series. Subject to local availability.

their tolerance is transient or permanent [12]. Patients undergoing OIT require careful monitoring. Various protocols have been described, some audacious and some prudent, and the procedure is very time consuming. For these reasons, OIT should be regarded at this time as experimental therapy and must only be undertaken by practitioners who have been trained in this procedure.

Follow-Up

The follow-up and re-evaluation of CMA is important. Follow-up assessments should include the following: adherence to diet, growth monitoring, the control of co-existing disorders, and the reinforcement of key educational messages, e.g. reading food labels and preparedness for emergencies. Periodic re-challenges should be conducted to monitor tolerance (every 6–12 months). In cases of IgE-mediated CMA, milk-specific IgE levels should also be monitored periodically. Declining levels of sIgE correlate well with the development of tolerance [23, 33]. Although an sIgE level for cow's milk protein of 2 kU/l has been reported to predict a 50% chance of passing a challenge test [34], systematic reviews have shown that this value is not universally applicable but is dependent on the patient population studied.

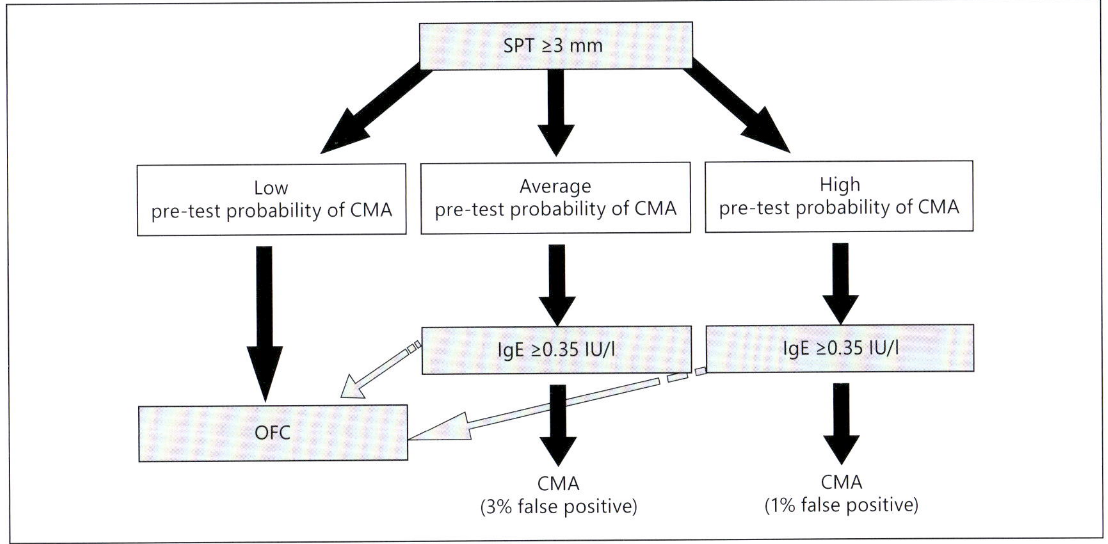

Fig. 1. A patient is reported with possible symptoms of IgE-mediated CMA. The probability of CMA is average, but the challenge is difficult to perform. Her SPT is positive. What can I get from an *in vitro* specific IgE determination? [36].

A Very Common Clinical Case

Adrian is a 6-month-old male infant born to a family of Albanian origin. He has lived in Asti – a small town 60 km southeast of Turin and 120 km southwest of Milan – since birth. His mother suffers from grass-induced allergic rhinitis. Exclusively breastfed, Adrian developed AD at 3 months of age. His eczema was kept under control with emollients, cetirizine for 5 days and then again for 20 days, and topical steroids (fluticasone furoate) for 7 days. When his mother went back to work, his grandmother fed him with his first CM formula meal. After 30 minutes, his grandmother reported urticaria and an AD flare-up after 1 hour for a duration of 12 hours. Adrian presented to his general practitioner (GP) with suspected CMA. At this point, the GP had the following five choices:

(1) To perform an SPT;
(2) To get an sIgE determination for milk;
(3) To perform a patch test;
(4) To propose an OFC; or

(5) To decide to treat Adrian with an alternative formula, a CM hydrolysate.

For this decision, the GP took into account the probability of the disease and the fact that in Asti, there are no facilities at which to perform OFCs. The probability of CMA was average in this patient; the reported 'milk reaction' involved a single organ (skin), it was not immediate, and the AD was of medium severity (SCORAD 25). Thus, according to the DRACMA guidelines, the GP had the following two choices:

(a) If the family agreed to spend time and resources in Turin or Milan for an OFC, they should be sent there without even performing an SPT as a triage or add-on test to establish a diagnosis; or

(b) If that is not possible for the family, a replacement test should be performed locally.

For the second case, atopy patch testing is not an option. The SPT and sIgE determination with ImmunoCAP have similar positive and negative predictive values. In the case of positivity, the combination of the two could minimize the need for an OFC (fig. 1) [35].

The decision for Adrian was to attempt to obtain sensitization data locally. The SPT turned out positive, but the sIgE determination was negative. Thus, he had to be sent to our clinic in Milan, where the OFC turned out to be positive after a cumulative dose of 44 ml of cow's milk.

At this point, Adrian was in need of a substitutive formula. No milk from other species could be considered because they are not nutritionally fit for a 6-month-old child. Thus, we had four choices:

(1) eHF (either casein or whey-based);
(2) rHF;
(3) AAF; or
(4) Soy formula.

This choice was based on allergenicity, nutritional values, availability, palatability, and formula price. Because this was not an anaphylactic reaction, AAF was not recommended. In Italy, where rHF is available and cheap, this may be the best option, and eHF can be considered. Where rHF is not available, eHF is the best option. In different settings, considerations of availability, price and individual choices could also lead to the selection of AAF or even soy formula [36]. Thus, these guidelines allow for a tailored choice of the best substitute.

Conclusions

CMA is one of the most frequent manifestations of food allergy and may present as an IgE- or non-IgE-mediated disease. Patients with IgE-mediated CMA and asthma are at the risk of potentially severe allergic reactions (anaphylaxis). The diagnosis of CMA relies primarily on clinical evaluation supported by SPT and the *in vitro* measurement of sIgE. CMA can be adequately treated with dietary manipulation, including the avoidance of cow's milk protein products. All cases of CMA must be managed in collaboration with an experienced dietician who has expertise in food allergy. The dietician's role is to provide advice/recipes/education (reading food labels, checking for hidden ingredients, etc.) and to ensure nutritional adequacy. Severe cases of CMA should be referred to a specialist with expertise in allergy.

References

1 Boyce JA, Assa'ad A, Burks AW, et al: Guidelines for the diagnosis and management of food allergy in the United States: report of the NIAID-sponsored expert panel. J. Allergy Clin Immunol 2010;126(6 suppl):S1–S58.
2 Urisu A, Ebisawa M, Mukoyama T, et al: Japanese guideline for food allergy. Allergol Int 2011;60:221–236.
3 Fiocchi A, Brozek J, Schunemann HJ, et al: World Allergy Organization (WAO) diagnosis and rationale for action against cow's milk allergy (DRACMA) guidelines. WAO Journal 2010;3:57–61.
4 Sackeyfio A, Senthinathan A, Kandaswamy P, et al: Diagnosis and assessment of food allergy in children and young people: summary of NICE guidance. BMJ 2011;342:d747.
5 Burks AW, Tang M, Sicherer S, et al: ICON: food allergy. J Allergy Clin Immunol 2012;129:906–920.
6 Steinke M, Fiocchi A, Kirchlechner V, et al: Food allergy in children and potential allergy medicine users in Europe. A randomised telephone survey of children in 10 European nations. Int Arch Allergy Immunol 2007;143:290–295.
7 Bahna SL: Cow's milk allergy versus cow milk intolerance. Ann Allergy Asthma Immunol 2002;89(6 suppl 1):56–60.
8 Johansson SG, Bieber T, Dahl R: Revised nomenclature for allergy for global use: report of the Nomenclature Review Committee of the World Allergy Organization, 2003. J Allergy Clin Immunol 2004;113:832–836.
9 International Union of Immunological Societies Allergen Nomenclature Sub-Committee: Allergen nomenclature. 2009. http://www.allergen.org/Allergen.aspx (accessed February 26, 2015).
10 Wal J-M: Cow's milk proteins/allergens. Ann Allergy Asthma Clin Immunol 2002;89(suppl 9):3–10.
11 Restani P, Ballabio C, Di Lorenzo C, et al: Molecular aspects of milk allergens and their role in clinical events. Anal Bioanal Chem 2009;395:47–56.
12 Fiocchi A, Bouygue GR, Albarini M, et al: Molecular diagnosis of cow's milk allergy. Curr Opin Allergy Clin Immunol 2011;11:216–221.
13 Leonard SA, Nowak-Węgrzyn A: Clinical diagnosis and management of food protein-induced enterocolitis syndrome. Curr Opin Pediatr 2012;24:739–745.

14 Lake AM, Whitington PF, Hamilton SR: Dietary protein-induced colitis in breast – fed infants. J Pediatr 1982;101:906–910.

15 Ngamphaiboon J, Chatchatee P, Thongkaew T: Cow's milk allergy in Thai children. Asian Pac J Allergy Immunol 2008;26:199–204.

16 Eigenmann PA, Sicherer SH, Borkowski TA, et al: Prevalence of IgE-mediated food allergy among children with atopic dermatitis. Pediatrics 1998;101:e8.

17 Kubota A, Kawahara H, Okuyama H, et al: Cow's milk protein allergy presenting with Hirschsprung's disease-mimicking symptoms. J Pediatr Surg 2006;41:2056–2058.

18 Berni Canani R, Ruotolo S, Auricchio L, et al: Diagnostic accuracy of the atopy patch test in children with food allergy-related gastrointestinal symptoms. Allergy 2007;62:738–743.

19 Høst A, Halken S, Jacobsen HP, et al: Clinical course of cow's milk protein allergy/intolerance and atopic diseases in childhood. Pediatr Allergy Immunol 2002;3:23–28.

20 García-Ara MC, Boyano-Martínez MT, Díaz-Pena JM, et al: Cow's milk-specific immunoglobulin E levels as predictors of clinical reactivity in the follow-up of the cow's milk allergy infants. Clin Exp Allergy 2004;34:866–870.

21 Fiocchi A, Terracciano L, Bouygue GR, et al: Incremental prognostic factors associated with cow's milk allergy outcomes in infant and child referrals: the Milan Cow's Milk Allergy Cohort study. Ann Allergy Asthma Immunol 2008;101:166–173.

22 Levy Y, Segal N, Garty B, et al: Lessons from the clinical course of IgE-mediated cow milk allergy in Israel. Pediatr Allergy Immunol 2007;18:589–593.

23 Skripak JM, Matsui EC, Mudd K, et al: The natural history of IgE-mediated cow's milk allergy. J Allergy Clin Immunol 2007;120:1172–1177.

24 Wood RA, Sicherer SH, Vickery BP, et al: The natural history of milk allergy in an observational cohort. J Allergy Clin Immunol 2013;131:805–812.

25 Savilahti EM, Rantanen V, Lin JS, et al: Early recovery from cow's milk allergy is associated with decreasing IgE and increasing IgG4 binding to cow's milk epitopes. J Allergy Clin Immunol 2010;125:1315–1321.

26 Nowak-Wegrzyn A, Bloom KA, Sicherer SH, et al: Tolerance to extensively heated milk in children with cow's milk allergy. J Allergy Clin Immunol 2008;122:342–347.

27 Skripak JM, Wood RA: Mammalian milk allergy: avoidance strategies and oral desensitization. Curr Opin Allergy Clin Immunol 2009;9:259–264.

28 Kim JS, Nowak-Węgrzyn A, Sicherer SH, et al: Dietary baked milk accelerates the resolution of cow's milk allergy in children. J Allergy Clin Immunol 2011;128:125–131.

29 Terracciano L, Bouygue G, Sarratud T, et al: Impact of dietary regimen on the duration of cow's milk allergy: a random allocation study. Clin Exp Allergy 2010;40:637–642.

30 Prescott SL, Bouygue GR, Videky D, et al: Avoidance or exposure to foods in prevention and treatment of food allergy? Curr Opin Allergy Clin Immunol 2010;10:258–266.

31 Kemp AS, Hill DJ, Allen KJ, et al: Guidelines for the use of infant formulas to treat cow's milk protein allergy: an Australian consensus panel opinion. Med J Aust 2008;188:109–112.

32 Fiocchi A, Schünemann HJ, Brozek J, et al: Diagnosis and Rationale for Action Against Cow's Milk Allergy (DRACMA): a summary report. J Allergy Clin Immunol 2010;126:1119–1128.

33 Celik-Bilgili S, Mehl A, Verstege A, et al: The predictive value of specific immunoglobulin E levels in serum for the outcome of oral food challenges. Clin Exp Allergy 2005;35:26–73.

34 Perry TT, Matsui EC, Kay Conover-Walker M, et al: The relationships of allergen-specific IgE levels and oral food challenge outcome. J Allergy Clin Immunol 2004;114:144–149.

35 Fiocchi A, Schunemann H, Terracciano L, Albarini M, Martelli A, Landi M, Compalati E, Canonica GW: DRACMA one year after: which changes have occurred in diagnosis and treatment of CMA in Italy? Ital J Pediatr 2011;37:53.

36 Terracciano L, Schünemann H, Brozek J, et al: How DRACMA changes clinical decision for the individual patient in CMA therapy. Curr Opin Allergy Clin Immunol 2012;12:316–322.

Alessandro Fiocchi, MD
Division of Allergy, Department of Pediatrics
Pediatric Hospital Bambino Gesù
IT–00100 Rome, Vatican City (Italy)
E-Mail agiovanni.fiocchi@opbg.net

Ebisawa M, Ballmer-Weber BK, Vieths S, Wood RA (eds): Food Allergy: Molecular Basis and Clinical Practice.
Chem Immunol Allergy. Basel, Karger, 2015, vol 101, pp 124–130 (DOI: 10.1159/000375416)

Hen's Egg Allergy

Atsuo Urisu[a] · Y. Kondo[a] · I. Tsuge[b]

[a]Department of Pediatrics, The Second Teaching Hospital, Fujita Health University, Nagoya,
[b]Department of Pediatrics, Fujita Health University School of Medicine, Toyoake, Japan

Abstract

Egg allergy is one of the most frequent food allergies in infants and young children. The prevalence of egg allergy is estimated to be between 1.8 and 2% in children younger than 5 years of age. The reactions are mainly mediated by IgE and partially by non-IgE or are a mix of both types. Egg white contains more than 20 different proteins and glycoproteins. Ovomucoid (Gal d 1), ovalbumin (Gal d 2), conalbumin (ovotransferrin) (Gal d 3) and lysozyme (Gal d 4) have been identified as major allergens in hen's egg. Alpha-livetin (Gal d 5) is thought to be a main egg yolk allergen responsible for bird-egg syndrome. The diagnosis of egg allergy is based on history taking, antigen-specific IgE measurements, such as the skin prick test, *in vitro* antigen-specific blood IgE tests and histamine release tests, and oral food challenges. The measurements of specific IgE to ovomucoid and its linear epitopes are more useful in the diagnosis of heated egg allergy and in the prediction of prognosis. Currently, the management of egg allergy is essentially minimal elimination based on the correct identification of the causative allergen. Although oral immunotherapy is promising as a tolerance induction protocol, several questions and concerns still remain, predominantly regarding safety.

© 2015 S. Karger AG, Basel

Introduction

Hen's egg is one of the most common allergenic foods in children. The estimated prevalence of egg allergy varies from 1.8 to 2% in children younger than 5 years of age [1], making it the second most common cause of food allergies in children. In several industrialized countries, such as Spain, France and Japan, egg allergy has in fact been reported to be the most prevalent food allergy in the pediatric population, exceeding that of cow's milk allergy [2]. In this article, we review recent advances in the diagnosis and management of egg allergy.

Allergen		Common name		MW (kDa)	IgE-binding activity		
					heat-treated	digestive enzyme-treated	allergenic activity
Gal d 1	Egg white	Ovomucoid	Egg white	28	stable	stable	+++
Gal d 2	Egg white	Ovalbumin	Egg white	45	unstable	unstable	++
Gal d 3	Egg white	Ovotransferrin/conalbumin	Egg white	76.6	unstable	unstable	+
Gal d 4	Egg white	Lysozyme	Egg white	14.3	unstable	unstable	++
Gal d 5	Egg yolk	α-Livetin	Egg yolk	65–70	unstable		+

Symptoms

The most common symptoms in children with egg allergy are IgE-mediated reactions, such as erythema, urticaria, eczematous rash, abdominal pain, diarrhea and vomiting. Anaphylactic reactions to egg are not commonly reported. In rare cases, egg has caused fatal reactions because of anaphylaxis [3]. In addition, it is one of the most common allergenic foods causing allergic eosinophilic esophagitis and allergic eosinophilic gastroenteritis, and reactions may be IgE-mediated, cell-mediated or both. Food protein-induced proctocolitis and food-induced enterocolitis are other gastrointestinal disorders that are also rarely caused by egg and appear to involve a non-IgE-mediated mechanism [4].

Allergenic Components of Egg White

The egg white of the domestic chicken (*Gallus domesticus*) represent the albumin fraction of the egg and contain more allergenic proteins than the yolk. Egg white contains more than 20 different proteins and glycoproteins. Ovomucoid (OVM) (Gal d 1, approximately 11%), ovalbumin (OVA) (Gal d 2, approximately 54%), conalbumin, also known as ovotransferrin (Gal d 3, approximately 12%) and lysozyme (Gal d 4, approximately 3%) [5] have been identified as the major allergens (table 1). Studies of human subjects utilizing serum IgE tests have reported the order of allergenicity as OVM > OVA > ovotransferrin > lysozyme [6]. OVM is a highly glycosylated molecule containing 186 amino acid residues. This protein consists of 3 tandem domains designated as DI, DII and DIII, and it belongs to a family of Kazal-type pancreatic secretory trypsin inhibitors [5]. OVM has several unique characteristics, such as stability against heat and digestion by proteinases. There have been a few studies on the IgE-binding epitopes in OVM [7 11], and the reported binding sites resemble each other (table 2) [12].

OVA, or Gal d 2, which has structural homology to the serpin (serine protease inhibitor) superfamily, comprises 54% of the total proteins in egg white. Its complete sequence of 385 amino acids has been determined [13]. In contrast to OVM, OVA is heat-labile and possibly less allergenic [5]. This means that the IgE-binding epitopes on OVA might be destroyed after heating, suggesting that children who have specific IgE primarily to OVA are likely to tolerate heated eggs [6].

Ovotransferrin (also called conalbumin) is a nonheme and iron-binding glycoprotein in egg white [5]. Although it is considered to be one of major allergens in egg white, the role of the specific IgE to ovotransferrin in the diagnosis of egg allergy has not been determined.

Lysozyme is a glycosidase commonly used as a food preservative due to its antibacterial proper-

Table 2. Sequential IgE-binding epitopes of ovomucoid (Gal d 1)

		Ref. no.	Year	IgE epitope				
Domain 1 AA 1–64	Cooke and Sampson	7	1997	AA 1–20				AA 49–56
	Besler et al.	8	1999					
	Holen et al.	10	2001	AA 1–14	AA 11–24	AA 31–44		AA 51–64
	Mine and Yang	5	2008			AA 32–42	AA 40–50	AA 56–66
	Järvinen et al.	9	2007	AA 1–10	AA 9–20			AA 47–56
	Martinez-Botas et al.	11	2013		AA 4–20			AA 46–59
Domain 2 AA 65–130	Cooke and Sampson	7	1997			AA 85–96		AA 115–122
	Besler et al.	8	1999				AA 90–121	
	Holen et al.	10	2001	AA 61–74			AA 101–114	AA 121–134
	Mine and Yang	5	2008	AA 71–75	AA 80–90		AA 101–105	AA 121–130
	Järvinen et al.	9	2007					AA 113–124
	Martinez-Botas et al.	11	2013				AA 91–104	AA 113–124
Domain 3 AA 131–186	Cooke and Sampson	7	1997			AA 175–186		
	Besler et al.	8	1999			AA 134–186		
	Holen et al.	10	2001					
	Mine and Yang	5	2008			AA 159–174	AA 179–186	
	Järvinen et al.	9	2007					
	Martinez-Botas et al.	11	2013					

ties in some pharmaceuticals and foods (e.g. eye drops and cheese) [5]. Egg-allergic individuals sensitized to lysozyme may therefore show hypersensitive reactions to such products.

Allergenic Components of Egg Yolk

Alpha-livetin (Gal d 5), or chicken serum albumin, is thought to be a main egg yolk allergen involved in bird-egg syndrome [14]. In this syndrome, the primary sensitization is induced by the inhalation of air-borne bird allergens with cross-reactivity with albumin in egg yolk (Gal d 5). These patients experience respiratory symptoms, such as rhinitis and/or asthma, upon bird exposure and an immediate allergic reaction to egg ingestion. The measurement of the specific IgE to Gal d 5 might therefore confirm the diagnosis of bird-egg syndrome. Several other potential allergens, such as vitellenin (apovitellenin I) and apoprotein B (apovitellenin VI), have been identified in egg yolk, although their roles in egg allergy remain unclear.

Diagnosis

Accurate history taking is the key element in the diagnostic process of food allergy. Its diagnosis is often assessed by positive IgE tests, such as the skin prick test, *in vitro* allergen-specific blood IgE tests and the histamine release test [15]. A significant percentage of children with high specific IgE levels to food allergens, especially those with atopic dermatitis, might show misleading positive tests because of sensitization in the absence of a clinical food allergy [16]. The presence of food allergen-specific IgE only indicates sensitization to an allergen; it does not necessarily confirm the clinical diagnosis of food allergy.

The skin prick test shows a good sensitivity but a poor specificity [17]. As a consequence, a negative test result essentially excludes an IgE-mediated egg allergy, whereas a positive test result does not predict clinical reactivity accurately.

These specific IgE tests always need to be correlated with a history of convincing symptoms after food exposure or verified by an oral food challenge. Recently, *in vitro* allergen-specific blood IgE tests have demonstrated a relationship between egg-specific IgE concentrations and the probability of reactions elicited by an oral food challenge. Threshold values of egg-specific IgE (cutoff values) for predicting the outcomes of challenge tests have been defined in several studies, showing various predictive values.

The studies by Sampson [18] have suggested that the diagnostic decision point for egg white-specific IgE is 7 kUA/l, with 95% of the children having a clinical reaction. A similar value, 7.4 kUA/l, has recently been reported by Ando et al. [19]. Although different values have been demonstrated in other studies, the predictive cutoff values are consistently lower in small children and increase with age [20]. The range of cutoff values observed might depend not only on differences in age but also on the types of symptoms, other clinical characteristics of the cohorts, such as prevalence and/or differing challenge procedures, and the type of food given during the challenge. Future studies utilizing patients with well-characterized clinical phenotypes and standardized challenge protocols, including food preparation, should give more comparable results and useful predictive information [21].

The measurement of OVM-specific IgE has been suggested to be more reliable in the diagnosis of a reaction to heated egg [19]. A concentration of specific IgE to OVM of higher than approximately 11 kUA/l (the positive decision point based on 95% clinical specificity) indicates a high risk of reacting to heated egg as well as raw egg. At the same time, a concentration of lower than approximately 1 kUA/l (the negative decision point based on 95% clinical sensitivity) means that there is a low risk of reacting to heated egg, even if the patient reacts well to raw egg [19]. OVM-specific IgE presents better diagnostic accuracy in the prediction of an allergic reaction to boiled egg than egg-white-specific IgE, even in infants [22].

Lemon-Mulé et al. [23] investigated immunologic changes associated with the ingestion of baked egg in children with egg allergy. Greater levels of specific IgE to OVM were found in children reacting to baked egg (baked with wheat flour in the form of a muffin or a waffle) compared with those who were tolerant to baked egg and lightly cooked egg (e.g. French toast). However, in this study, only very high levels of specific IgE to OVM (>50 kUA/l) were highly predictive of heated egg reactivity. This finding might be explained by the so-called matrix effect because the egg was baked with wheat matrix. Kato et al. [24] have previously shown the decreased solubility of OVM when egg is mixed with wheat flour and wheat gluten and heated, suggesting that OVM forms complexes or chemical bonds with gluten, leading to aggregation and insolubility and potentially decreased digestibility.

Natural History

The prognosis of egg allergy is generally considered to be good because it is thought that most children will outgrow it as they become older. Egg allergy usually develops within the first 2 years of life and resolves in 52% of individuals by 3 years of age and in 66% by 5 years of age [25]. However, in a study of a referral population, Savage et al. [26] have reported an increased persistence of egg allergy. Egg was tolerated by only 4% of individuals by 4 years, 12% by 6 years, 37% by 10 years and 68% by 16 years of age. These figures are far lower than those reported by Boyano-Martinez et al. [25]. Moreover, children with egg-specific IgE greater than 50 kUA/l are unlikely to develop egg tolerance before the age of 18 years, which is the highest age that was studied [26].

According to a study by Montesinos [27], 50% of children develop tolerance at around 4 years of age, and only 26% remain allergic at 5 years. This rate of acquiring tolerance is similar to that reported by Boyano [25]. Montesinos et al. [27] have speculated that atopic dermatitis is associated with the persistence of egg allergy, and the different rates of this disease explain the differences in the egg allergy resolution rates reported by previous studies.

There are a number of laboratory correlates that may predict or be associated with the persistence or resolution of egg allergy. Monitoring egg-specific IgE levels is useful in the prediction of the prognosis of allergic disease. A relationship between the degree of decrease in egg-specific IgE levels over time and the likelihood of developing tolerance has been demonstrated, showing that a greater decrease in egg-specific IgE levels over a shorter period of time is indicative of a greater likelihood of tolerance development [28]. Application of this model might help clinicians in the timing of food challenge tests and in providing prognostic information to patients and their families.

OVM is a better predictor for the natural history of an egg allergy as well as the diagnosis of the disease. Children with a persistent egg allergy have significantly higher levels of IgE specific for OVM than those who outgrow their reactivity [29]. Additionally, subjects with high IgE-binding activity to pepsin-digested OVM are unlikely to outgrow their egg allergy compared to those who develop tolerance [30], and a small, 4.5 kDa fragment of pepsin-digested OVM has been found to contain an IgE epitope that appears to be associated with the persistence of egg allergy [31]. Moreover, IgE from children with persistent egg allergy recognizes more linear epitopes on OVM. Four sequential IgE-binding sites on OVM have been identified (table 2), allowing for the differentiation of children with persistent egg allergy from those with transient egg allergy [9]. The presence of IgE specific to sequential epitopes may therefore be useful as a screening tool for persistent egg allergy.

Management and Therapy

Currently, the mainstay of treatment for food allergy is minimal avoidance of the offending food based on the correct diagnosis of the causative food and education regarding the use of emergency medication in cases of accidental ingestion or exposure. This therapy places a burden, to a greater or lesser extent, on food-allergic patients and their parents if they are children. These individuals always face the probable risk of an unexpected accident resulting from the intake of causative foods, particularly compound food products. Therefore, once the causative food has been identified by an exact diagnosis, the strict avoidance of offending foods is an essential principle for dietary therapy.

Oral Immunotherapy to Egg Allergy

Many studies on oral immunotherapy (OIT) have provided encouraging results, showing increased tolerance to the offending food. Although encouraging, several questions and concerns still remain, predominantly regarding safety. Early reports on oral desensitization to different foods were based on a limited number of patients and showed inconsistent tolerance achievement. In recent years, more convincing studies have been performed and published, showing promising results on achieving clinical tolerance to egg by OIT [32]. Mild to severe side effects associated with OIT are, to some extent, inevitable in any protocol using food antigens. Lemon-Mule et al. [23] have performed large clinical trials using extensively heated egg in children with egg allergy. They have effectively increased tolerance by providing muffins including extensively heated egg. Furthermore, the children had no increase in acute allergic reactions or in the severity of underlying atopic diseases, such as asthma and atopic dermatitis. We need to develop novel modified antigens, such as hypoallergenic antigens, for a safer OIT for food allergy [33].

Clinical Case

A 7-year-old boy with egg allergy developed wheezing and generalized urticaria after accidental ingestion of a half-boiled egg and was injected auto-administered adrenaline (epinephrine) by his mother before visiting the emergency room. He was advised to strictly eliminate all egg-containing foods by a physician in the emergency room. Then, he was referred to an allergy specialist. His egg-white- and OVM-specific IgE titers were 20.0 and <0.35 kUA/l, respectively. He received an oral challenge test with a 15-minute boiled egg and showed a negative result. This patient was permitted to eat hard-boiled egg and processed products, including heated egg, but to avoid raw and half-boiled eggs by a dietician.

Acknowledgments

This study is partially supported by the Health and Labor Sciences Research Grants for Research on Allergic Disease and Immunology from the Ministry of Health, Labor and Welfare.

References

1 Sicherer SH: Epidemiology of food allergy. J Allergy Clin Immunol 2011;127: 594–602.

2 Benhamou AH, Caubet JC, Eigenmann PA, Nowak-Węgrzyn A, Marcos CP, Reche M, Urisu A: State of the art and new horizons in the diagnosis and management of egg allergy. Allergy 2010;65:283–289.

3 Sampson HA, Mendelson L, Rosen JP: Fatal and near-fatal anaphylactic reactions to food in children and adolescents. N Eng J Med 1992;327:380–384.

4 Nowak-Węegrzyna A, Muraro A: Food protein-induced enterocolitis syndrome. Curr Opin Allergy Clin Immunol 2009;9: 371–377.

5 Mine Y, Yang M: Recent advances in the understanding of egg allergens: basic, industrial, and clinical perspectives. J Agric Food Chem 2008;56:4874–4900.

6 Urisu A, Ando H, Morita Y, Wada E, Yasaki T, Yamada K, Komada K, Torii S, Goto M, Wakamatsu T: Allergenic activity of heated and ovomucoid-depleted egg white. J Allergy Clin Immunol 1997; 100:171–176.

7 Cooke SK, Sampson HA: Allergenic properties of ovomucoid in man. J Immunol 1997;159:2026–2032.

8 Besler M, Petersen A, Steinhart H, Paschke A: Identification of IgE-binding peptides derived from chemical and enzymatic cleavage of ovomucoid (Gal d 1). Internet Symposium on Food Allergens 1999;1:1–12.

9 Järvinen KM, Beyer K, Vila L, Bardina L, Mishoe M, Sampson HA: Specificity of IgE antibodies to sequential epitopes of hen's egg ovomucoid as a marker for persistence of egg allergy. Allergy 2007; 62:758–765.

10 Holen E, Bolann B, Elsayed S: Novel B and T cell epitopes of chicken ovomucoid (Gal d 1) induce T cell secretion of IL-6, IL-13, and IFN-gamma. Clin Exp Allergy 2001;31:952–964.

11 Martínez-Botas J, Cerecedo I, Zamora J, Vlaicu C, Dieguez MC, Gómez-Coronado D, de Dios V, Terrados S, de la Hoz B: Mapping of the IgE and IgG4 sequential epitopes of ovomucoid with a peptide microarray immunoassay. Int Arch Allergy Immunol 2013;161:11–20.

12 Caubet JC, Kondo Y, Urisu A, Nowak-Węgrzyn A: Molecular diagnosis of egg allergy. Curr Opin Allergy Clin Immunol 2011;11:210–215.

13 Nisbet AD, Saundry RH, Moir AJ, Fothergill LA, Fothergill JE: The complete amino-acid sequence of hen ovalbumin. Eur J Biochem 1981;115:335–345.

14 Quirce S, Marañón F, Umpiérrez A, de las Heras M, Fernández-Caldas E, Sastre J: Chicken serum albumin (Gal d 5) is a partially heat-labile inhalant and food allergen implicated in the bird-egg syndrome. Allergy 2001;56:754–762.

15 Sato S, Tachimoto H, Shukuya A, Ogata M, Komata T, Imai T, Tomikawa M, Ebisawa M: Utility of the peripheral blood basophil histamine release test in the diagnosis of hen's egg, cow's milk, and wheat allergy in children. Int Arch Allergy Immunol 2011;155(suppl 1):96–103.

16 Eigenmann PA, Sicherer SH, Borkowski TA, Cohen BA, Sampson HA: Prevalence of IgE-mediated food allergy among children with atopic dermatitis. Pediatrics 1998;101:e8.

17 Sampson HA, Ho DG: Relationship between food-specific IgE concentration and the risk of positive food challenges in children and adolescents. J Allergy Clin Immunol 1997;100:444–451.

18 Sampson HA: Utility of food-specific IgE concentrations in predicting symptomatic food allergy. J Allergy Clin Immunol 2001;107:891–896.

19 Ando H, Movérare R, Kondo Y, Tsuge I, Tanaka A, Borres M, Urisu A: Utility of ovomucoid-specific IgE concentrations in predicting symptomatic egg allergy. J Allergy Clin Immunol 2008;122:583–588.

20 Komata T, Soderstrom L, Borres MP, Tachimoto H, Ebisawa M: The predictive relationship of food-specific serum IgE concentrations to challenge outcomes for egg and milk varies by patient age. J Allergy Clin Immunol 2007;119: 1272–1274.

21 Eigenmann PA: Are specific immunoglobulin E titres reliable for prediction of food allergy? Clin Exp Allergy 2005; 35:247–249.

22 Haneda Y, Kando N, Yasui M, Kobayashi T, Maeda T, Hino A, Hasegawa S, Ichiyama T, Ito K: Ovomucoids IgE is a better marker than egg white-specific IgE to diagnose boiled egg allergy. J Allergy Clin Immunol 2012;129:1681–1682.

23 Lemon-Mulé H, Sampson HA, Sicherer SH, Shreffler WG, Noone S, Nowak-Wegrzyn A: Immunologic changes in children with egg allergy ingesting extensively heated egg. J Allergy Clin Immunol 2008;122:977–983.

24 Kato Y, Oozawa E, Matsuda T: Decrease in antigenic and allergenic potentials of ovomucoid by heating in the presence of wheat flour: dependence on wheat variety and intermolecular disulfide bridges. J Agric Food Chem 2001;49:3661–3665.

25 Boyano-Martinez T, Garcia-Ara C, Diaz-Pena JM, Martin-Esteban M: Prediction of tolerance on the basis of quantification of egg white-specific IgE antibodies in children with egg allergy. J Allergy Clin Immunol 2002;110:304–309.

26 Savage JH, Matsui EC, Skripak JM, Wood RA: The natural history of egg allergy. J Allergy Clin Immunol 2007; 120:1413–1417.

27 Montesinos E, Martorell A, Félix R, Cerdá JC: Egg white specific IgE levels in serum as clinical reactivity predictors in the course of egg allergy follow-up. Pediatr Allergy Immunol 2010;21:634–639.

28 Shek LPC, Soderstrom L, Ahlstedt S, Beyer K, Sampson HA: Determination of food specific IgE levels over time can predict the development of tolerance in cow's milk and hen's egg allergy. J Allergy Clin Immunol 2004;114:387–391.

29 Bernhisel-Broadbent J, Dintzis HM, Dintzis RZ, Sampson HA: Allergenicity and antigenicity of chicken egg ovomucoid (Gal d III) compared with ovalbumin (Gal d I) in children with egg allergy and in mice. J Allergy Clin Immunol 1994;93:1047–1059.

30 Urisu A, Yamada K, Tokuda R, Ando H, Wada E, Kondo Y, Morita Y: Clinical significance of IgE-binding activity to enzymatic digests of ovomucoid in diagnosis and prediction of outgrow of egg white hypersensitivity. Int Arch Allergy Appl Immunol 1999;120:192–198.

31 Takagi K, Teshima R, Okunuki H, Itoh S, Kawasaki N, Kawanishi T, Hayakawa T, Kohno Y, Urisu A, Sawada J: Kinetic analysis of pepsin digestion of chicken egg white ovomucoid and allergenic potential of pepsin fragments. Int Arch Allergy Immunol 2005;136:23–32.

32 Staden U, Rolinck-Werninghaus C, Brewe F, Wahn U, Niggemann B, Beyer K: Specific oral tolerance induction in food allergy in children: efficacy and clinical patterns of reaction. Allergy 2007;62:1261–1269.

33 Urisu A, Tanaka K, Ogura K, Naruse N, Hirata N, Nakajima Y, Inuo C, Suzuki S, Ando H, Kondo Y, Tsuge I, Yamada K, Kimura M: New approach for improving the safety of oral immunotherapy for food allergy. Clin Exp Allergy Rev 2012; 12:25–28.

Atsuo Urisu, MD, PhD
Department of Pediatrics, The Second Teaching Hospital
Fujita Health University
3-6-10 Otobashi Nakagawa-ku, Nagoya 454-8509 (Japan)
E-Mail urisu@fujita-hu.ac.jp

Ebisawa M, Ballmer-Weber BK, Vieths S, Wood RA (eds): Food Allergy: Molecular Basis and Clinical Practice.
Chem Immunol Allergy. Basel, Karger, 2015, vol 101, pp 131–144 (DOI: 10.1159/000375417)

Peanut and Tree Nut Allergy

Amanda Cox · Scott H. Sicherer

Division of Allergy and Clinical Immunology, Department of Pediatrics, Jaffe Food Allergy Institute,
Icahn School of Medicine at Mount Sinai, New York, N.Y., USA

Abstract

Allergy to peanut and tree nuts is a major worldwide health concern. The prevalence of these allergies may be increasing, but the reasons for these increases remain unclear. This group of foods accounts for a large proportion of severe and fatal food-allergic reactions. These allergies present most often during childhood but can occur at any age. Resolution is possible but uncommon, and frequent lifetime reactions caused by accidental ingestion are a serious problem. The major allergens of peanut and most tree nuts have been identified, allowing for insights into patient diagnoses, clinical outcomes, and potential future immunotherapies.   © 2015 S. Karger AG, Basel

Introduction

Allergies to peanuts, a legume, and tree nuts are common and have become an important health problem in children and adults [1]. The prevalence of peanut and tree nut allergies appears to have increased, particularly in westernized countries [2]. Peanuts and tree nuts are common ingredients in many cuisines and in processed foods, making avoidance difficult for those with allergies. Additionally, these foods account for many of the most severe and fatal food-allergic reactions. For most, allergies to peanut and tree nuts are permanent. Living with peanut and tree nut allergy has significant burdensome effects on quality of life [3, 4].

Epidemiology

The prevalence of peanut allergy varies in different regions worldwide. Westernized countries, including the US, the UK, Canada, and Australia, have reported prevalence rates of 1–2% for children and 0.6% for adults [2]. Lower rates have been reported in France (0.3–0.7%), Denmark (0.2–0.6%) and Israel (0.04–0.17%) and in Asian countries, where peanut allergy is actually rare [5–9].

Nine tree nuts account for most tree nut allergies: almond, Brazil nut, cashew, English walnut, hazelnut, macadamia nut, pecan, pine nut, and pistachio [10]. The overall prevalence of tree nut allergy has been found to be similar to that of peanut allergy in several general population surveys conducted in the US. However, the most likely tree nut to trigger allergic reactions may vary in different regions. Among 5,149 participants in a US registry who mainly included children with parent-reported peanut and/or tree nut allergies, the most common reported tree nut allergies were to walnut (34%), followed by cashew (20%), almond (15%), pecan (9%), pistachio (7%) and the other tree nuts (<5% each) [11]. In another US study of 101 patients with a history of reactions to tree nuts, the reaction rates were 30% for walnut, 30% for cashew, 14% for pecan, 8% for almond, 5% for hazelnut, and less than 5% for Brazil nut, macadamia nut, pine nut and pistachio [12]. A publication from the UK has demonstrated that Brazil nut allergy is the most common tree nut allergy in the UK, followed by almond, hazelnut and walnut [13].

Patients are in some cases co-allergic to peanut and tree nuts and may be allergic to multiple tree nuts. Studies have shown rates of co-sensitization (the presence of specific IgE) and co-allergy to both peanut and tree nuts ranging from approximately 20–70% [11–16]. Peanut allergy may precede the onset of tree nut allergies, and several studies have reported that reactions to peanut occur at much earlier ages than those to tree nuts. However, this pattern may simply be due to the age of children at the time of initial exposure. Individuals may become sensitized and clinically allergic to multiple tree nut types with increasing age [17].

Studies have indicated rising prevalences of both peanut and tree nut allergies over the last two decades, especially amongst children. Three nationwide, cross-sectional random-calling telephone surveys designed to assess the self-reported prevalence of peanut and tree nut allergies in the US were conducted in 1997, 2002, and 2008 [18–20]. In 1997, 1.4% of the participants reported a peanut allergy, tree nut allergy or both. The rates of peanut and tree nut allergy in adults (0.7 and 0.4%, respectively) were higher than those in

children younger than 18 years of age (0.4 and 0.2%, respectively). The 2002 and 2008 surveys showed similar overall peanut and tree nut allergy prevalences of 1.2 and 1.4%, respectively. However, significant increases in the prevalences of both peanut and tree nut allergies were found among children younger than 18 years of age in the two subsequent surveys. The prevalences of self-reported peanut allergy for this population were found to be 0.8% in 2002 and 1.2% in 2008, while the prevalences of self-reported tree nut allergy were 0.5% in 2002 and 1.1% in 2008. Similar rates of peanut and tree nut allergy have been demonstrated in studies conducted in Canada, the UK and Australia [21–23].

Clinical Reactions

Clinical reactions to peanut and tree nuts are almost always IgE mediated and can range from mild to severe. Peanut and tree nuts are among the most common causes of food-induced anaphylaxis and have been demonstrated to be the most common causes of fatal food-induced anaphylaxis in several series [24–26]. Reactions may occur with skin contact but are generally limited to the site of contact for peanut or tree nuts [27–29]. Contact reactions rarely lead to systemic symptoms. While many individuals worry about airborne exposure to peanut butter, peanut butter is an oily substance, and reactions to its odor are extremely unlikely [28]. However, peanut and tree nuts can trigger allergic reactions when sensitive patients are exposed to aerosolized proteins or dust [30, 31]. Peanut and tree nuts can also cause localized oropharyngeal symptoms, or oral allergy syndrome, due to peanut protein components that cross-react with plant or tree allergens, such as those of the birch tree.

Predictors of clinical reactivity and diagnostic tests for peanut and tree nut allergy are described in other chapters in this volume and will not be emphasized here.

Age of Presentation or First Reaction to Peanut and Tree Nuts

While peanut and tree nut allergies can develop at any age, peanut allergy most often presents by the second year of life. US studies performed in the last 15 years have suggested that the first exposure to peanut occurs at 12–22 months of age and that the first reaction occurs at 14–24 months [14, 32, 33]. Interestingly, the first reaction to peanut commonly occurs with the first known exposure (75–80%) [11, 14, 34].

Overall, tree nut allergy seems to present later in childhood than peanut allergy. US studies have suggested that the initial tree nut reaction occurs at 36–62 months of age [11, 14]. With increasing age, children who are diagnosed with at least one tree nut allergy may become multi-nut-sensitized and develop clinically allergies to multiple tree nuts [17]. The presentation and diagnosis of tree nut allergy later in childhood is associated with an increased rate of multiple tree nut sensitizations (19% at 2 years of age versus 85% at 5–14 years of age) [17].

Co-Allergy to Peanut and Tree Nuts and Allergy to Multiple Tree Nuts

Several studies of selected populations of allergic individuals have indicated that the rate of co-allergy to peanut and tree nuts is between 23 and 68%, although the pathogenesis of this phenomenon is still not well understood [11–16]. Peanuts and tree nuts are potentially cross-reactive because there are major allergens in peanut (2S albumins, vicilin, legumins, and profilins) that have homologs in many tree nuts [10]. Nonetheless, plant taxonomic classifications are poor predictors of allergic cross-reactivity, and even some highly homologous peanut and tree nut proteins do not demonstrate *in vitro* immunologic cross-reactivity or IgE binding [35]. Moreover, the presence of tree nut-specific serum IgE and posi-

tive tree nut skin test results in a peanut-allergic individual does not necessarily indicate clinical cross-reactivity or the presence of co-existing peanut and tree nut allergies [36]. Patients for which these allergies co-exist are likely sensitized separately to peanut and tree nuts. The relationship between homologous allergens in peanut and tree nuts with the development of both sensitization and clinical allergy is an area of ongoing investigation.

Subsequent Reactions

While patients are instructed to avoid peanut and tree nuts following a diagnosis of allergy, their inadvertent ingestion is common [32]. Accidental exposure to peanut and tree nuts may occur for many reasons, including inadequate patient instruction or implementation of allergen avoidance strategies, the misreading of food product labels, or the mislabeling of food allergens in products by manufacturers. A wide variation in the rate of subsequent reactions has been reported, likely due to issues involving patient age, referral patterns, changes in awareness, allergy severity, threshold tolerance, the use of educational programs and other factors. Studies conducted in the US and Canada have demonstrated a 14–33% annual incidence rate of accidental peanut ingestion among peanut-allergic individuals and a 55–75% rate of accidental exposure over a 5-year period [11, 36–38]. A 5-year US follow-up telephone survey has found that 66% of individuals with a self-reported peanut or tree nut allergy have experienced more than five lifetime reactions to peanut or tree nuts [19]. A British study of the efficacy of a management plan and educational intervention for tree nut allergy has found that 21% of participants have a subsequent reaction to tree nuts after diagnosis, but severe reactions are rare [15]. In a US referral population, lower rates of post-diagnosis accidental exposure to peanut (4.7% per year) and severe reactions to peanut (1.6% per year) have been demonstrated [39]. These findings suggest that expert care, avoidance counseling, and comprehensive allergy management plans may reduce the incidence of subsequent reactions to peanut and tree nuts.

There have been conflicting findings regarding whether subsequent exposures and reactions to peanut or tree nuts tend to be more severe. Some studies have demonstrated trends toward more severe reactions with repeat exposures [11, 22, 36, 40], while others have demonstrated similar or decreased severity of subsequent reactions [15, 37]. Adulthood, as well as the severity of co-existing chronic atopic diseases, including rhinitis, asthma and eczema, may also be predictive of more severe, life-threatening reactions to peanut and tree nuts [27, 39].

Resolution of Peanut Allergy

Most patients do not experience resolution of peanut allergy, and little information about the natural history of this allergy in adults is available. Studies conducted in the US and the UK have demonstrated that between 15 and 20% of young children with a peanut allergy will become tolerant to peanut by school age [16, 41]. The potential for the resolution of peanut allergy is the highest for children who have reduced skin prick test responsiveness, a lower peanut-specific IgE level, a less certain clinical history of allergy or past mild reactions to peanut, and fewer additional allergies [42, 43]. Those with a trend of low or declining peanut-specific IgE levels during the first few years after diagnosis also have a better prognosis. In a study of 80 patients subjected to oral food challenge (OFC) to confirm peanut allergies at two US pediatric allergy clinics, 80 children (median age of 6 years) with peanut-specific IgE levels of 5 kU_A/l or less were evaluated. Fifty-five percent passed the peanut challenges overall, and 63% of those who had peanut-specific IgE levels of 2 kU_A/l or less passed the OFCs [43]. Of note, this group and others have shown that a small number of patients (8–14%) will develop a recurrent peanut allergy or become intolerant to peanut, even after demonstrating tolerance [44, 45]. This finding generally occurs if peanut is rarely eaten or is never incorporated into the diet following a successful OFC.

Resolution of Tree Nut Allergy

There are limited data on the long-term natural history and resolution of tree nut allergy; however, the dogma that tree nut allergy is permanent has been dispelled. In one study of 278 tree nut-allergic patients evaluated at an allergy referral center, approximately 9% became tolerant of tree nuts, including some who had experienced previous severe reactions to these nuts [12]. Predictors of outgrowing tree nut allergy in this study included a low tree nut-specific IgE level, a lack of other food or tree nut allergies, and a history of a resolved peanut allergy. Tree nut allergy recurrence has not been reported or studied to date.

Peanut and Tree Nut Allergens

The identification and characterization of the proteins in peanuts and tree nuts have provided insights regarding their potential cross reactivity, and have allowed for enhanced diagnostics and improved prospects for future therapeutics.

Peanut
The peanut *(Arachis hypogaea)* belongs to the Leguminosae (legume) family of plants and is native to South America. While there are multiple peanut varieties, the allergenic proteins are conserved among them and are found in the cotyledon [46]. For peanut and tree nuts, the allergenic proteins have particular functions in the plant.

Table 1. Peanut (*Arachis hypogaea*) allergens

Allergen designation	Biochemical name/function
Ara h 1	Cupin (vicilin-type, 7S globulin)
Ara h 2	Conglutin (2S albumin)
Ara h 3	Cupin (legumin-type, 11S globulin, glycinin)
Ara h 5	Profilin
Ara h 6	Conglutin (2S albumin)
Ara h 7	Conglutin (2S albumin)
Ara h 8	Pathogenesis-related protein, PR-10, Bet v 1 family member
Ara h 9	Nonspecific lipid-transfer protein 1
Ara h 10	16 kDa oleosin
Ara h 11	14 kDa oleosin
Ara h 12	Defensin
Ara h 13	Defensin

Extracted from the International Union of Immunological Societies, Allergen Nomenclature Subcommittee website, http://www.allergen.org [48].

For instance, vicilin seed storage proteins may inhibit fungal growth and deter insect predators. 2S albumins and lipid transfer proteins (LTPs) are considered to be plant defense-related proteins. LTPs are involved in the biosynthesis of cutin in plants. Profilins, heveins, and LTPs are considered to be panallergens, and they contribute to IgE-mediated cross-reactivity among peanut and a variety of pollens, seeds, fruits, and vegetables. The biological plant-protective functions of many of these proteins contribute to their resistance to degradation as well as to their overall allergenicity [47].

There are nine major and minor allergenic proteins in peanut that have been identified over the past 2 decades and are thought to be responsible for IgE-mediated responses. They are designated Ara h 1–9 and have homologies to different plant seed proteins. The currently recognized peanut allergens listed on the World Health Organization/International Union of Immunological Studies Allergen Nomenclature Sub-committee website (http://www.allergen.org) are shown in table 1 [48]. In most populations, the seed storage proteins Ara h 1 (vicilin), Ara h 2 (conglutin), and Ara h 3 (glycinin) are considered to be the dominant allergens among patients with primary sensitization to peanut. In the US and UK populations, more than 90% of peanut-allergic patients have specific IgE to Ara h 1 and 2 [49, 50], and 45–95% have specific IgE to Ara h 3 [51, 52]. Furthermore, IgE binding to Ara h 2 is emerging as a sensitive predictor of clinical reactions to peanut in the US, European, and Asian pediatric populations [53–56].

Ara h 4 is a member of the glycinin family and is an isoform of Ara h 3 (www.allergen.org), and Ara h 6 and Ara h 7 are conglutinins that are highly homologous to Ara h 2. Ara h 6 may be an important allergen in some patients with severe reactions [57]. Ara h 5, Ara h 8, and Ara h 9 are proteins associated with pollen-food allergy syndrome (or oral allergy syndrome), and specific IgE to these proteins are often found in individuals who have birch pollen sensitization. Ara h 5 is a profilin, and Ara h 8 is a Bet v 1 (birch pollen allergen) homolog. Ara h 8 is a labile protein that is poorly stable to roasting and gastric digestion and is not usually associated with severe peanut allergy [58]. Ara h 9, an LTP, has also been associated with systemic peanut allergy symptoms and appears to be unique to the Mediterranean population. Ara h 9 sensitization likely follows primary sensitization to Pru p 3, the major peach allergen, or to LTPs in other fruits [59]. There are other molecules in peanut, including the oleosins Ara h 10 and Ara h 11, for which clinical relevance is yet to be established.

Sensitization to different peanut proteins, as well as binding to diverse combinations of peanut proteins or even several specific regions (epitopes) within a specific peanut allergen, confer varying likelihoods of clinical reactivity [60]. These patterns may also be predictive, in some cases, of the severity of a reaction to peanut, as well as the potential for resolution [42]. Moreover, patterns of binding to peanut allergens may vary in different regions of the world. In one study comparing peanut-allergic patients from Spain, the US, and Sweden, differences were found in peanut allergen-binding patterns, the severity of symptoms, and the timing of the onset of peanut allergy [61]. These differences reflected sensitization to LTPs (Spain) and birch pollen (Sweden) and primary sensitization to peanut Ara h 2 (US). These regional distinctions in sensitization patterns also had ramifications for the severity of the clinical reactions to peanut. Further research on sensitization patterns to specific peanut allergens will likely reveal additional regional clinical and immunologic differences.

Case Study

A 2-year-old child had anaphylaxis to peanut and a serum peanut IgE level of 4.7 kIU$_A$/l. Her family was informed that she had a low chance of 'outgrowing' the allergy. She was retested at 4 years of age and showed a level of 3.2 kIU$_A$/l, and at 5 years of age, it was 2.1 kIU$_A$/l. The family was offered an oral food challenge (OFC) because of the patient's increasing odds of tolerance, but they deferred. They had her retested at age 10, and her level was 13.2 kIU$_A$/l. This ap-

peared to be a disheartening result, but the allergist discovered that she had developed seasonal allergies, and birch pollen testing revealed a strongly positive result. Component testing to peanut allergens was undertaken and revealed that IgE did not bind to Ara h 1, Ara h 2 or Ara h 3, only to Ara h 8. The child successfully ingested peanut butter during an OFC. The increase in peanut-specific IgE was simply reflective of her increasing pollen sensitization.

Tree Nut Allergens

There are 12 major types of edible tree nuts, including almond, English walnut, pecan, cashew, pistachio, hazelnut (filbert), Brazil nut, macadamia nut, pine nut, chestnut, black walnut, and coconut [62]. English walnut, hazelnut, almond, cashew, and Brazil nut are the most frequent causes of tree nut-allergic reactions [11, 13, 20]. Tree nut allergens are not as well characterized as those of peanut. Both native and recombinant tree nut allergens have been identified, and for some nut allergens, IgE-reactive epitopes have been mapped. The major tree nut allergens that have been identified to date are seed storage proteins, such as vicilins (7S globulins), legumins (11S globulins), and 2S albumins [47]. Vicilins and legumins are members of the cupin superfamily of plant proteins. 2S albumins are members of the prolamin superfamily. Vicilins and 2S albumins are also considered to have plant defense-related properties. Additional tree nut allergens are pan-allergens, including LTPs, profilins, and heveins. These are found in a wide variety of pollens, tree nuts, seeds, fruits, and vegetables and are associated with significant IgE-mediated cross-reactivity [63]. Similar to many of the allergens responsible for peanut allergy, many of the proteins responsible for severe reactions to tree nuts (vicilins, legumin-like proteins, LTPs, and heveins) are resistant to proteolysis and denaturation [64, 65]. Table 2 lists the recognized tree nut allergens

Table 2. Tree nut allergens

Tree nut name	Allergen designation	Biochemical name/function
Almond *(Prunus dulcis)*	Pru du 1	Pathogenesis-related protein, PR-10, Bet v 1 family
	Pru du 3	Nonspecific lipid transfer protein type 1
	Pru du 4	Profilin
	Pru du 5	60s acidic ribosomal protein P2
	Pru du 6	Amandin, 11S globulin legumin-like protein
Brazil nut *(Bertholletia excelsa)*	Ber e 1	2S sulfur-rich seed storage albumin
	Ber e 2	11S globulin seed storage protein
Cashew *(Anacardium occidentale)*	Ana o 1	Vicilin-like protein
	Ana o 2	Legumin-like protein
	Ana o 3	2S albumin
Hazelnut *(Corylus avellana)*	Cor a 1	Pathogenesis-related protein, PR-10, Bet v 1 family member
	Cor a 2	Profilin
	Cor a 6	Isoflavone reductase homologue
	Cor a 8	Nonspecific lipid transfer protein type 1
	Cor a 9	11S seed storage globulin (legumin-like)
	Cor a 10	Luminal binding protein
	Cor a 11	7S seed storage globulin (vicilin-like)
	Cor a 12	17 kDa oleosin
	Cor a 13	14–16 kDa oleosin
	Cor a 14	2S albumin
Pecan *(Carya illinoinensis)*	Car i 1	2S albumin seed storage protein
	Car i 4	Legumin seed storage protein
Pistachio *(Pistacia vera)*	Pis v 1	2S albumin
	Pis v 2	11S globulin subunit
	Pis v 3	Vicilin
	Pis v 4	Manganese superoxide dismutase
	Pis v 5	11S globulin subunit
Black walnut *(Juglans nigra)*	Jug n 1	2S albumin seed storage protein
	Jug n 2	Vicilin seed storage protein
English walnut *(Juglans regia)*	Jug r 1	2S albumin seed storage protein
	Jug r 2	Vicilin seed storage protein
	Jug r 3	Nonspecific lipid transfer protein type 1
	Jug r 4	11S globulin seed storage protein
Chestnut *(Castanea sativa)*	Cas s 1	Pathogenesis-related protein, PR-10, Bet v 1 family member
	Cas s 5	Chitinase
	Cas s 8	Nonspecific lipid transfer protein type 1
	Cas s 9	Cytosolic class I small heat shock protein

Extracted from the International Union of Immunological Societies, Allergen Nomenclature Subcommittee website, http://www.allergen.org [48].

extracted from the World Health Organization/International Union of Immunological Studies Allergen Nomenclature website [48].

Hazelnut (Corylus avellana)
The hazelnut tree is a member of the Betulaceae family, which also includes the birch and alder trees. Hazelnut sensitization may primarily be directed toward unique hazelnut proteins, or it may be secondary to a birch tree pollen allergy, or both. Cor a 1 is a pathogenesis-related (PR-10) family protein and a homolog of Bet v 1, the major birch pollen allergen, and it has generally been implicated in oral allergy symptoms to hazelnut. Less is known about Cor a 2, a profilin that is homologous to birch pollen Bet v 2 and can also cause oral allergy symptoms in individuals sensitized to birch pollen and grass pollen, sometimes in the absence of Cor a 1 sensitization [66].

Several other allergens in hazelnut may account for hazelnut allergy in non-pollen-sensitized individuals. Cor a 8 (an LTP) is a heat-stable seed storage protein that is homologous to allergens in peanut and other tree nuts and is not cross-reactive with pollen allergens. Several studies have shown that Cor a 8 is associated with severe allergic reactions to hazelnut [66, 67]. Cor a 9, an 11S (legumin-like) globulin that is homologous to allergens in cashew, peanut, and soybean, has been found in 87% of subjects with systemic reactions to hazelnut in one study, most of whom were children [68]. Another study has found sensitization to Cor a 11 (7S vicilin) among patients with systemic reactions to hazelnut [69]. Sensitization to 2S albumins and oleosins in hazelnut may also be clinically relevant; however, more data are needed [66, 70]. Cor a 9 and Cor a 14 are heat stable storage proteins in hazelnut. A study of patients who underwent double-blind placebo-controlled hazelnut food challenges showed highly specific sensitizations to Cor a 9 and Cor a 14 as markers of a more severe hazelnut allergic phenotype [71].

Regional and age-related differences in sensitization to different hazelnut allergens have been demonstrated, especially in birch tree-endemic areas. One Belgian study has found that preschool and school-aged children are disproportionately sensitized to Cor a 9, with systemic reactions to hazelnut, whereas adults are sensitized to Cor a 1 and primarily exhibit oral allergy symptoms caused by hazelnut [72]. Even within Europe, substantially different hazelnut component sensitization and clinical reactivity patterns have been demonstrated among different geographical regions, as has been demonstrated in one study comparing sera from hazelnut-allergic patients in Denmark, Switzerland, and Spain. In this study, all of the patients (100%) in the northern European countries of Switzerland and Denmark were sensitized to recombinant rCor a 1, and only 15% and 5%, respectively, were sensitized to rCor a 8. Among the hazelnut-allergic patients in Spain, however, rCor a 8 sensitization prevailed, affecting 71% of the patients, while only 18% possessed IgE specific to Cor a 1 [73].

Walnut (Juglans regia) and Pecan (Carya illinoinensis)
There are about 20 recognized species of walnut trees worldwide. *Juglans nigra* and *Juglans californica* are common trees in North America, but the nuts are rarely eaten. Most walnut allergies are related to English walnut *(Juglans regia)*, which is more widely consumed [47]. In a voluntary US registry of peanut and tree nut allergy, walnut has been determined to be the most common tree nut allergy [11]. Four English walnut allergens have been described and cloned, including Jug r 1 (2S albumin), Jug r 2 (7S vicilin-like protein), Jug r 3 (LTP), and Jug r 4 (legumin-like 11S seed storage protein). Jug r 1 and Jug r 2 IgE binding have been demonstrated in walnut-allergic patient sera [74].

There is considerable *in vitro* immunogenic cross-reactivity between walnut and pecan, another member of the Juglandaceae family [75]. Pecans are widely grown and are popular in the southern

US. Among self-reported tree nut-allergic individuals in the US, 9% have reported a pecan allergy [11]. Two major pecan allergens have been identified, Car i 1 (2S albumin) and Car i 4 (11S legumin), which show cross-reactivity with walnut Jug r 1 and Jug r 4, respectively [75, 76]. Jug r 4 also shows cross-reactivity with hazelnut Cor a 9.

Cashew (Anacardium occidentale) and Pistachio (Pistacia vera)

Cashew and pistachio are closely related tree nuts of the Anacardiaceae family. Cashew nut allergy is the second most commonly reported IgE-mediated tree nut allergy, and it has been reported by 44% of 82 tree nut-allergic individuals in a US survey and 22% of those reporting a pistachio allergy [19]. Cashew has been identified as causing more severe reactions than peanut in a case-matched comparison of cashew- and peanut-allergic children performed in the UK [77]. Patients are often co-sensitized to cashew and pistachio, and significant homology to cashew allergens has been demonstrated for pistachio.

The major cashew allergens include Ana o 1 (7S vicilin), Ana o 2 (11S globulin), and Ana o 3 (2S albumin), which are all seed storage proteins [78–80]. In a study of 20 cashew-allergic patient serum samples, 50% recognized Ana o 1 [78]. Pistachio demonstrates *in vitro* cross-reactivity with cashew and mango [81]. Pis v 1 (2S albumin) and Pis v 2 (11S globulin) have been identified and are homologous to Ana o 3 and Ana o 2, respectively. Both recombinant Pis v 1 and Pis v 2 have shown significant binding in the sera of pistachio-allergic patients [82]. IgE reactivity in cashew- and pistachio-allergic patients has also been demonstrated to another allergen isolated from pistachio, Pis v 3, (7S vicilin), which shares cross-reactivity with Ana o 1 from cashew [83].

Almond (Prunus dulcis)

Almond is one of the most commonly consumed tree nuts in the world, with the US and Spain leading in world production [84]. Almond aller-gy is the third most common tree nut allergy in the US, with 15% of tree nut-allergic patients reporting reactivity [11]. Eight groups of allergenic proteins have been identified in almond; however, only a few have been linked to clinical reactivity, including Pru du 1 (PR-10 allergen), Pru du 3 (nsLTP), Pru du 4 (profilin), Pru du 5, and Pru du 6 (11S globulin) [84]. Almond is a member of the Rosaceae family, and an allergy to this tree nut may present as oral allergy symptoms due to cross-reactivity between the PR-10 protein, Pru du 1, and Bet v 1 from birch pollen, although these same allergens may cause severe allergic reactions. In Mediterranean countries, sensitization to Pru du 3 can trigger severe reactions to almond as well as to other Rosaceae fruits [85]. Pru du 4 is a panallergen that shares homology with profilins from many plant sources. Pru du 4 is not stable to heat or gastric digestion; thus, reactivity to this allergen is most often associated with symptoms limited to the oral cavity or with no symptoms at all [86]. Pru du 5 has shown IgE binding in the sera of almond-allergic patients; however, further study is needed to determine the clinical ramifications of sensitization to this allergen [87]. Pru du 6 (amandin) has been identified as a major almond allergen that accounts for approximately 65–75% of the total proteins in almond. This allergen is a storage protein [88] that is highly resistant to heat and processing treatments [89]. Roux et al. have reported that 50% of serum samples from patients with a severe allergy to almond demonstrate IgE binding to Pru du 6 [47].

Other Tree Nuts

Allergens in other less commonly consumed tree nuts, such as pine nut, Brazil nut, chestnut, and macadamia, have also been identified and classified (see table 2) [48]. Allergy to coconut, typically classified as a fruit (a one-seeded drupe), is rare, although IgE binding to coconut proteins has been shown in sera from walnut-allergic patients, indicating the existence of some cross-reactivity between walnut and coconut [90]. There are also some tree nuts that are not common to the western diet, such as nangai nut from Micronesia and acorn, which have been associated with clinical allergies, but limited relevant data are available [91, 92]. Shea nut, which is distantly related to Brazil nut and cross-reacts with almond, hazelnut, walnut and peanut, is widely used in foods and topical cosmetic products, often in the form of shea butter [93]. Allergic reactions to shea nut or shea butter have not been reported to date, and the allergenicity of shea nut is still not known. In a study seeking to determine whether IgE from the sera of peanut- or tree nut-allergic patients recognizes shea nut (processed by water/salt extraction) or shea butter proteins, no IgE binding was detected by Western blot or ELISA, and it was suggested that shea nut and shea nut butter contain low levels of protein [93]. Furthermore, there are many other edible tree nuts that have not been thoroughly studied nor associated with a significant allergy risk.

Pathogenesis
Allergy to peanut and tree nuts may develop via primary sensitization directly to the foods themselves or by secondary sensitization to plant or other cross-reactive allergens. Peanut and tree nuts may be more allergenic than other food allergens for several reasons. Seed storage proteins, the major allergens in peanut and tree nuts, are glycosylated proteins that contain disulfide bonds. These features confer stability to the protein structures under conditions of high temperature and extreme pH, such as those occurring during gastric digestion [63]. There is a genetic predisposition to peanut allergy, with a 7% sibling risk, but the apparent increase in prevalence may be attributed to environmental factors [1]. Theories regarding this increase are numerous.

Furthermore, there may be factors in the harvesting and processing of peanuts that contribute to their increased allergenicity. For example, Ara h 1 can be extracted at increased concentrations under conditions of curing and drying at higher temperatures [94]. The high heat of roasting results in a Maillard reaction, whereby the glycosylation of amino groups forms stable advanced glycation end products [95]. Extractable Ara h 1 has been shown to be 22-fold higher in peanuts roasted for 10–15 min compared with raw peanuts [96]. Frying or boiling peanuts produces fewer allergenic peanut products in comparison [97]. Additionally, most manufactured peanut butters are homogenized such that the peanut proteins are emulsified in vegetable oils. This process may also increase the immunogenicity of the peanut proteins that are ingested [98]. Additional factors that promote the allergenicity of peanut and tree nuts may include food matrices and other processes in the manufacture of peanut and tree nuts for consumption.

The timing of ingestion of peanut has also been considered to be a potential risk factor for the development of peanut allergy, as illustrated by the observation that Jews in Israel have an approximately 10% lower rate of peanut allergy compared with Jews in the UK, with the primary difference in exposure being a significantly later oral introduction in the UK cohort [99]. Recent theories and data suggest that the increased rates of peanut allergy may be attributed to the bypassing of oral tolerance due to the delay in its introduction to childrens' diets during periods of frequent environmental exposure to peanut, thereby promoting sensitization [100].

Conclusion

Peanut and tree nuts are popular in diets around the world and have emerged as important food allergens in many regions. Allergic reactions to peanut and tree nuts are often severe and can be fatal; thus, sensitization and allergies to peanut and tree nuts have become major health issues. Much research has been performed in recent years to determine the clinically relevant allergens in peanut and in individual tree nuts; however, more research is needed. In most cases, these are life-long food allergies; however, natural history studies have demonstrated that some individuals will outgrow their peanut and/or tree nut allergies. Diagnostic modalities, management, and promising therapeutic interventions for peanut and tree nut allergies are evolving and are discussed in detail elsewhere in this volume.

References

1 Sicherer SH, Sampson HA: Peanut allergy: emerging concepts and approaches for an apparent epidemic. J Allergy Clin Immunol 2007;120:491–503.
2 Sicherer SH: Epidemiology of food allergy. J Allergy Clin Immunol 2011;127:594–602.
3 Lieberman JA, Sicherer SH: Quality of life in food allergy. Curr Opin Allergy Clin Immunol 2011;11:236–242.
4 King RM, Knibb RC, Hourihane JO: Impact of peanut allergy on quality of life, stress and anxiety in the family. Allergy 2009;64:461–468.
5 Morisset M, Moneret-Vautrin DA, Kanny G, Allergo-Vigilance Network: Prevalence of peanut sensitization in a population of 4,737 subjects – an Allergo-Vigilance Network enquiry carried out in 2002. Eur Ann Allergy Clin Immunol 2005;37:54–57.
6 Osterballe M, Hansen TK, Mortz CG, Høst A, Bindslev-Jensen C: The prevalence of food hypersensitivity in an unselected population of children and adults. Pediatr Allergy Immunol 2005;16:567–573.
7 Dalal I, Binson I, Reifen R, Amitai Z, Shohat T, Rahmani S, et al: Food allergy is a matter of geography after all: sesame as a major cause of severe IgE-mediated food allergic reactions among infants and young children in Israel. Allergy 2002;57:362–365.
8 Orhan F, Karakas T, Cakir M, Aksoy A, Baki A, Gedik Y: Prevalence of immunoglobulin E-mediated food allergy in 6–9-year-old urban schoolchildren in the eastern Black Sea region of Turkey. Clin Exp Allergy 2009;39:1027–1035.
9 Shek LP, Lee BW: Food allergy in Asia. Curr Opin Allergy Clin Immunol 2006;6:197–201.
10 Teuber SS, Comstock SS, Sathe SK, Roux KH: Tree nut allergy. Curr Allergy Asthma Rep 2003;3:54–61.
11 Sicherer SH, Furlong TJ, Munoz-Furlong A, Burks AW, Sampson HA: A voluntary registry for peanut and tree nut allergy: characteristics of the first 5149 registrants. J Allergy Clin Immunol 2001;108:128–132.
12 Fleischer DM, Conover-Walker MK, Matsui EC, Wood RA: The natural history of tree nut allergy. J Allergy Clin Immunol 2005;116:1087–1093.
13 Ewan PW: Clinical study of peanut and tree nut allergy in 62 consecutive patients: new features and associations. BMJ 1996;312:1074–1078.
14 Sicherer SH, Burks AW, Sampson HA: Clinical features of acute allergic reactions to peanut and tree nuts in children. Pediatrics 1998;102:e6.
15 Ewan PW, Clark AT: Long-term prospective observational study of patients with peanut and nut allergy after participation in a management plan. Lancet 2001;357:111–115.
16 Skolnick HS, Conover-Walker MK, Koerner CB, Sampson HA, Burks W, Wood RA: The natural history of peanut allergy. J Allergy Clin Immunol 2001;107:367–374.
17 Clark AT, Ewan PW: The development and progression of allergy to multiple nuts at different ages. Pediatr Allergy Immunol 2005;16:507–511.
18 Sicherer SH, Munoz-Furlong A, Burks AW, Sampson HA: Prevalence of peanut and tree nut allergy in the US determined by a random digit dial telephone survey. J Allergy Clin Immunol 1999;103:559–562.
19 Sicherer SH, Munoz-Furlong A, Sampson HA: Prevalence of peanut and tree nut allergy in the United States determined by means of a random digit dial telephone survey: a 5-year follow-up study. J Allergy Clin Immunol 2003;112:1203–1207.
20 Sicherer SH, Munoz-Furlong A, Godbold JH, Sampson HA: US prevalence of self-reported peanut, tree nut, and sesame allergy: 11-year follow-up. J Allergy Clin Immunol 2010;125:1322–1326.
21 Ben-Shoshan M, Kagan RS, Alizadehfar R, Joseph L, Turnbull E, St Pierre Y, et al: Is the prevalence of peanut allergy increasing? A 5-year follow-up study in children in Montreal. J Allergy Clin Immunol 2009;123:783–788.
22 Mullins RJ, Dear KB, Tang ML: Characteristics of childhood peanut allergy in the Australian Capital Territory, 1995 to 2007. J Allergy Clin Immunol 2009;123:689–693.
23 Venter C, Hasan AS, Grundy J, Pereira B, Bernie CC, Voigt K, et al: Time trends in the prevalence of peanut allergy: three cohorts of children from the same geographical location in the UK. Allergy 2010;65:103–108.
24 Bock SA, Munoz-Furlong A, Sampson HA: Further fatalities caused by anaphylactic reactions to food, 2001–2006. J Allergy Clin Immunol 2007;119:1016–1018.
25 Bock SA, Munoz-Furlong A, Sampson HA: Fatalities due to anaphylactic reactions to foods. J Allergy Clin Immunol 2001;107:191–193.
26 Pumphrey RS, Gowland MH: Further fatal allergic reactions to food in the United Kingdom, 1999–2006. J Allergy Clin Immunol 2007;119:1018–1019.
27 Summers CW, Pumphrey RS, Woods CN, McDowell G, Pemberton PW, Arkwright PD: Factors predicting anaphylaxis to peanuts and tree nuts in patients referred to a specialist center. J Allergy Clin Immunol 2008;121:632–638.e2.
28 Simonte SJ, Ma S, Mofidi S, Sicherer SH: Relevance of casual contact with peanut butter in children with peanut allergy. J Allergy Clin Immunol 2003;112:180–182.

29 Wainstein BK, Kashef S, Ziegler M, Jelley D, Ziegler JB: Frequency and significance of immediate contact reactions to peanut in peanut-sensitive children. Clin Exp Allergy 2007;37:839–845.

30 Eigennman PA, Zamora S: An internet-based survey on the circumstances of food-induced reactions following the diagnosis of IgE-mediated food allergy. Allergy 2002;57:449–453.

31 Furlong TJ, DeSimone J, Sicherer SH: Peanut and tree nut allergic reactions in restaurants and other food establishments. J Allergy Clin Immunol 2001; 108:867–870.

32 Green TD, LaBelle VS, Steele PH, Kim EH, Lee LA, Mankad VS, et al: Clinical characteristics of peanut-allergic children: recent changes. Pediatrics 2007; 120:1304–1310.

33 Hourihane JO, Aiken R, Briggs R, Gudgeon LA, Grimshaw KE, DunnGalvin A, et al: The impact of government advice to pregnant mothers regarding peanut avoidance on the prevalence of peanut allergy in United Kingdom children at school entry. J Allergy Clin Immunol 2007;119:1197–1202.

34 Hourihane JO, Kilburn SA, Dean P, Warner JO: Clinical characteristics of peanut allergy. Clin Exp Allergy 1997; 27:634–639.

35 Rosenfeld L, Shreffler W, Bardina L, Niggemann B, Wahn U, Sampson HA, et al: Walnut allergy in peanut-allergic patients: significance of sequential epitopes of walnut homologous to linear epitopes of Ara h 1, 2 and 3 in relation to clinical reactivity. Int Arch Allergy Immunol 2012;157:238–245.

36 Bock SA, Atkins FM: The natural history of peanut allergy. J Allergy Clin Immunol 1989;83:900–904.

37 Yu JW, Kagan R, Verreault N, Nicolas N, Joseph L, St Pierre Y, et al: Accidental ingestions in children with peanut allergy. J Allergy Clin Immunol 2006;118: 466–472.

38 Vander Leek TK, Liu AH, Stefanski K, Blacker B, Bock SA: The natural history of peanut allergy in young children and its association with serum peanut-specific IgE. J Pediatr 2000;137:749–755.

39 Neuman-Sunshine DL, Eckman JA, Keet CA, Matsui EC, Peng RD, Lenehan PJ, et al: The natural history of persistent peanut allergy. Ann Allergy Asthma Immunol 2012;108:326–331.e3.

40 Chiang WC, Pons L, Kidon MI, Liew WK, Goh A, Burks AW: Serological and clinical characteristics of children with peanut sensitization in an Asian community. Pediatr Allergy Immunol 2010; 21(2p2):e429–e438.

41 Hourihane JO, Roberts SA, Warner JO: Resolution of peanut allergy: case-control study. BMJ 1998;316:1271–1275.

42 Sicherer SH, Wood RA: Advances in diagnosing peanut allergy. J Allergy Clin Immunol Pract 2013;1:1–13.

43 Fleischer DM: The natural history of peanut and tree nut allergy. Curr Allergy Asthma Rep 2007;7:175–181.

44 Fleischer DM, Conover-Walker MK, Christie L, Burks AW, Wood RA: Peanut allergy: recurrence and its management. J Allergy Clin Immunol 2004;114:1195–1201.

45 Busse PJ, Nowak-Wegrzyn AH, Noone SA, Sampson HA, Sicherer SH: Recurrent peanut allergy (correspondence). N Engl J Med 2002;347:1535–1536.

46 Scurlock AM, Burks AW: Peanut allergenicity. Ann Allergy Asthma Immunol 2004;93(5 suppl 3):S12–S18.

47 Roux KH, Teuber SS, Sathe SK: Tree nut allergens. Int Arch Allergy Immunol 2003;131:234–244.

48 International Union of Immunological Societies Allergen Nomenclature Subcommittee: Allergen nomenclature. http://www.allergen.org (accessed April 20, 2013).

49 Burks AW, Sampson HA, Bannon GA: Peanut allergens. Allergy 1998;53:725–730.

50 Clarke MC, Kilburn SA, Hourihane JO, Dean KR, Warner JO, Dean TP: Serological characteristics of peanut allergy. Clin Exp Allergy 1998;53:1251–1257.

51 Restani P, Ballabio C, Corsini E, Fiocchi A, Isoardi P, Magni C, et al: Identification of the basic subunit of Ara h 3 as the major allergen in a group of children allergic to peanuts. Ann Allergy Asthma Immunol 2005;94:262–266.

52 Koppelman SJ, Wensing M, Ertmann M, Knulst AC, Knol EF: Relevance of Ara h1, Ara h2 and Ara h3 in peanut-allergic patients, as determined by immunoglobulin E Western blotting, basophil-histamine release and intracutaneous testing: Ara h2 is the most important peanut allergen. Clin Exp Allergy 2004; 34:583–590.

53 Flinterman AE, van Hoffen E, den Hartog Jager CF, Koppelman S, Pasmans SG, Hoekstra MO, et al: Children with peanut allergy recognize predominantly Ara h2 and Ara h6, which remains stable over time. Clin Exp Allergy 2007;37: 1221–1228.

54 Keet CA, Johnson K, Savage JH, Hamilton RG, Wood RA: Evaluation of Ara h2 IgE thresholds in the diagnosis of peanut allergy in a clinical population. J Allergy Clin Immunol Pract 2013;1: 101–103.

55 Pedrosa M, Boyano-Martinez T, Garcia-Ara MC, Caballero T, Quirce S: Peanut seed storage proteins are responsible for clinical reactivity in Spanish peanut-allergic children. Pediatr Allergy Immunol 2012;23:654–659.

56 Lin YT, Wu CT, Cheng JH, Huang JL, Yeh KW: Patterns of sensitization to peanut allergen components in Taiwanese preschool children. J Microbiol Immunol Infect 2012;45:90–95.

57 Asarnoj A, Glaumann S, Elfström L, Lilja G, Lidholm J, Nilsson C, et al: Anaphylaxis to peanut in a patient predominantly sensitized to Ara h6. Int Arch Allergy Immunol 2012;159:209–212.

58 Mittag D, Akkerdaas J, Ballmer-Weber BK, Vogel L, Wensing M, Becker WM, et al: Ara h 8, a Bet v 1-homologous allergen from peanut, is a major allergen in patients with combined birch pollen and peanut allergy. J Allergy Clin Immunol 2004;114:1410–1417.

59 Krause S, Reese G, Randow S, Zennaro D, Quaratino D, Palazzo P, et al: Lipid transfer protein (Ara h 9) as a new peanut allergen relevant for a Mediterranean allergic population. J Allergy Clin Immunol 2009;124:771–778.e5.

60 Shreffler WG, Beyer K, Chu TH, Burks AW, Sampson HA: Microarray immunoassay: association of clinical history, in vitro IgE function, and heterogeneity of allergenic peanut epitopes. J Allergy Clin Immunol 2004;113:776–782.

61 Vereda A, van Hage M, Ahlstedt S, Ibanez MD, Cuesta-Herranz J, van Odijk J, et al: Peanut allergy: Clinical and immunologic differences among patients from 3 different geographic regions. J Allergy Clin Immunol 2011;127:603–607.

62 Burket S: Industry & Trade Summary: Edible Nuts. Washington, DC, United States International Trade Commission, 2000.

63 Breiteneder H, Mills ENC: Food allergens: molecular and immunological characteristics; in Metcalfe DD, Sampson HA, Simon RA (eds): Food Allergy: Adverse Reactions to Foods and Food Additives, ed 4. Oxford, UK, Blackwell Publishing Ltd., 2009, pp 43–61.

64 Astwood JD, Leach JN, Fuchs RL: Stability of food allergens to digestion in vitro. Nat Biotechnol 1996;14:1269–1273.

65 Taylor SL, Lehrer SB: Principles and characteristics of food allergens. Crit Rev Food Sci Nutr 1996;36(suppl):S91–S118.

66 Pastorello EA, Vieths S, Pravettoni V, Farioli L, Trambaioli C, Fortunato D, et al: Identification of hazelnut major allergens in sensitive patients with positive double-blind, placebo-controlled food challenge results. J Allergy Clin Immunol 2002;109:563–570.

67 Flinterman AE, Akkerdaas JH, den Hartog Jager CF, Rigby NM, Fernandez-Rivas M, Hoekstra MO, et al: Lipid transfer protein-linked hazelnut allergy in children from a non-Mediterranean birch-endemic area. J Allergy Clin Immunol 2008;121:423–428.

68 Beyer K, Grishina G, Bardina L, Grishin A, Sampson HA: Identification of an 11S globulin as a major hazelnut food allergen in hazelnut-induced systemic reactions. J Allergy Clin Immunol 2002;110:517–523.

69 Lauer I, Foetisch K, Kolarich D, Ballmer-Weber BK, Conti A, Altmann F, et al: Hazelnut (Corylus avellana) vicilin Cor a 11: molecular characterization of a glycoprotein and its allergenic activity. Biochem J 2004;383:327–334.

70 Akkerdaas JH, Schocker F, Vieths S, Versteeg S, Zuidmeer L, Hefle SL, et al: Cloning of oleosin, a putative new hazelnut allergen, using a hazelnut cDNA library. Mol Nutr Food Res 2006;50:18–23.

71 Masthoff LJ, Mattsson L, Zuidmeer-Jongejan L, Lidholm J, Andersson K, Akkerdaas JH, et al: Sensitization to Cor a 9 and Cor a 14 is highly specific for a hazelnut allergy with objective symptoms in Dutch children and adults. J Allergy Clin Immunol 2013;132:393–399.

72 De Knop KJ, Verweij MM, Grimmelikhuijsen M, Philipse E, Hagendorens MM, Bridts CH, et al: Age-related sensitizatio profiles for hazelnut (Corylus avellana) in a birch-endemic region. Pediatr Allergy Immunol 2011;22:e139–e149.

73 Hansen KS, Ballmer-Weber BK, Sastre J, Lidholm J, Andersson K, Oberhofer H, et al: Component-resolved in vitro diagnosis of hazelnut allergy in Europe. J Allergy Clin Immunol 2009;123:1134–1141.

74 Bannon GA, Ling M, Cockrell G, Sampson HA: Cloning, expression and characterization of two major allergens, Jug n 1 and Jug n 2, from the black walnut, Juglans niger. J Allergy Clin Immunol 2001;107(S):140.

75 Sharma GM, Irsigler A, Dhanarajan P, Ayuso R, Bardina L, Sampson HA, et al: Cloning and characterization of an 11S legumin, Car i 4, a major allergen in pecan. J Agric Food Chem 2011;59:9542–9552.

76 Sharma GM, Irsigler A, Dhanarajan P, Ayuso R, Bardina L, Sampson HA, et al: Cloning and characterization of 2S albumin, Car i 1, a major allergen in pecan. J Agric Food Chem 2011;59:4130–4139.

77 Clark AT, Anagnostou K, Ewan PW: Cashew nut causes more severe reactions than peanut: case-matched comparison in 141 children. Allergy 2007;62:913–916.

78 Wang F, Robotham JM, Teuber SS, Tawde P, Sathe SK, Roux KH: Ana o 1, a cashew (Anacardium occidental) allergen of the vicilin seed storage protein family. J Allergy Clin Immunol 2002;110:160–166.

79 Wang F, Robotham JM, Teuber SS, Sathe SK, Roux KH: Ana o 2, a major cashew (Anacardium occidentale L.) nut allergen of the legumin family. Int Arch Allergy Immunol 2003;132:27–39.

80 Robotham JM, Wang F, Seamon V, Teuber SS, Sathe SK, Sampson HA, et al: Ana o 3, an important cashew nut (Anacardium occidentale L.) allergen of the 2S albumin family. J Allergy Clin Immunol 2004;115:821–830.

81 Fernandez C, Fiandor A, Martinez-Garate A, Martinez Quesada J: Allergy to pistacho: cross-reactivity between pistachio nut and other Anacardiaceae. Clin Exp Allergy 1995;25:1254–1259.

82 Ahn K, Bardina L, Grishina G, Beyer K, Sampson HA: Identification of two pistachio allergens, Pis v 1 and Pis v 2, belonging to the 2S albumin and 11S globulin family. Clin Exp Allergy 2009;39:926–934.

83 Willison LN, Tawde P, Robotham JM, Penney IV RM, Teuber SS, Sathe SK, et al: Pistachio vicilin, Pis v 3, is immunoglobulin E-reactive and cross-reacts with the homologous cashew allergen, Ana o 1. Clin Exp Allergy 2008;38:1229–1238.

84 Costa J, Mafra I, Carrapatoso I, Oliveira MB: Almond allergens: molecular characterization, detection, and clinical relevance. J Agric Food Chem 2012;60:1337–1349.

85 Fernandez-Rivas M, van Ree R, Cuevas M: Allergy to Rosaceae fruits without related pollinosis. J Allergy Clin Immunol 1997;100:728–733.

86 Wensing M, Akkerdaas JH, van Leeuwen WA, Stapel SO, Bruijnzeel-Koomen CA, Aalberse RC, et al: IgE to Bet v 1 and profilin: cross-reactivity patterns and clinical relevance. J Allergy Clin Immunol 2002;110:435–442.

87 Abolhassani M, Roux KH: cDNA cloning, expression and characterization of an allergenic 60s ribosomal protein of almond (Prunus dulcis). Iran J Allergy Asthma Imunol 2009;8:77–84.

88 Sathe SK, Wolf WJ, Roux KH, Teuber SS, Venkatachalam M, Sze-Tao KW: Biochemical characterization of amandin, the major storage protein in almond (Prunus dulcis L.). J Agric Food Chem 2002;50:4333–4341.

89 Venkatachalam M, Teuber SS, Roux KH, Sathe SK: Effects of roasting, blanching, autoclaving, and microwave heating on antigenicity of almond (Prunus dulcis L.). J Ag 2002;50:3544–3548.

90 Teuber SS, Peterson WR: Systemic allergic reaction to coconut (Cocos nucifera) in 2 subjects with hypersensitivity to tree nut and demonstration of cross-reactivity to legumin-like seed storage proteins: new coconut and walnut food allergens. J Allergy Clin Immunol 1999;103:1180–1185.

91 Sten E, Stahl Skov P, Andersen SB, Torp AM, Olesen A, Bindslev-Jensen U, et al: Allergenic components of a novel food, Micronesian nut Nangai (Canarium indicum), shows IgE cross-reactivity in pollen allergic patients. Allergy 2002;57:398–404.

92 Vega A, Domínguez C, Cosmes P, Martínez A, Bartolomé B, Martínez J, et al: Anaphylactic reaction to ingestion of Quercus ilex acorn nut. Clin Exp Allergy 1998;28:739–742.

93 Chawla KK, Bencharitiwong R, Ayuso R, Grishina G, Nowak-Węgrzyn A: Shea butter contains no IgE-binding soluble proteins. J Allergy Clin Immunol 2011; 127:680–682.

94 Chung SY, Butts CL, Maleki SJ, Champagne ET: Linking peanut allergenicity to the processes of maturation, curing, and roasting. J Agric Food Chem 2003; 51:4273–4277.

95 Chung SY, Champagne ET: Allergenicity of Maillard reaction products from peanut proteins. J Agric Food Chem 1999; 47:5227–5231.

96 Pomés A, Butts CL, Chapman MD: Quantification of Ara h1 in peanuts: why roasting makes a difference. Clin Exp Allergy 2006;36:824–830.

97 Mondoulet L, Paty E, Drumare MF, Ah-Leung S, Scheinmann P, Willemot RM, et al: Influence of thermal processing on the allergenicity of peanut proteins. J Agric Food Chem 2005;53:4547–4553.

98 Audibert F, Chedid L: [Increase of immuneresponse by administration of metabolizable vegetable oil emulsions]. C R Acad Sci Hebd Seances Acad Sci D 1975; 280:1629–1632.

99 Du Toit G, Katz Y, Sasieni P, Mesher D, Maleki SJ, Fisher HR, et al: Early consumption of peanuts in infancy is associated with a low prevalence of peanut allergy. J Allergy Clin Immunol 2008;122:984–991.

100 Fox AT, Sasieni P, du Toit G, Syed H, Lack G: Household peanut consumption as a risk factor for the development of peanut allergy. J Allergy Clin Immunol 2009;123:417–423.

Amanda Cox, MD
Brooklyn Pediatric Allergy and Immunology
ProHEALTH Care Associates, LLP
330 Court Street
Brooklyn, NY 11231 (USA)
E-Mail acox@prohealthcare.com

Ebisawa M, Ballmer-Weber BK, Vieths S, Wood RA (eds): Food Allergy: Molecular Basis and Clinical Practice.
Chem Immunol Allergy. Basel, Karger, 2015, vol 101, pp 145–151 (DOI: 10.1159/000375468)

Grain and Legume Allergy

Komei Ito

Department of Allergy, Aichi Children's Health and Medical Center, Aichi, Japan

Abstract

Among grains and legumes, wheat and soybean are the most frequent and well-characterized allergenic foods. Wheat proteins are divided into water/salt-soluble and water/salt-insoluble (gluten) fractions. The most dominant allergen in the former is α-amylase/trypsin inhibitor, which acts as an inhaled allergen causing baker's asthma. Gluten allergens, including ω-5 gliadin and high- and low-molecular-weight glutenins, contribute to wheat-dependent exercise-induced anaphylaxis in adults and immediate-type wheat allergies, including anaphylaxis, in children. Recently, wheat allergies exclusively caused by hydrolyzed wheat proteins or deamidated glutens have been reported, and the presence of unique IgE-binding epitopes has been suggested. Soybean allergens contributing to immediate-type allergic reactions in children are present in seed storage proteins, namely Gly m 5, Gly m 6 and Gly m 8. However, pollen-related soybean allergy in adults is caused by the Bet v 1 homolog of soybeans, Gly m 4. Taken together, the varying clinical manifestations of wheat and soybean allergies are predominantly caused by their different allergen components.

© 2015 S. Karger AG, Basel

Grain (Wheat) Allergies

General Description of Wheat Allergens

Grains are cultivated and consumed all over the world and consist of major dietary and nutritional components. Among grains, wheat is a staple food consumed in Western countries, and people in Asian countries consume wheat products in addition to rice in their daily meals.

Wheat flour contains 8% (weak flour) to 12% (strong flour) proteins. These proteins are classified as water/salt-soluble (albumin/globulin) and water/salt-insoluble (gluten), the latter of which comprises 80% of the total wheat proteins. Gluten is composed of large disulfide-linked polymers of gliadin and glutenin, which gives viscoelasticity to dough and a chewy texture to the final food product. Gliadins are characterized as glutamine-rich, alcohol-soluble cereal storage prolamins and are categorized as α/β-, γ-, and ω-gliadins. Glutenins are alcohol-insoluble, acid/base-soluble proteins that are classified as high molecular weight [1] or low molecular weight [2].

Table 1. Nominated wheat allergens and related clinical manifestations

Groups/ Allergen	Biochemical name	MW (SDS-PAGE)	Baker's asthma	Anaphylaxis	WDEIA	HWPEIA
Alpha-amylase/trypsin inhibitor family						
Tri a 15	Monomeric alpha-amylase inhibitor 0.28		●			
Tri a 28	Dimeric alpha-amylase inhibitor 0.19	13	●			
Tri a 29	Tetrameric alpha-amylase inhibitor CM1/CM2	13	●			
Tri a 30	Tetrameric alpha-amylase inhibitor CM3	16	●			
Glutens						
Tri a 21	Alpha-beta-gliadin					●
Tri a 19	Omega-5 gliadin	65		●	●	
Tri a 26	High-molecular-weight glutenin	88		●	●	
Tri a 36	Low-molecular-weight glutenin	40		●	●	
Pan-allergens						
Tri a 12	Profilin	14				
Tri a 14	Non-specific lipid transfer protein 1	9.5	●			
Others						
Tri a 18	Agglutinin isolectin 1	21.2				
Tri a 25	Thioredoxin	13.3	●			
Tri a 37	Alpha purothionin	12	●			
Tri a 27	Thiol reductase homologue	27	●			
Tri a 31	Triosephosphate isomerase	26.8	●			
Tri a 32	1-Cys peroxiredoxin	23.9	●			
Tri a 33	Serpin	43.2	●	●		
Tri a 39	Serine protease inhibitor-like protein		●			
Tri a 34	Glyceraldehyde-3-phosphate dehydrogenase	36.5	●			
Tri a 35	Dehydrin	12.4	●			

IUIS Allergen Nomenclature database, February 2013.

Allergenic components are present in each fraction, and several components contribute to the different clinical manifestations of allergic reactions (table 1).

Baker's Asthma

Occupational sensitization to inhaled wheat allergens with the subsequent elicitation of bronchial asthma upon exposure to airborne wheat flour is known as baker's asthma. Most cases of baker's asthma occur in Western countries; however, some cases have also been reported in Korean bakery workers [3].

The α-amylase/trypsin inhibitor has been identified to be the major allergen contributing to baker's asthma. Monomeric, dimeric and tetrameric forms of the glycosylated subunits have been recognized to be equally allergenic [4]. Nonspecific lipid transfer protein (nsLTP) [5], profilin, serine protease inhibitor (serpin) [6] and other water/salt-soluble proteins have also been identified as wheat allergens causing baker's asthma.

Immediate-Type Food Allergy to Wheat

Immediate-type wheat allergy is common in children in Japan as well as in the US [7], and it sometimes causes anaphylaxis. Based on the results of oral wheat challenge tests conducted at our institute, cutaneous symptoms are provoked in 88% of patients, followed by respiratory symptoms in

Table 2. Provoked symptoms observed in oral wheat challenges

Numbers of positive OFCs	136
Age at OFC: mean ± SD (range)	4.0 ± 2.5 (1.0–12.4) years
sIgE to wheat: median (range)	23.2 (0.36–100<) kU_A/l
Sensitivity (>0.34 kU_A/l)	100%
sIgE to ω-5 gliadin: median (range)	1.38 (<0.34–100<) kU_A/l
Sensitivity (>0.34 kU_A/l)	83.3%
Cumulative dose: median (range)	221 (7.8–2,600) mg protein
Cutaneous/mucosal symptoms	119 (88%)
Respiratory symptoms	100 (74%)
Gastrointestinal symptoms	26 (19%)
Cardiovascular symptoms	7 (5%)
Administration of epinephrine	9 (6.6%)

Based on a total of 177 open wheat challenges using udon noodles conducted at the Aichi Children's Health and Medical Center between April 2011 and November 2012.

74% (table 2). ω-5 Gliadin has been identified as the primary wheat allergen [8], and fitted predicted probability curves for ω-5 gliadin [9] are available for clinical use. The α-amylase/trypsin inhibitor, nsLTP and low-molecular-weight glutenin have also been identified to be important allergens in adult patients with wheat allergy in Europe [10].

Children with immediate-type wheat allergies are expected to achieve resolution. Based on a report of 103 cases, the rate of resolution is 29% by the age of 4 years, 56% by 8 years and 65% by 12 years. Higher wheat IgE levels are associated with poorer outcomes [11]. Decreased specific IgE (sIgE) levels of ω-5 gliadin, even those <0.35 kU_A/l, can be predictive of the outgrowing of wheat allergies over approximately 2 years of follow-up [12].

Wheat-Dependent Exercise-Induced Anaphylaxis
Wheat is the predominant food causing food-dependent exercise-induced anaphylaxis, also designated as wheat-dependent exercise-induced anaphylaxis (WDEIA). The major contributing allergens to WDEIA have been identified to be ω-5 gliadin and high-molecular-weight glutenin [13]. Exercise and/or nonsteroidal anti-inflam-

matory drugs facilitate allergen absorption from the gastrointestinal tract, and immunoreactive gliadin is detected in the sera of affected patients during positive challenge tests [14].

Allergies to Hydrolyzed Wheat Proteins or Deamidated Gluten
A new subtype of WDEIA has been reported among patients who have used soap containing acid-hydrolyzed wheat protein (HWP) [15]. The predominant symptom is angioedema of the eyelids during anaphylaxis, and almost half of the patients also develop contact allergies to the soap, suggesting that they are sensitized to HWP via percutaneous and/or rhinoconjunctival routes [16]. sIgE antibodies to HWP are detected in the sera, whereas sIgE to ω-5 gliadin is almost always negative.

In addition, patients exclusively allergic to deamidated gluten but tolerant to wheat have been reported. Deamidated gluten is a product of the acid or alkali treatment of gluten for the purpose of improving water solubility. Deamidation removes the amide group from glutamine (Q) residues, resulting in the formation of corresponding glutamic acid (E) residues. The sera of affected patients display sIgE binding to deamidated γ- and ω2-gliadins. A consensus epitope, QPQQPFPQ, has been repeatedly found within the sequences of native γ- and ω2-gliadins, and the substitution of three glutamines, QPEEPFPE, best increases its recognition [17].

Allergies to Other Grains

In Asian countries, especially Korea and Japan, buckwheat *(Fagopyrum esculentum)* is a well-known allergenic food that causes anaphylactic reactions. However, limited information about buckwheat allergens is currently available. Fag e 2 (2S albumin) and Fag e 3 (vicilin) have been included in the IUIS allergen database; however, the sample sizes and diagnostic procedures used in clinical studies have not been sufficient to obtain conclusive knowledge regarding the primary buckwheat allergens contributing to anaphylaxis.

Sensitization to rice, corn and other plant foods is common in patients with atopic dermatitis; however, few convincing cases of allergic reactions have been reported. A 16 kD rice protein has been reported to be a cross-reactive IgE binding protein [18] between cereal grains, although the subjects in that study were not clinically allergic to rice or other cereals.

A Case of Successful Oral Immunotherapy for Wheat Allergy

A 12-year-old boy decided to undergo oral immunotherapy (OIT) for food allergy to wheat. His first episode of anaphylaxis to wheat occurred at 5 months of age, and an oral wheat challenge at 5 years of age resulted in anaphylaxis featuring systemic erythema, wheezing and colic after eating 3 g of udon noodles (78 mg of wheat protein). Before the OIT was administered at 12 years of age, the consumption of 8.5 g of udon noodles was again found to provoke abdominal pain and urticaria. The patient's sIgE levels to wheat and ω-5 gliadin were >100 and 5.47 kU$_A$/l, respectively, before OIT.

Following a rush OIT protocol during 2 weeks of admission, the patient was able to consume 50 g of udon noodles without symptoms. He kept eating the noodles and increased the dose at home, and he passed a 200-g udon challenge after 6 months of therapy. Since then, he has continued to eat wheat products almost freely, and his sIgE titers to wheat and ω-5 gliadin have decreased to 77.9 and 1.63 kU$_A$/l after 1 year and to 52.4 and 1.32 kU$_A$/l after 2 years, respectively.

Legume (Soybean) Allergies

General Description of Legume Allergens

A legume refers to a plant in the family Fabaceae (or Leguminosae) or a fruit of these species. Typical edible legumes and their nominated allergens are listed in table 3. Respiratory allergens from soybean shells (Gly m 1 and Gly m 2) are not included and are not discussed in this chapter.

The major food allergens present in legumes are seed storage proteins. These proteins are traditionally separated by ultracentrifugation into 2S albumin, 7S globulin and 11S globulin. The amino acid sequences of vicilins (7S, Gly m 5) and glycinins (11S, Gly m 6) in soybeans are approximately 50% identical to those of other legume proteins. The sequence of soybean 2S albumin (Gly m 8) is less similar to that of peanuts (34–28%) and even less similar to those of other tree nut allergens.

Gly m 4 is the Bet v 1-homologous allergen in soybean, and it is functionally classified as a pathogenesis-related protein 10 [19]. Profilin (Gly m 3) and nsLTPs also have the potential to cause allergic reactions to soybean.

Cross-reactive carbohydrate determinant (CCD) is present in a wide range of glycoproteins of legumes and tree nuts, and it leads to cross-allergenicity between these foods. The typical structure of CCD is an N-linked glycan composed of a mannose framework, and the presence of xylose and fucose residues contributes to IgE binding [20]. Due to its reduced potential to induce

Table 3. Officially accepted food allergens from legumes

Common name	Scientific name	Seed storage proteins			Pan-allergens			
		2S albumin	7S globulin β-conglycinin, vicilin	11S globulin glycinin, legumin	Bet v 1 homolog PR-10	Profilin	nsLTP	Oleosin
Soybean	*Glycine max*	Gly m 8	Gly m 5	Gly m 6	Gly m 4	Gly m 3		
Peanut	*Arachis hypogaea*	Ara h 2, Ara h 6, Ara h 7	Ara h 1	Ara h 3, Ara h 4	Ara h 8	Ara h 5	Ara h 9	Ara h 10, Ara h 11
Pea	*Pisum sativum*		Pis s 1	Pis s 2 (convicilin)				
Lentil	*Lens culinaris*		Len c 1 (gamma-vicilin subunit)				Len c 3	
Common bean, kidney bean, green bean, French bean	*Phaseolus vulgaris*						Pha v 3	
Mung bean, green gram	*Vigna radiata*	Vig r 4	Vig r 2		Vig r 1, Vig r 6			
Lupin	*Lupinus angustifolius*		Lup an 1					

IUIS allergen nomenclature database, January 2015.

histamine release from mast cells and basophils, sIgE to CCD causes almost no allergic reactions in sensitized patients [21].

Immediate-Type Food Allergy to Soybean
Soybeans are one of the eight common foods causing immediate-type allergic reactions that require emergency visits in Japan. The allergic manifestations observed in 33 children have included cutaneous symptoms in 91% and respiratory symptoms in 36% [22]. The natural history of soybean allergies [23] shows that resolution is obtained in 25% of affected patients by 4 years of age, 45% by 6 years of age and 69% by 10 years of age.

Gly m 5 and Gly m 6 have been identified to be the major allergenic components involved in immediate-type soybean allergies in children [24]; however, the specificity of tests evaluating sIgE to Gly m 5/6 is limited because of the existence of children with nonsymptomatic sensitization [22]. Soybean 2S albumin (Gly m 8) has also been identified as a major allergen in soybean with a high diagnostic value [25].

Pollen-Related Soybean Allergies
Adult patients with soybean allergies in Japan [26], as well as in Europe [19], are predominantly sensitized to Gly m 4, but not Gly m 5/6. Such patients are primarily sensitized to birch or alder pollen, belonging to the Betulaceae family. The most frequent symptom is oral allergy syndrome; however, lower respiratory symptoms, gastrointestinal symptoms and anaphylaxis have also been reported. Soymilk is the most allergy-provoking food, while fermented soy products, such as natto, miso and soy sauce, rarely provoke symptoms.

Other Legume Allergies
Except for peanut (see Cox and Sicherer, pp. 131–144) there is little information about allergies to other legumes. Among 44 Spanish children with legume allergies [27], allergies to lentils were the most frequent (80%), followed by chickpeas (59%). Allergic reactions to more than one legume (median: three legumes) have been observed in 69% of children, suggesting the presence of cross-reactivity between these foods.

Conclusions

The variable clinical manifestations of wheat and soybean allergies are predominantly caused by different allergen components. Component-resolved diagnostics may contribute to obtaining more precise clinical diagnoses of these plant food allergies.

Acknowledgments

This review was partially supported by a research grant from the Ministry of Health, Labor and Welfare of Japan.

References

1 Matsuo H, Kohno K, Niihara H, Morita E: Specific IgE determination to epitope peptides of omega-5 gliadin and high molecular weight glutenin subunit is a useful tool for diagnosis of wheat-dependent exercise-induced anaphylaxis. J Immunol 2005;175:8116–8122.

2 Baar A, Pahr S, Constantin C, Scheiblhofer S, Thalhamer J, Giavi S, Papadopoulos NG, Ebner C, Mari A, Vrtala S, Valenta R: Molecular and immunological characterization of Tri a 36, a low molecular weight glutenin, as a novel major wheat food allergen. J Immunol 2012;189:3018–3025.

3 Hur GY, Koh DH, Kim HA, Park HJ, Ye YM, Kim KS, Park HS: Prevalence of work-related symptoms and serum-specific antibodies to wheat flour in exposed workers in the bakery industry. Respir Med 2008;102:548–555.

4 Sander I, Rozynek P, Rihs HP, van Kampen V, Chew FT, Lee WS, Kotschy-Lang N, Merget, R, Bruning T, Raulf-Heimsoth M: Multiple wheat flour allergens and cross-reactive carbohydrate determinants bind IgE in baker's asthma. Allergy 2011;66:1208–1215.

5 Palacin A, Quirce S, Armentia A, Fernandez-Nieto M, Pacios LF, Asensio T, Sastre J, Diaz-Perales A, Salcedo G: Wheat lipid transfer protein is a major allergen associated with baker's asthma. J Allergy Clin Immunol 2007;120:1132–1138.

6 Mameri H, Denery-Papini S, Pietri M, Tranquet O, Larre C, Drouet M, Paty E, Jonathan AM, Beaudouin E, Moneret-Vautrin DA, Moreau T, Briozzo P, Gaudin JC: Molecular and immunological characterization of wheat Serpin (Tri a 33). Mol Nutr Food Res 2012;56:1874–1883.

7 Ellman LK, Chatchatee P, Sicherer SH, Sampson HA: Food hypersensitivity in two groups of children and young adults with atopic dermatitis evaluated a decade apart. Pediatr Allergy Immunol 2002;13:295–298.

8 Ito K, Futamura M, Borres MP, Takaoka Y, Dahlstrom J, Sakamoto T, Tanaka A, Kohno K, Matsuo H, Morita E: IgE antibodies to omega-5 gliadin associate with immediate symptoms on oral wheat challenge in Japanese children. Allergy 2008;63:1536–1542.

9 Ebisawa M, Shibata R, Sato S, Borres MP, Ito K: Clinical utility of IgE antibodies to omega-5 gliadin in the diagnosis of wheat allergy: a pediatric multicenter challenge study. Int Arch Allergy Immunol 2012;158:71–76.

10 Pastorello EA, Farioli L, Conti A, Pravettoni V, Bonomi S, Iametti S, Fortunato D, Scibilia J, Bindslev-Jensen C, Ballmer-Weber B, Robino AM, Ortolani C: Wheat IgE-mediated food allergy in European patients: alpha-amylase inhibitors, lipid transfer proteins and low-molecular-weight glutenins. Allergenic molecules recognized by double-blind, placebo-controlled food challenge. Int Arch Allergy Immunol 2007;144:10–22.

11 Keet CA, Matsui EC, Dhillon G, Lenehan P, Paterakis M, Wood RA: The natural history of wheat allergy. Ann Allergy Asthma Immunol 2009;102:410–415.

12 Shibata R, Nishima S, Tanaka A, Borres MP, Morita E: Usefulness of specific IgE antibodies to omega-5 gliadin in the diagnosis and follow-up of Japanese children with wheat allergy. Ann Allergy Asthma Immunol 2011;107:337–343.

13 Morita E, Matsuo H, Chinuki Y, Takahashi H, Dahlstrom J, Tanaka A: Food-dependent exercise-induced anaphylaxis -importance of omega-5 gliadin and HMW-glutenin as causative antigens for wheat-dependent exercise-induced anaphylaxis. Allergol Int 2009;58:493–498.

14 Matsuo H, Morimoto K, Akaki T, Kaneko S, Kusatake K, Kuroda T, Niihara H, Hide M, Morita E: Exercise and aspirin increase levels of circulating gliadin peptides in patients with wheat-dependent exercise-induced anaphylaxis. Clin Exp Allergy 2005;35:461–466.

15 Chinuki Y, Morita E: Wheat-dependent exercise-induced anaphylaxis sensitized with hydrolyzed wheat protein in soap. Allergol Int 2012;61:529–537.

16 Fukutomi Y, Itagaki Y, Taniguchi M, Saito A, Yasueda H, Nakazawa T, Hasegawa M, Nakamura H, Akiyama K: Rhinoconjunctival sensitization to hydrolyzed wheat protein in facial soap can induce wheat-dependent exercise-induced anaphylaxis. J Allergy Clin Immunol 2012;127:531–533.e1–e3.

17 Denery-Papini S, Bodinier M, Larre C, Brossard C, Pineau F, Triballeau S, Pietri M, Battais F, Mothes T, Paty E, Moneret-Vautrin DA: Allergy to deamidated gluten in patients tolerant to wheat: specific epitopes linked to deamidation. Allergy 2012;67:1023–1032.

18 Urisu A, Yamada K, Masuda S, Komada H, Wada E, Kondo Y, Horiba F, Tsuruta M, Yasaki T, Yamada M: 16-kilodalton rice protein is one of the major allergens in rice grain extract and responsible for cross-allergenicity between cereal grains in the Poaceae family. Int Arch Allergy Appl Immunol 1991;96:244–252.

19 Kleine-Tebbe J, Vogel L, Crowell DN, Haustein UF, Vieths S: Severe oral allergy syndrome and anaphylactic reactions caused by a Bet v 1- related PR-10 protein in soybean, SAM22. J Allergy Clin Immunol 2002;110:797–804.

20 van Ree R, Cabanes-Macheteau M, Akkerdaas J, Milazzo JP, Loutelier-Bourhis C, Rayon C, Villalba M, Koppelman S, Aalberse R, Rodriguez R, Faye L, Lerouge P: Beta(1,2)-xylose and alpha(1,3)-fucose residues have a strong contribution in IgE binding to plant glycoallergens. J Biol Chem 2000;275: 11451–11458.

21 Ito K, Morishita M, Ohshima M, Sakamoto T, Tanaka A: Cross-reactive carbohydrate determinant contributes to the false positive IgE antibody to peanut. Allergol Int 2005;54:387–392.

22 Ito K, Sjolander S, Sato S, Moverare R, Tanaka A, Soderstrom L, Borres M, Poorafshar M, Ebisawa M: IgE to Gly m 5 and Gly m 6 is associated with severe allergic reactions to soybean in Japanese children. J Allergy Clin Immunol 2011; 128:673–675.

23 Savage JH, Kaeding AJ, Matsui EC, Wood RA: The natural history of soy allergy. J Allergy Clin Immunol 2010; 125:683–686.

24 Holzhauser T, Wackermann O, Ballmer-Weber BK, Bindslev-Jensen C, Scibilia J, Perono-Garoffo L, Utsumi S, Poulsen LK, Vieths S: Soybean (Glycine max) allergy in Europe: Gly m 5 (beta-conglycinin) and Gly m 6 (glycinin) are potential diagnostic markers for severe allergic reactions to soy. J Allergy Clin Immunol 2009;123:452–458.

25 Ebisawa M, Brostedt P, Sjölander S, Sato S, Borres MP, Ito K: Gly m 2S albumin is a major allergen with a high diagnostic value in soybean-allergic children. J Allergy Clin Immunol 2013;132:976–978.

26 Fukutomi Y, Sjolander S, Nakazawa T, Borres MP, Ishii T, Nakayama S, Tanaka A, Taniguchi M, Saito A, Yasueda H, Nakamura H, Akiyama K: Clinical relevance of IgE to recombinant Gly m 4 in the diagnosis of adult soybean allergy. J Allergy Clin Immunol 2012;129:860–863.e3.

27 Martinez San Ireneo M, Ibanez MD, Sanchez JJ, Carnes J, Fernandez-Caldas E: Clinical features of legume allergy in children from a Mediterranean area. Ann Allergy Asthma Immunol 2008; 101:179–184.

Komei Ito, MD, PhD
Department of Allergy, Aichi Children's Health and Medical Center
7-426, Morioka, Obu, Aichi 474-8710 (Japan)
E-Mail koumei_itoh@mx.achmc.pref.aichi.jp

Ebisawa M, Ballmer-Weber BK, Vieths S, Wood RA (eds): Food Allergy: Molecular Basis and Clinical Practice.
Chem Immunol Allergy. Basel, Karger, 2015, vol 101, pp 152–161 (DOI: 10.1159/000375508)

Fish and Shellfish Allergy

Meera Thalayasingam[a] · Bee-Wah Lee[a, b]

[a]Department of Paediatrics, Khoo Teck Puat National University Children's Medical Institute,
National University Hospital, Singapore, [b]Department of Paediatrics, Yong Loo Lin School of Medicine,
National University of Singapore, Singapore, Singapore

Abstract

Fish and shellfish consumption has increased worldwide, and there are increasing reports of adverse reactions to fish and shellfish, with an approximate prevalence of 0.5–5%. Fish allergy often develops early in life, whilst shellfish allergy tends to develop later, from adolescence onwards. Little is known about the natural history of these allergies, but both are thought to be persistent. The clinical manifestations of shellfish allergy, in particular, may vary from local to life-threatening 'anaphylactic' reactions within an individual and between individuals. Parvalbumin and tropomyosin are the two major allergens, but several other allergens have been cloned and described. These allergens are highly heat and biochemically stable, and this may in part explain the persistence of these allergies. Diagnosis requires a thorough history, skin prick and in-vitro-specific IgE tests, and oral challenges may be needed for diagnostic confirmation. Strict avoidance of these allergens is the current standard of clinical care for allergic patients, and when indicated, an anaphylactic plan with an adrenaline auto-injector is prescribed. There are no published clinical trials evaluating specific oral immunotherapy for fish or shellfish allergy.

© 2015 S. Karger AG, Basel

Introduction

There has been a worldwide increase of fish and shellfish consumption, possibly in part due to the health concerns associated with red meat and its high levels of dietary fat. Traditionally, seafood has been seen as a healthy alternative, providing a good source of protein, anti-oxidants and, in particular, omega-3 fatty acids. However, the increase in seafood consumption may have partly led to an increase in adverse reactions to these foods. This chapter aims to highlight the varying clinical presentation, the involved allergens, the potential allergenic cross-reactivity within the fish family and between shellfish and other arthropods (arachnids and insects), the specific diagnostic approach of crude vs. commercial extracts, and the natural course and clinical predictive index for transient vs. persistent allergies.

Prevalence

Despite the ubiquity of fish in the diet, the prevalence of fish allergy in Asia and in the rest of the world is relatively low. In a recent population-

Table 1. Classification of shellfish and fish species

Common reference	Phyla	Subphyla	Class	Orders	Common name
Shellfish (Invertebrates)	Arthropoda	Crustacea	Malacostraca		Shrimps (Caridea), prawns (Penaeidea), crabs, lobsters, crayfish
	Mollusca		Gastropoda		Abalone
					Snails (escargot)
			Bivalvia		Mussels, oysters, clams, scallops, cockles
			Cephalopoda		Squids (calamari), octopus, cuttlefish
Fish	Chordata		Agnatha		Lampreys, hagfishes
			Chondrichthyes (cartilaginous fish)		Shark, rays, fins
			Osteichthyes	Gadiformes	Cod, haddock, hake
			(bony fish)	Salmoniformes	Trout, salmon, pike
				Perciformes	Snapper, mackerel, tuna, bonito, grouper, pomfret, threadfin
				Pleuronect-formes	Sole, flounder, halibut, plaice
				Clupeiformes	Indian anchovy

based study, fish allergy in late childhood was more prevalent in the Philippines (2.29%) compared to Singapore (0.26%) and Thailand (0.29%) [1], and the authors speculated that food processing, dietary habits and cultural practices may have accounted for these differences. The figures are similarly low in the West, where a telephone survey done in the US reported a prevalence of fish allergy of 0.2% in children and of 0.5% in adults [2]. On the other hand, shellfish allergy is more prevalent, especially in adolescents and adults, but it has a wide geographical variation. A population survey of teenagers in the Philippines and Singapore reported prevalence rates of 5.12% and 5.23%, respectively, to shellfish [3], and it was reported as the top allergenic food in Hong Kong, accounting for more than a third of all self-reported food allergy reactions [4]. In contrast to the reports from Asia, a similar survey done in the US reported a prevalence of 0.7% in 6–17-year-olds [2]. This phenomenon may not be entirely due to the amount of shellfish being consumed in Asia, as other countries with high seafood consumption rates report a lower prevalence of shellfish allergy. Indeed, it raises the possibility that other factors may be contributory, such as whether there is any correlation between house dust mite and shellfish allergies [5]. Shellfish is also an important cause of food-induced anaphylaxis, which has been predominantly reported in most Asian countries [6].

Classification of Seafood Species

Edible seafood can be categorized into 3 phyla – Mollusca, Arthropoda (crustaceans) and Chordata (fish), which are then divided into multiple subclasses and species [7]. The term 'Shellfish' refers to the two invertebrate groups: the crustaceans and the molluscs (table 1).

Fish species can be divided into two main groups: the bony fish and cartilaginous fish, as outlined in table 1. Bony fish are further subdivided into 45 orders. The most commonly consumed bony fish belong to the orders Salmoniformes (salmon and trout), Cypriniformes (carp), Gadiformes (cod, hake and whiting), Perciformes (perch, mackerel, threadfin, pomfret, tengirri pappan and tuna), and Clupeiformes (Indian anchovy, herring and sardine). The threadfin, pomfret, tengirri and Indian anchovy are commonly consumed in tropical Asia.

Case I

JR is a 19-year old Chinese girl with moderate childhood eczema, symptomatic chronic persistent asthma and allergic rhinitis. She developed several episodes of intermittent throat itchiness and urticarial rash after eating shrimp and took anti-histamines to relieve her symptoms. Her parents cautioned her to avoid eating shellfish altogether, and she obliged. She had no known fish allergy. Two years later, she was helping her mother prepare for a barbecue and was de-shelling crab. Within minutes of peeling off the shell of a crab, she felt her throat itch and lips swell and felt flushed. She then developed an intractable cough and had chest tightness. Her parents alerted the emergency services, and she was administered intramuscular adrenaline and taken to the hospital for observation for possible biphasic reactions.

At the allergy clinic, she underwent SPTs to house dust mites, cockroaches and an extensive panel of shellfish allergens, which revealed strongly positive reactions to prawn, crab and house dust mites. Her allergen-specific IgE level to shrimp was 23 kU/l, to crab was 20 kU/l, to squid was 10.5 kU/l, to octopus was 8 kU/l, to scallop was 5 kU/l, to clam was 4.4 kU/l, to mackerel was 2.9 kU/l, to tuna was 2.3 kU/l, and to oyster was 1 kU/l; and the specific IgE levels to *Dermatophagoides farina* and *D. pteronyssinus* were >100.

Case Discussion
This case illustrates the varying severity of reactions in the same individual to shellfish. Initially, JR's reactions were mild and localized, involving mainly the cutaneous system. However, this was not a reliable predictor of the subsequent reaction, which was a severe, IgE-mediated reaction resulting in bronchospasm, i.e. anaphylaxis. Interestingly, although the most common route of exposure is gastrointestinal, contact and inhalant routes are also well described.

Clinical Manifestations

The clinical features of fish and shellfish allergies are classically IgE-mediated and can range from trivial to fatal reactions. The typical symptoms of fish allergy are gastrointestinal and include vomiting, diarrhea and abdominal pain. In contrast, the symptoms of shellfish allergy are usually cutaneous and include throat and lip pruritus, flushing, urticaria and localized angioedema. However, both fish and shellfish can cause severe and life-threatening reactions such as laryngeal edema, asthma and fatal anaphylaxis [8, 9].

There are two relatively unique clinical manifestations of shellfish allergy seen in the Asian-Pacific area, as reviewed by Lee et al. [10]. First, the isolated oral symptoms are confined to the lip and mucosa, which may be reminiscent of the oral allergy syndrome (pollen-food) that occurs when pollen allergy cross-reacts with allergens in fruits and nuts in subjects (see case I). Second is the varying severity of reaction within an individual. The factors responsible for this are not well understood;

however, it has been hypothesized that differences exist in the allergenicity of consumed species of prawns/shrimps and are dependent on which part of the prawn was eaten as well as the method of preparation. Rosa et al. [11] highlighted 3 cases where there was a clinical reaction only to the cephalothorax and not to the abdomen of prawn.

Non-IgE-mediated mechanisms are much less common, and in these cases, patients may experience symptoms of food protein-induced enterocolitis, with predominant gastrointestinal symptoms in children [12] and rarely in adults [13].

An important aspect of fish and shellfish allergy is that clinical symptoms result not only from ingestion but also by inhaling cooking vapors and/or handling of seafood either at home or at work. Occupational fish and shellfish allergy is a well-described entity [14]. Exposures through the inhalation of dust, steam, vapors and seafood proteins generated during cutting, scrubbing, cleaning, degutting, cooking, boiling and drying may be multiple. The most common clinical manifestations are contact urticaria and occupational

	Parvalbumin	Collagen	Enolase	Aldolase	Tropomyosin	Vitellogenin	Calcitonin
Fish							
Clupea harengus (Atlantic Herring)	Clu h 1						
Cyprinus carpio (Common carp)	Cyp c 1						
Gadus callarias (Baltic cod)	Gad c 1	#Gad c Elastin					
Gadus morhua (Atlantic cod)	Gad m 1	#Gad m Gelatin	Gad m 2	Gad m 3			
#Katsuwonus pelamis (Skipjack tuna)	Kat p 1						
Lates calcarifer (Barramundi)	Lat c 1						
Lepidorhombus whiffiagonis (Megrim, Whiff, Gallo)	Lep w 1						
Oncorhynchus keta (Chum Salmon)						Onc k 5	
Oncorhynchus mykiss (Rainbow trout)	Onc m 1						
Oreochromis mossambicus (Mozambique tilapia)					Ore m 4		
#Pampus chinensis (Chinese pomfret)	Pam c 1						
#Polynemus indicus (Threadfin)	Lep l 1						
Salmo salar (Atlantic salmon)	Sal s 1	#Sal s Gelatin	Sal s 2	Sal s 3	#Sal s 4	#Sal s 5	#Sal s
Sardinops sagax	Sar sa 1						
#Scomber japonicus (Chub mackerel)	Sco j 1						
#Scomber australasicus (Blue mackerel)	Sco a 1						
#Scomber scrombrus (Atlantic mackerel)	Sco s 1						
#Scomberomorus guttatus (Tengirri)	Sco g 1						
Sebastes marinus (Ocean perch, redfish, snapper)	Seb m 1						
#Stolephorus indicus (Indian anchovy)	Sto l 1						
#Thunnus obesus (Big eye tuna)	Thu 0 1	#Thu 0					
Thunnus albacares (Yellow fin tuna)	Thu a 1	#Thu a	Thu a 2	Thu a 3			
Xiphias gladius (Swordfish)	Xip g 1						

Allergen nomenclature obtained from the official International Union of Immunological Societies database (http://www.allergen.org); # Allergome database (http://www.allergome.com).

asthma [15]. Although there is no known cross-reactivity between fish and shellfish, concurrent fish and shellfish allergies have been described [9].

Fish and Shellfish Allergens

Many allergens have been described in fish and shellfish allergy. These allergens have been listed in the official database of the International Union of Immunological Societies Allergen Nomenclature Subcommittee (http://www.allergen.org); however, an increasing number of allergens have also been identified using the Allergome database (http://www.allergome.com). The major fish allergen is parvalbumin, a 12-kDa sarcoplasmic protein; however, other proteins have been iden-

tified (table 2). The most extensively studied parvalbumin is Gad c 1 (the major allergen in cod fish) that regulates calcium switching in muscular skeletal cells and is distributed universally in the white muscle of fish. White muscle is used for short bouts of swimming and is more prevalent in cod and flounder compared to tuna and skipjack, which are therefore less allergenic [16]. This protein is heat-resistant and has 2 distinct isoform lineages: α and β.

Currently, only the following four major crustacean allergens have been identified and cloned (table 3): Group 1 – tropomyosin, Group 2 – arginine kinase (AK), Group 3 – myosin light chain 2 (MLC), and Group 4 – sarcoplasmic calcium-binding protein (SCP). Tropomyosin is found as 34–36-kDa protein bands and is the major aller-

Table 3. Shellfish allergens and allergen nomenclature

	Tropomyosin	Arginine kinase	Myosin light chain	Sarcoplasmic calcium binding protein	Others
Crustaceans					
Artemia franciscana (Brine shrimp)					Art fr 5 (Myosin l light chain 1)
Crangon crangon (North Sea shrimp)	Cra c 1	Cra c 2		Cra c 4	Cra c 5 (Myosin light chain 1) Cra c 6 (Troponin C) Cra c 8 (Triose phosphate isomerase)
#Fenneropenaeus chinensis (Prawn, fleshy)	Fen c 1	Fen c 2			
#Fenneropenaeus merguiensis	Fen me 1	Fen me 1			
Machrobrachium rosenbergii (Prawn, giant fresh water)	Mac r 1				Mac ro hemocyanin
#Marsupenaeus japonicus (Prawn, tiger)	Mar j 1	Mar j 2			
Melicertus latisulcatus (King prawn)	Mel l 1				
Metapenaeus ensis (Prawn, sand)	Met e 1				
Litopenaeus vannamei (Shrimp, white leg Pacific)	Lit v 1	Lit v 2	Lit v 3	Lit v 4	
Pandalus borealis (Northern shrimp)	Pan b 1				
Penaeus aztecus (Shrimp, brown)	Pen a 1				
Penaeus indicus (Shrimp)	Pen i 1				
Penaeus monodon (Shrimp, Black tiger)	Pen m 1	Pen m 2	Pen m 3	Pen m 4	Pen m 6 (troponin C)
#Penaeus orientalis (Prawn, fleshy)	Fen c 1				
Charybdis feriatus (Crab)	Cha f 1				
#Chionoecetes opilio (Crab, Snow)	Chi o 1	Chi o 2		Chi o 4	
#Euphausia superba (Krill, Antarctic)	Eup s 1				
#Euphausia pacifica (Krill, Pacific)	Eup p 1				
Homarus americanus (Lobster, American)	Hom a 1		Hom a 3		Hom a 6 (troponin c)
#Jasus lalandii (Lobster, Rock)	Jas la 1				
Panulirus stimpsoni (Spiny lobster)	Pan s 1				
Pontastacus leptodactylus (Narrow-clawed crayfish)				Pon l 4	Pon l 7 (troponin 1)
Portunus pelagicus (Blue swimmer crab)	Por p 1				
#Scylla paramamosai (Crab, Mud)	Scy pa 1	Scy pa 2			
Molluscs					
#Buccinum undatum (Common whelk)	Buc u 1				
#Chlamys nipponensis (Scallop, Japanese)	Chl n 1				
#Crassostrea gigas (Oyster, Pacific)	Cra g 1				
#Enis macha (Clam, Razor)	Ens m 1				
#Haliotis discus (Abalone)	Hal d 1				
Haliotis midae (Abalone)	Hal m 1				
#Haliotis rufescens (Abalone)	Hal r 1				
#Helix aspersa (Brown garden snail)	Hel as 1				
#Octopus vulgaris (Octopus, common)	Oct v 1				
#Patinopecten yessoensis (Scallop, Giant)	Pat y 1				
#Perna viridis (Mussel, Tropical green)	Per v 1				
#Todarodes pacificus (Squid)	Tod p 1				
#Venerupis philippinarum (Cockles, Japanese)	Ven ph 1				

Allergen nomenclature obtained from the official International Union of Immunological Societies database (http://www.allergen.org); # Allergome database (http://www.allergome.com).

gen of shellfish [17]. Tropomyosin is highly cross-reactive [18] and is considered a pan-allergen, as it is a well-conserved protein in the invertebrate family. Tropomyosin is essential for muscle contraction [7], but these allergens are not only found in crustaceans (Pen a 1, Pen m 1, Lit v 1, etc.) but also in other invertebrate species such as arachnids (e.g. dust mites), insects (e.g. cockroach) and molluscs. Nomenclature is given according to the species in which the tropomyosin was identified. More than 85% of shrimp-allergic individuals show reactivity to Pen a 1 [19]; likewise, the major allergen in molluscs such as oyster (Cra g 1, Cra g 2), abalone (Hal m 1), snail (Tur c 1) and squid (Tod p 1) is also tropomyosin (table 3).

The Group 2 allergen arginine kinase, a 40-kDa protein, was identified in both the black tiger prawn [20] and subsequently in the white leg Pacific prawn [21]. Arginine kinase is also a pan-allergen and has been identified in other invertebrates such as the moth, cockroach and lobster (ref). Group 3 (myosin light chain) and Group 4 (sarcoplasmic calcium-binding proteins) appear to be especially important in the pediatric age group [22, 23].

However, in addition to these 4 allergens, other IgE-binding proteins have been described, such as that in the North Sea shrimp *(Crangon crangon)* [24]. Further work is therefore necessary to identify the complete panel of crustacean allergens in order to facilitate further clinical evaluation through component-resolved diagnostics and immune therapies.

Allergenic Cross-Reactivity

Parvalbumin within the Fish Group and Frog
Parvalbumin is the major allergen identified in fish and frog muscles. It has been best characterized in cod but also in Atlantic salmon, mackerel and carp, with a deduced amino acid sequence homology of up to 78%. Furthermore, this major allergen was also identified in four tropical fish (threadfin, Indian anchovy, pomfret and tengirri) and has been implicated in tropical fish allergy in Singapore [25]. This observation has clinical relevance when advising fish-allergic patients regarding the ingestion of other fish unless there is already established clinical tolerance. However, Van Do et al.'s study on 9 commonly edible fish challenges this notion and suggests that fish allergy may have species-specific allergenic epitopes [26] (see case II). Cross-reactivity is dependent not only on the expression and distribution of parvalbumin but also on the homology and similarity of shared binding epitopes [27, 28]. There have also been reports of clinical cross-reactivity between parvalbumin of fish and frog [29].

Within the Shellfish Group
It is well reported that tropomyosin is the major allergen responsible for cross-reactions between the Mollusca, Crustacea and Echinodermata phyla [30]. There is a high degree of molecular homology (98%) within the crustacean species and a similar intra-class homology within the molluscs [31]. This unique amino acid homology between the tropomyosin allergens is why blanket shellfish avoidance should be prescribed in all patients with shellfish allergy in the absence of clinical tolerance.

Between Shellfish and Other Arthropods
Shellfish are phytogenetically related to arachnids and insects and belong to the same phylum, *Arthropoda* (fig. 1). Of these, house dust mites (arachnids) and cockroaches (insects) have been best studied in relation to shellfish allergy, with particular reference to the pan-allergen tropomyosin. A unique study amongst Orthodox Jews who suffered from atopy (allergic rhinitis with known dust mite/cockroach sensitivity) and who, by virtue of their religion, were prohibited from consuming shellfish demonstrated skin prick positivity to shrimp [32]. Likewise, similar studies have shown a positive correlation be-

Case II

JA is a 10-month-old Caucasian girl with severe atopic dermatitis who was on a very restrictive diet. Her parents had excluded milk, eggs, soy, wheat, fish and peanuts and noticed dramatic improvement. However, unknown to them, her maternal grandmother had gradually introduced fish into her diet, specifically pomfret, Indian anchovy and tengirri. One morning, grandma decided that she would introduce threadfin into JA's diet, as she had tolerated the other fishes well. After a teaspoon of the threadfin porridge, JA broke out in a perioral rash with generalized hives and later had a flare of her atopic dermatitis.

At the allergy clinic, SPTs and specific IgE tests to cod, threadfin, Indian anchovy, pomfret and tengirri were done. Her SPTs were positive for cod and threadfin and were negative for the other fish. Her total IgE was 2,500, and her specific IgE to cod was 13 kU/l, to threadfin was 60 kU/l, to Indian anchovy was 13 kU/l, to pomfret was 27 kU/l, and to tengirri was 15 kU/l.

Case Discussion
This toddler had an IgE-mediated reaction to threadfin. Generally, most fish-allergic individuals are unable to tolerate most species of fish because of cross-reactivity of the major fish allergen, parvalbumin. However, there are some patients who have species-specific fish allergy. Approximately one-third of children with severe atopic dermatitis may have a food allergy; however, specific IgE to food in atopic dermatitis should be interpreted with caution, as false-positive rates are relatively common.

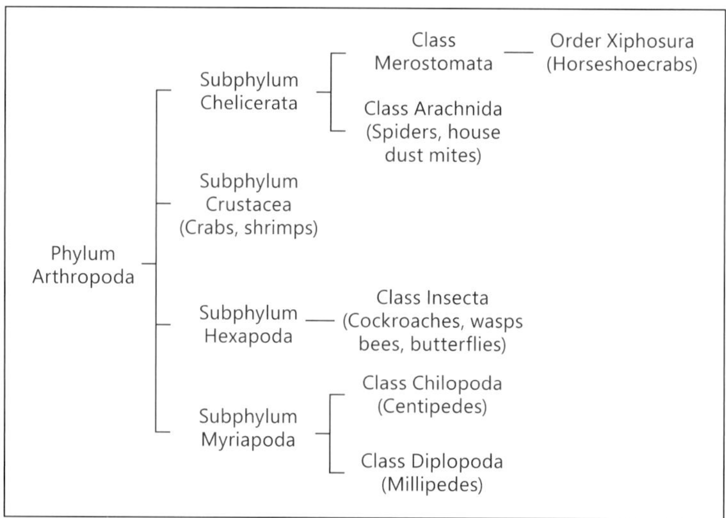

Fig. 1. Phylogenetic relationships of major arthropod species.

tween IgE specific to shrimp, with cockroach and dust-mite exposure demonstrating sensitization, which might or might not correlate with clinical reactivity [33, 34]. The primary sensitization here is possibly through inhalation of these environmental allergens, which may possibly impact food-induced reactions to shellfish; however, this warrants further epidemiological studies.

Differential Diagnosis for Fish and Shellfish Allergy

Adverse reactions to seafood may in fact be secondary to food contamination, toxins (e.g. scombroid poisoning) or preservatives, especially in the presence of negative allergy tests [35]. An astute clinician should consider the possibilities outlined in table 4.

Type of poisoning	Type of toxins	Source	Symptom onset	Clinical syndrome
Scombroid	Histamine	Tuna, mahi-mahi, bonita, marlin, bluefish, wahoo, mackerel, salmon	Minutes–4 hours	Severe headache, dizziness, nausea, vomiting, flushed skin, urticaria and wheezing
Ciguatera	Ciguatoxins	Coral reef fish, amberjack, snappers, grouper, goat fish, barracuda, sea bass, surgeon fish, ulua and paio	30 minutes–4 hours	Abdominal pain, diarrhea, vomiting, paresthesias, cold to hot sensory reversal, weakness and myalgias
Puffer fish poisoning	Tetrodotoxin	Ocean, Sunfishes, porcupine fishes and fugu	10–45 minutes	Paresthesias, headache, vomiting, diaphoresis, and respiratory paralysis
Paralytic fish	Saxitoxins	Mussels, clams, oysters	5–30 minutes	Vomiting diarrhea, facial paresthesia and respiratory symptoms
Neurotoxin	Brevetoxins	Mussels, clams	30 minutes–3 hours	Diarrhea, vomiting, abdominal pain, myalgias, paresthesia and ataxia
Amnesic shellfish	Domoic acid	Mussels, clams, crabs and anchovies	15 minutes–38 hours	Vomiting, diarrhea, headache, myoclonus, loss of short-term memory, seizures, coma and hemiparesis
Diarrhetic shellfish	Okadaic acid, Dinophysis toxins, pectenotoxins, yessotoxin	Mussels, clams and scallops	30 minutes–6 hours	Diarrhea, nausea, vomiting and abdominal pain

Adapted from Chegini and Metcalfe [41].

Diagnosis

History is key to the diagnostic process. Skin prick tests (SPTs) for the shellfish in question as well as for cross-reacting arthropods should be undertaken. An SPT is an inexpensive and relatively easy way for screening patients with a suspected hypersensitivity. SPTs can be initially performed using commercial extracts; however, crude extracts may have better sensitivity and specificity [36]. In addition, shrimp- and fish-specific IgE, in conjunction with a positive SPT, have been found to be useful predictors of a positive challenge [37]. Except for tropomyosin, component-resolved diagnostics have not been widely utilized in clinical practice, and their clinical value has not been widely studied.

Natural History and Treatment

Shellfish allergy tends to persist into adulthood and may be life-threatening. Possible reasons for this may be that these proteins are resistant to heat, denaturing chemicals and proteolytic enzymes. Current guidelines recommend that individuals with shellfish allergy observe strict avoidance, and if reactions are severe, they should be armed with an anaphylactic plan and an adrenaline auto-injector. There are few studies on the natural history of shellfish and fish allergy [38]. A recent paper [39] highlighted that shrimp sensitization decreased with age, with greater epitope recognition in childhood compared to adulthood. There may, therefore, be a possibility that clinical tolerance may develop in some individuals. With regards to fish allergy, recombinant hypoallergenic parvalbumin may represent an interesting candidate vaccine for immunotherapy of fish allergy in the future [40].

Conclusions

Shellfish and fish are considered common food allergens but are less prevalent than allergy to hen's eggs, cow's milk, peanuts or tree nuts. Shellfish allergy tends to occur in adults and older children and is a common cause of anaphylaxis that requires emergency room visits. In contrast, fish allergy tends to occur in young children and seems to be less prevalent than shellfish allergy. There is a paucity of data on the natural history of these allergies, and further work is required to provide a better understanding and to delineate the predictive factors of persistence of the allergy.

References

1　Connett GJ, Gerez I, Cabrera-Morales EA, Yuenyongviwat A, Ngamphaiboon J, Chatchatee P, Sangsupawanich P, Soh SE, Yap GC, Shek LP, Lee BW: A population-based study of fish allergy in the Philippines, Singapore and Thailand. Int Arch Allergy Immunol 2012;159:384–390.

2　Sicherer SH, Munoz-Furlong A, Sampson HA: Prevalence of seafood allergy in the United States determined by a random telephone survey. J Allergy Clin Immunol 2004;114:159–165.

3　Shek LP, Cabrera-Morales EA, Soh SE, Gerez I, Ng PZ, Yi FC, Ma S, Lee BW: A population-based questionnaire survey on the prevalence of peanut, tree nut, and shellfish allergy in 2 Asian populations. J Allergy Clin Immunol 2010;126: 324–331.e1–e7.

4　Ho MH, Lee SL, Wong WH, Ip P, Lau YL: Prevalence of self-reported food allergy in Hong Kong children and teens–a population survey. Asian Pac J Allergy Immunol 2012;30:275–284.

5　Klaewsongkram J: High prevalence of shellfish and house dust mite allergies in Asia-Pacific: probably not just a coincidence. Asian Pac J Allergy Immunol 2012;30:247–248.

6　Yang MS, Lee SH, Kim TW, Kwon JW, Lee SM, Kim SH, Kwon HS, Park CH, Park HW, Kim SS, Cho SH, Min KU, Kim YY, Chang YS: Epidemiologic and clinical features of anaphylaxis in Korea. Ann Allergy Asthma Immunol 2008; 100:31–36.

7　Lehrer SB, Ayuso R, Reese G: Seafood allergy and allergens: a review. Mar Biotechnol (NY) 2003;5:339–348.

8　Wu AY, Williams GA: Clinical characteristics and pattern of skin test reactivities in shellfish allergy patients in Hong Kong. Allergy Asthma Proc 2004;25: 237–242.

9　Turner P, Ng I, Kemp A, Campbell D: Seafood allergy in children: a descriptive study. Ann Allergy Asthma Immunol 2011;106:494–501.

10　Lee AJ, Gerez I, Shek LP, Lee BW: Shellfish allergy–an Asia-Pacific perspective. Asian Pac J Allergy Immunol 2012;30: 3–10.

11　Rosa S, Prates S, Piedade S, Marta CS, Pinto JR: Are there shrimp allergens exclusive from the cephalothorax? Allergy 2007;62:85–87.

12　Zapatero Remon L, Alonso Lebrero E, Martín Fernández E, Martínez Molero MI: Food-protein-induced enterocolitis syndrome caused by fish. Allergol Immunopathol (Madr) 2005;33:312–316.

13　Fernandes BN, Boyle RJ, Gore C, Simpson A, Custovic A: Food protein-induced enterocolitis syndrome can occur in adults. J Allergy Clin Immunol 2012; 130:1199–1200.

14　Jeebhay MF, Lopata AL: Occupational allergies in seafood-processing workers. Adv Food Nutr Res 2012;66:47–73.

15　Jeebhay MF, Cartier A: Seafood workers and respiratory disease: an update. Curr Opin Allergy Clin Immunol 2010;10: 104–113.

16　Kobayashi A, Tanaka H, Hamada Y, Ishizaki S, Nagashima Y, Shiomi K: Comparison of allergenicity and allergens between fish white and dark muscles. Allergy 2006;61:357–363.

17　Ayuso R: Update on the diagnosis and treatment of shellfish allergy. Curr Allergy Asthma Rep 2011;11:309–316.

18　Shanti KN, Martin BM, Nagpal S, Metcalfe DD, Rao PV: Identification of tropomyosin as the major shrimp allergen and characterization of its IgE-binding epitopes. J Immunol 1993;151:5354–5363.

19　Wild LG, Lehrer SB: Fish and shellfish allergy. Curr Allergy Asthma Rep 2005; 5:74–79.

20　Yu CJ, Lin YF, Chiang BL, Chow LP: Proteomics and immunological analysis of a novel shrimp allergen, Pen m 2. J Immunol 2003;170:445–453.

21　Garcia-Orozco KD, Aispuro-Hernández E, Yepiz-Plascencia G, Calderón-de-la-Barca AM, Sotelo-Mundo RR: Molecular characterization of arginine kinase, an allergen from the shrimp Litopenaeus vannamei. Int Arch Allergy Immunol 2007;144:23–28.

22　Ayuso R, Grishina G, Bardina L, Carrillo T, Blanco C, Ibáñez MD, Sampson HA, Beyer K: Myosin light chain is a novel shrimp allergen, Lit v 3. J Allergy Clin Immunol 2008;122:795–802.

23　Ayuso R, Grishina G, Ibáñez MD, Blanco C, Carrillo T, Bencharitiwong R, Sánchez S, Nowak-Wegrzyn A, Sampson HA: Sarcoplasmic calcium-binding protein is an EF-hand-type protein identified as a new shrimp allergen. J Allergy Clin Immunol 2009;124:114–120.

24 Bauermeister K, Wangorsch A, Garoffo LP, Reuter A, Conti A, Taylor SL, Lidholm J, Dewitt AM, Enrique E, Vieths S, Holzhauser T, Ballmer-Weber B, Reese G: Generation of a comprehensive panel of crustacean allergens from the North Sea Shrimp Crangon crangon. Mol Immunol 2011;48:1983–1992.

25 Lim DL, Neo KH, Yi FC, Chua KY, Goh DL, Shek LP, Giam YC, Van Bever HP, Lee BW: Parvalbumin–the major tropical fish allergen. Pediatr Allergy Immunol 2008;19:399–407.

26 Van Do T, Elsayed S, Florvaag E, Hordvik I, Endresen C: Allergy to fish parvalbumins: studies on the cross-reactivity of allergens from 9 commonly consumed fish. J Allergy Clin Immunol 2005;116:1314–1320.

27 Griesmeier U, Vázquez-Cortés S, Bublin M, Radauer C, Ma Y, Briza P, Fernández-Rivas M, Breiteneder H: Expression levels of parvalbumins determine allergenicity of fish species. Allergy 2010;65: 191–198.

28 Lee PW, Nordlee JA, Koppelman SJ, Baumert JL, Taylor SL: Measuring parvalbumin levels in fish muscle tissue: relevance of muscle locations and storage conditions. Food Chem 2012;135:502–507.

29 Hilger C, Thill L, Grigioni F, Lehners C, Falagiani P, Ferrara A, Romano C, Stevens W, Hentges F: IgE antibodies of fish allergic patients cross-react with frog parvalbumin. Allergy 2004;59:653–660.

30 Pascal M, Grishina G, Yang A, Ayuso R: A sea urchin roe tropomyosin-like protein is recognized in vitro by shrimp-allergic individuals. J Investig Allergol Clin Immunol 2012;22:306–307.

31 Taylor SL: Molluscan shellfish allergy. Adv Food Nutr Res 2008;54:139–177.

32 Fernandes J, Reshef A, Patton L, Ayuso R, Reese G, Lehrer SB: Immunoglobulin E antibody reactivity to the major shrimp allergen, tropomyosin, in unexposed Orthodox Jews. Clin Exp Allergy 2003;33:956–961.

33 Wang J, Calatroni A, Visness CM, Sampson HA: Correlation of specific IgE to shrimp with cockroach and dust mite exposure and sensitization in an inner-city population. J Allergy Clin Immunol 2011;128:834–837.

34 Ayuso R, Reese G, Leong-Kee S, Plante M, Lehrer SB: Molecular basis of arthropod cross-reactivity: IgE-binding cross-reactive epitopes of shrimp, house dust mite and cockroach tropomyosins. Int Arch Allergy Immunol 2002;129:38–48.

35 Woo CK, Bahna SL: Not all shellfish 'allergy' is allergy! Clin Transl Allergy 2011;1:3.

36 Jirapongsananuruk O, Sripramong C, Pacharn P, Udompunturak S, Chinratanapisit S, Piboonpocanun S, Visitsunthorn N, Vichyanond P: Specific allergy to Penaeus monodon (seawater shrimp) or Macrobrachium rosenbergii (freshwater shrimp) in shrimp-allergic children. Clin Exp Allergy 2008;38:1038–1047.

37 Daul CB, Morgan JE, Hughes J, Lehrer SB: Provocation-challenge studies in shrimp-sensitive individuals. J Allergy Clin Immunol 1988;81:1180–1186.

38 Daul CB, Morgan JE, Lehrer SB: The natural history of shrimp hypersensitivity. J Allergy Clin Immunol 1990;86:88–93.

39 Ayuso R, Sánchez-Garcia S, Lin J, Fu Z, Ibáñez MD, Carrillo T, Blanco C, Goldis M, Bardina L, Sastre J, Sampson HA: Greater epitope recognition of shrimp allergens by children than by adults suggests that shrimp sensitization decreases with age. J Allergy Clin Immunol 2010; 125:1286–1293.e3.

40 Swoboda I, Bugajska-Schretter A, Linhart B, Verdino P, Keller W, Schulmeister U, Sperr WR, Valent P, Peltre G, Quirce S, Douladiris N, Papadopoulos NG, Valenta R, Spitzauer S: A recombinant hypoallergenic parvalbumin mutant for immunotherapy of IgE-mediated fish allergy. J Immunol 2007;178: 6290–6296.

41 Chegini S, Metcalfe DD: Seafood toxins; in Sampson HA, Simon RA (eds): Food Allergy: Adverse Reactions to Foods and Food Additives, ed 4. Malden, MA, Blackwell Publishing, 2008, vol 41, pp 524.

Bee-Wah Lee, MD
Department of Paediatrics, Yong Loo Lin School of Medicine
National University of Singapore, NUHS Tower Block, Level 12
1E Kent Ridge Road
Singapore 119228 (Singapore)
E-Mail paeleebw@nus.edu.sg

Ebisawa M, Ballmer-Weber BK, Vieths S, Wood RA (eds): Food Allergy: Molecular Basis and Clinical Practice.
Chem Immunol Allergy. Basel, Karger, 2015, vol 101, pp 162–170 (DOI: 10.1159/000375469)

Fruit and Vegetable Allergy

Montserrat Fernández-Rivas

Allergy Department, Hospital Clínico San Carlos, IdISSC, Madrid, Spain

Abstract

Fruit and vegetable allergies are the most prevalent food allergies in adolescents and adults. The identification of the allergens involved and the elucidation of their intrinsic properties and cross-reactivity patterns has helped in the understanding of the mechanisms of sensitisation and how the allergen profiles determine the different phenotypes. The most frequent yet contrasting fruit and vegetable allergies are pollen-food syndrome (PFS) and lipid transfer protein (LTP) syndrome. In PFS, fruit and vegetable allergies result from a primary sensitisation to labile pollen allergens, such as Bet v 1 or profilin, and the resulting phenotype is mainly mild, consisting of local oropharyngeal reactions. In contrast, LTP syndrome results from a primary sensitisation to LTPs, which are stable plant food allergens, inducing frequent systemic reactions and even anaphylaxis. Although much less prevalent, severe fruit allergies may be associated with latex (latex-fruit syndrome). Molecular diagnosis is essential in guiding the management and risk assessment of these patients. Current management strategies comprise avoidance and rescue medication, including adrenaline, for severe LTP allergies. Specific immunotherapy with pollen is not indicated to treat pollen-food syndrome, but sublingual immunotherapy with LTPs seems to be a promising therapy for LTP syndrome.

© 2015 S. Karger AG, Basel

Introduction

The first description of fruit and vegetable allergies and their association with pollen allergy was reported in 1942. In the 1970s, an association between ragweed pollinosis and allergy to melon and watermelon was described in the USA, while in Scandinavia, fruit and vegetable allergies were reported in birch pollen-allergic patients who typically experienced mild oropharyngeal symptoms. These studies were followed by a boom of publications across Europe that confirmed the initial findings and revealed new associations of plant food allergies with different pollen sources and with latex, and the terms pollen-food syndrome (PFS) and latex-fruit syndrome (LFS) were coined. In the late 1990s, the first publications on lipid transfer proteins (LTPs) by Spanish and Italian groups challenged the current knowledge by showing that primary allergy to fruits could exist. The identification of the allergens involved in fruit and vegetable allergies and the elucidation of their intrinsic properties and cross-reactivity patterns has helped in the understanding of the different mechanisms of sensitisation and how allergen profiles determine phenotypes. Furthermore, the application of individual allergens has improved diagnosis and management and may lead to new therapeutic options.

Epidemiology

Fruit and vegetable allergies are the most common food allergies in adolescents and adults. They are more frequently found in females and pollen-allergic subjects. In a systematic review [1], 2.2–11.5% of children 0–6 years of age and 0.4–6.6% of adults reported adverse reactions to fruits. The figures for perceived vegetable allergy in the same age groups were lower, totalling 0.7–3.3% and 0.5–2.2%, respectively. There are very few population-based studies that have confirmed clinical reactivities to fruits and vegetables by oral food challenges [1–5]. In a study performed in Germany [2, 3], Rosaceae fruits, kiwi, pineapple and carrot were the foods most commonly involved in challenge-proven allergic reactions, with the highest prevalence estimates (for all ages) calculated for carrot (2.7%) and apple (1.7%). In this study, the highest prevalence of food allergy – 4.3% – was found in the subjects aged 20–39 years, and 61% of them were females. The most common eliciting foods in the children and adults were plant foods, including fruits, nuts and vegetables, with apple and hazelnut being the most frequent elicitors of allergic reactions.

A general population-based study carried out in Denmark [4] has also shown that the prevalence of challenge-confirmed primary food allergy in adults is higher (3.2%) than that in children, and the most common foods are fruits and vegetables, with an overall prevalence of 2.7%. Interestingly, in Danish adults sensitised to pollen, the prevalence of allergy to plant foods rose to 32%, and those of allergies to apple, kiwi, celery and tomato were 16.7, 13.3, 7.6 and 5%, respectively. The probability of having PFS is higher in patients with a symptomatic pollen allergy, especially in those allergic to birch pollen who are either monosensitised or who also have grass and/or mugwort pollen allergies [5].

Studies performed in Southern Europe have also confirmed the relevant roles of fruits and vegetables, although the allergens involved and the allergy severities are different from those of Northern and Central Europe due to frequent sensitisations to LTPs. In a multicentre, nationwide, cross-sectional study performed in Spain on 4,991 patients (children and adults) recruited in outpatient clinics, food allergy was diagnosed in 7.4% of the patients. Fruits accounted for 33% of the reactions and were the most common offenders in patients over 5 years of age [6]. In a multicentre, cross-sectional study performed in outpatient clinics across Italy, food allergy was diagnosed in 8.5% of 25,601 adult subjects screened. A total of 55% of the cases corresponded to PFS, and 19.5% involved a primary LTP allergy [7]. The fruits most commonly involved in allergic reactions in Southern Europe are Rosaceae fruits (with peach more frequent than apple, in contrast to Northern and Central Europe), followed by kiwi and Cucurbitaceae (melon and watermelon). Among vegetables, lettuce and tomato are common offenders [6, 7].

The prevalence of LFS in the general population has not been established. Up to 50% of patients who are allergic to latex present allergic reactions to plant-derived foods, especially fresh fruits, such as kiwi, banana, and avocado [8].

Pathogenesis: Allergen Sensitisation

Most fruit and vegetable allergies are associated with pollen allergies, but they can exist independently, such as those mediated by LTPs. When a plant food allergy results from a primary sensitisation occurring through inhalation of a pollen allergen that has a homologous counterpart in the plant food, it is called PFS. The IgE antibodies initially directed towards the pollen allergen react with the homologous allergen present in the fruit or

Table 1. Associations of pollen and plant food allergies described in different geographical areas and the allergens involved

Area	Pollen	Food	Allergens
Central-Northern EU	Birch	Rosaceae, Apiaceae, kiwi, soybean, tree nuts (hazelnut)	Bet v 1 homologues, profilin
Central EU	Mugwort	Apiaceae	Profilin, CCDs, 40–60 kDa
Central EU	Birch, mugwort	Apiaceae	Bet v 1 homologues, profilin, CCDs, 40–60 kDa
USA	Ragweed	Cucurbitaceae, banana	Profilin[#]
Spain	Mugwort	Compositae, Rosaceae, Brasicaceae, tree nuts	LTPs, profilin
Spain, Italy	Grass	Rosaceae	Profilin, CCDs
Spain	Plantain, grass	Cucurbitaceae	Profilin; 31, 40–70 kDa
Italy	Parietaria	Pistachio	Unknown
Spain	Plane tree	Rosaceae and other fruits, peanut, tree nuts, vegetables	Profilin, LTPs

EU = Europe; and [#] probably (not identified).

vegetable when it is eaten and elicit the reaction. This type of food allergy is also known as a type II food allergy, and the allergens involved are considered incomplete because they are able to elicit reactions but cannot induce sensitisation by the oral route. The allergens most frequently involved are Bet v 1 homologues and profilins (table 1) [9–12]. Bet v 1 sensitisation arises from exposure to birch pollen, whereas profilin sensitisation is related to grass and weed (mugwort and ragweed) pollen allergies [9–12]. Both Bet v 1 homologues and profilins are labile, and their IgE-binding epitopes (mostly conformational) are altered by the high temperatures of food processing and by the proteolytic enzymes of the digestive tract [10]. For these reasons, reactions are only elicited by fresh fruits and vegetables, and they are usually restricted to the oropharyngeal mucosa, with infrequent systemic involvement [13]. However, some cases of PFS have been reported in association with mugwort pollen with more severe clinical presentations, suggesting that stable allergens are involved, although

they have not been fully elucidated [11]. Several associations have been described in various geographical areas of PFS with different allergens (table 1) [11, 12], reflecting the local aerobiology and dietary habits. With the elucidation of the allergens involved, it is more appropriate to look at them from an allergen-based perspective (table 2).

Fruit and vegetable allergies linked to LTPs have been described predominantly in the Mediterranean area, where they are major plant food allergens. LTPs are stable allergens that resist heat treatment and enzymatic digestion (table 2) and therefore have the intrinsic potential of behaving like complete food allergens, inducing sensitisation and eliciting reactions through the oral route (i.e. type I food allergies) [9–12]. The peach LTP Pru p 3 seems to be the primary sensitiser [14–16]. Sensitisation may occur through the oral route and through the skin. The latter is suggested by the frequent observation of peach contact urticaria, which can even precede the onset of reactions that occurs upon peach ingestion [15]. The abundance of Pru

Table 2. Summary of the main fruit and vegetable allergens

Allergen family	Representative allergens	MW (kDa)	Characteristics
Bet v 1 homologues	Mal d 1 (apple) Pru av 1 (cherry) Pru p 1 (peach) Api g 1 (celery) Dau c 1 (carrot) Gly m 4 (soybean)	18	Plant defence proteins: PR10 Labile allergens: altered by thermal treatment and proteolytic enzymes
Lipid transfer proteins	Pru p 3 (peach) Mal d 3 (apple) Vit v 1 (grape) Cit s 3 (orange) Lyc e 3 (tomato) Lac s 1 (lettuce) Bra o 3 (cabbage)	9	Plant defence proteins: PR14 Conserved cysteine residues involved in 4 disulphide bonds confer stability to heat treatment, low pH and proteolytic digestion
Profilins	Pru p 4 (peach) Mal d 4 (apple) Cuc m 2 (melon) Lyc e 1 (tomato) Mus a 1 (banana) Api g 4 (celery) Dau c 4 (carrot)	12–15	Cytosolic proteins found in all eukaryotic cells (including pollens, plant foods and latex) Regulate actin polymerization during cell movement, cytokinesis, and signalling Labile allergens: sensitive to heat and proteases
Chitinases and proteins with hevein-like domain	Pers a 1 (avocado) Act d chitinase (kiwi) Mus a 2 (banana) Bra r 2 (turnip)*	32 20*	Plant defence proteins: PR3, 4, 8 Heat-sensitive: ethylene-induced Sensitive to proteolytic digestion, although the resultant peptides maintain IgE binding capacity
Thaumatin-like proteins	Act d 2 (kiwi) Mal d 2 (apple) Pru av 2 (cherry) Cap a 1 (pepper)	23	Plant defence proteins: PR5 Presence of 8 disulphide bonds confers stability to low pH and resistance to heat and proteolytic digestion
β-1,3-glucanases	Mus a 5 (banana) Identified in tomato, potato, grape and bell pepper	33–39	Plant defence proteins: PR2 Glycoproteins with IgE-binding N-linked glycans May be involved in cross-reactivity between latex (Hev b 2), pollen (Ole e 9) and foods
Proteases Cysteine proteases	Act d 1, actinidin (kiwi)	30	Major kiwi allergen associated with severe kiwi allergy and marker of isolated kiwi allergy
Serine proteases	Cuc m 1, cucumisin (melon)	66	Major melon allergen; stable to heat and pepsin digestion

MW = Molecular weight; PR = pathogenesis-related. * Bra r 2 has a MW of 20 kDa.

p 3 in peach skin, together with its peculiar vellous aspect, might favour cutaneous sensitisation.

LTPs have been described as allergens in the pollens of mugwort (Art v 3), plane tree (Pla a 3), olive (Ole e 7), pellitory (Par j 1–2), cypress and ragweed (Amb a 6) [16]. These findings have led to the hypothesis that plant food LTP allergy may result from a primary sensitisation to pollen LTPs, which may explain geographical differences in LTP sensitisation. There is no evidence to support the allergenic roles of olive, pellitory and ragweed LTPs, but there are some contradictory findings regarding those of mugwort and plane tree [17, 18]. In cross-sectional studies performed in the Mediterranean coastal areas of Spain with prevalent plane tree and mugwort pollinosis, an association has been found between sensitisation to plant foods linked to LTPs and Art v 3 and Pla a 3. However, in a cross-sectional study on plant food allergies performed across Spain, the frequency of LTP sensitisation was similar, despite striking differences in pollen exposure. In addition, about 20% of patients who were allergic to LTPs did not have an associated pollen allergy [16–19]. Accordingly, a study performed in Italy has not found a role of Art v 3 in peach allergy. Furthermore, IgE inhibition experiments have shown a dominant role of Pru p 3 over Art v 3 or Pla a 3 in most cases. However, there are a few publications reporting that in some areas and for some patients, sensitisation to Pru p 3 may be secondary to inhalant sensitisation to Art v 3. It has also been shown that in patients sensitised to Pru p 3, if they are also sensitised to Art v 3, the number of plant food allergies is higher, indicating that the additional sensitisation to Art v 3 may have broadened the LTP epitope repertoire [16].

In summary, LTP syndrome cannot be considered a PFS for the majority of patients. According to the current evidence, LTP syndrome may be a type I food allergy driven by Pru p 3, the peach LTP, although in a subset of patients, additional sensitisation to pollen LTPs may broaden the epitope recognition pattern. It is also possible that high exposure to some pollen LTPs (Pla a 3 and Art v 3) may induce a primary sensitisation in some patients with the later onset of a linked plant food allergy [16]. Mechanistic animal models of sensitisation and longitudinal studies of clinical cohorts are needed to establish the chronology of sensitisation to different LTPs and the onset of clinical food allergy.

LFS is a cross-reactive syndrome that results (in most cases) from primary sensitisation to latex allergens by skin contact or inhalation. Several latex allergens are involved in latex-food cross-reactivity, such as Hev b 2 (β1,3-glucanase), Hev b 6.02 (hevein), Hev b 7 (patatin-like protein), Hev b 8 (profilin), and Hev b 12 (LTP). Class I chitinases, which have a hevein N-terminal domain, are considered to be the main allergens responsible for LFS, although their role in this syndrome has been recently questioned [8–10, 20].

Allergens

The main allergens involved in fruit and vegetable allergies are summarised in table 2 [10], and detailed information can be found in the chapter on food allergens (see Lorenz et al., pp. 18–29). Bet v 1 homologues, profilins, and LTPs are the most important allergens in terms of frequency of sensitisation and clinical relevance, although there are geographical differences across Europe [12, 14]. Thaumatin-like proteins are stable allergens with the potential for inducing sensitisation and eliciting reactions, but their clinical relevance has not been fully elucidated [8]. The thiol proteases actinidin and cucumisin have been described as major allergens in kiwi and melon allergies [8, 21].

Clinical Symptoms

The term oral allergy syndrome (OAS) has been used in different ways in the medical literature. Some authors use OAS to refer to oropharyngeal symptoms induced by IgE- mediated food allergy, whereas some others use it as a synonym of PFS. Oropharyngeal symptoms are very frequently found in PFS. However, they are also elicited by any plant food, independent of pollen sensitisation, and by animal foods. For this reason, in this chapter, OAS refers exclusively to oropharyngeal symptoms.

In PFS, in which the main allergens involved are Bet v 1 homologues and profilins, the ingestion of fresh fruits and vegetables very often induces local reactions in the oropharynx, characterised by the itching of the lips, mouth and throat with or without local angioedema (OAS). These reactions are mild and self-limited and normally appear within the first 15 minutes following ingestion. Some patients also report mild rhinitis (itching and sneezing), and in some subjects, severe pharyngeal swelling has been described. Processed fruits and vegetables are well tolerated [14, 22]. However, some patients with celery allergy present systemic reactions and may react to cooked celery [23]. Additionally, severe reactions to soybean caused by the Bet v 1 homologue Gly m 4 have been described [13].

The clinical presentation of LTP syndrome is more severe, and reactions are induced by both fresh and processed foods. Peeled fruits are better tolerated because LTPs accumulate in the skin. In Rosaceae fruit allergy linked to LTP, approximately two-thirds of the patients present with OAS exclusively, and one-third experience systemic reactions with or without associated OAS. Peach-allergic patients frequently present with contact urticaria [14, 15]. It has been shown that LTP-allergic subjects with an associated pollen allergy who are co-sensitised to profilin or Bet v 1 homologues present milder reactions than those who are not allergic to pollen [24]. The latter accounts for approximately 20% of LTP-allergic patients, who present very frequently with systemic involvement and even anaphylaxis [19]. It has also been shown that exercise or the intake of nonsteroidal anti-inflammatory drugs enhances

the severity of reactions [25]. In the Mediterranean area, plant food allergies linked to LTP are most commonly involved in anaphylactic reactions [26].

A total of 30–50% (depending on the series) of individuals with LFS present with reactions to plant foods, and chestnut, avocado, banana, and kiwi are the most frequently involved. Although latex allergy precedes hypersensitivity to foods in most patients, the opposite may also occur. Patients may experience OAS but they can also have systemic reactions. The proportion of reactions with anaphylaxis ranges from 5 to 50%. Banana, avocado and kiwi are frequently associated with anaphylaxis, while potato frequently induces mild local reactions [8].

Diagnosis

The diagnosis of fruit and vegetable allergies comprises the collection of a detailed medical history to establish the relationship between food intake and the onset of symptoms, the type of symptoms experienced by the patient, the need for treatment, the presence of associated cofactors and how the food was eaten (raw or processed). The subsequent intake of the food in a different presentation should be investigated, as well as the subsequent intake of related plant foods. The presence of a pollen, latex or other associated respiratory allergy or asthma should always be studied. Sensitisation to the food, as shown by either skin prick tests (SPTs) or serum IgE (sIgE) determinations, should be investigated. The sensitivities of SPTs and sIgE to whole fruit and vegetable extracts are often low when labile allergens, such as Bet v 1 homologues and profilins, are involved. To overcome this problem, a prick-prick test with the fresh food is often needed, or recombinant allergen can be used for the assessment of sIgE. On the other hand, IgE cross-reactivity among allergens reduces specificity, which can only be overcome by performing oral food challenges [27].

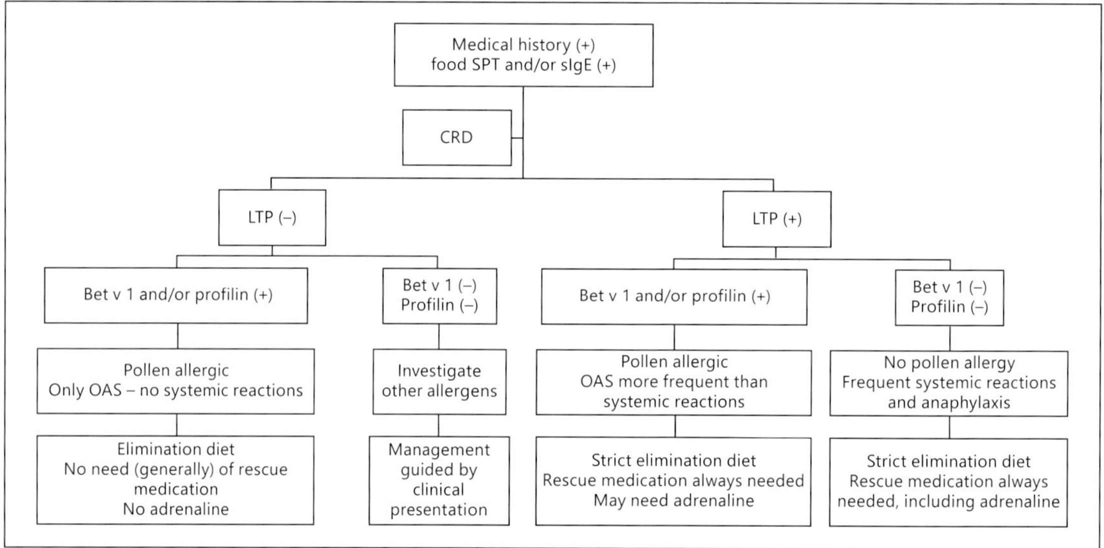

Fig. 1. Proposed algorithm for an allergen-based diagnosis and management of patients with allergy to Rosaceae fruits in the Mediterranean area. It can be 'adapted' to other plant foods and to other geographical areas depending on the local molecular epidemiology.

Patients may be consulted after the first clinical reaction or after having experienced several reactions to different plant foods, and they may also experience new reactions during follow-up. Therefore, clinically relevant cross-reactivity should always be investigated by carefully evaluating medical history, including the detailed intake of related plant foods after a given reaction, SPT and/or sIgE testing, and oral food challenges [27, 28].

Molecular diagnosis (also known as component-resolved diagnosis, CRD) is currently the cornerstone in the diagnosis of fruit and vegetable allergies. CRD has a higher sensitivity than the use of whole extracts [29], and most importantly, it provides a risk assessment for guiding patient management. The assessment of IgE sensitisation to the three key allergens – Bet v 1 homologues, LTPs and profilins – is of paramount importance, especially in the Mediterranean area (fig. 1). The knowledge of local molecular epidemiology is essential to guide allergists in choosing the components to test in their population [17, 18]. CRD is performed by the testing of sIgE binding to either individual allergens or to multiple allergens with a microarray test. In Spain, it is also possible to perform CRD by SPT because profilin (nPho d 2) and LTP (nPru p 3) diagnostic materials have been commercialised [30].

Management

The current management of fruit and vegetable allergies relies on the avoidance of the offending food and on rescue medication (fig. 1). The accurate identification of the culprit food(s) is essential to ensure for an adequate diet. Patients may also react to foods that share homologous allergens; thus, if tolerance to cross-reactive foods has not been assessed, the patient should be instructed of the possible dangers of related cross-reactivity. This warning is obviously more relevant to those patients with previous severe reactions and in those sensitised to allergens with the intrinsic risk of eliciting severe reactions. The need for rescue medication depends on the previous reactions and the allergens involved. For patients with PFS who have only experienced mild self-limited OAS and are only sensitised to PR10 proteins or profilins, rescue medication is not generally recommended. For patients with LTP syndrome and LFS and in those with previous systemic reactions, rescue medication should always be given and may include adrenaline auto-injectors [6, 8, 19, 22, 25, 26, 28].

Fruit and vegetable allergies have negative impacts on both nutrition and quality of life. They are persistent, and patients often react to a wide variety of foods and need to follow extensive elimination diets. Additionally, patients with LTP syndrome are at risk of severe systemic reactions due to accidental exposure or the presence of co-factors. Therefore, there is a need for specific immunotherapy (IT). The effects of birch pollen IT on associated food allergies, mainly involving apple, have been investigated, but the results are controversial, and it cannot be recommended for the treatment of associated plant food allergies. In contrast, sublingual IT with a Pru p 3-quantified extract has shown promise as a therapy for LTP syndrome because it is able to modify the clinical reactivity of patients to the intake of peach and the underlying immunological responses with an overall good tolerance [31].

References

1 Zuidmeer L, Goldhahn K, Rona RJ, Gislason D, Madsen C, Summers C, Sodergren E, Dahlstrom J, Lindner T, Sigurdardottir ST, McBride D, Keil T: The prevalence of plant food allergies: a systematic review. J Allergy Clin Immunol 2008;121:1210–1218.

2 Zuberbier T, Edenharter G, Worm M, Ehlers I, Reimann S, Hantke T, Roehr CC,Bergmann KE, Niggemann B: Prevalence of adverse reactions to food in Germany- a population study. Allergy 2004;59:338–345.

3 Roehr CC, Edenharter G, Reimann S, Ehlers I, Worm M, Zuberbier T, Niggemann B: Food allergy and non-allergic food hypersensitivity in children and adolescents. Clin Exp Allergy 2004;34: 1534–1541.

4 Osterballe M, Hansen TK, Mortz CG, Høst A, Bindslev-Jensen C: The prevalence of food hypersensitivity in an unselected population of children and adults. Pediatr Allergy Immunol 2005; 16:567–573.

5 Osterballe M, Hansen TK, Mortz CG, Bindslev-Jensen C: The clinical relevance of sensitisation to pollen-related fruits and vegetables in unselected pollen-sensitized adults. Allergy 2005;60: 218–225.

6 Fernández Rivas M: Food allergy in Alergológica 2005. J Investig Allergol Clin Immunol 2009;19(suppl 2):37–44.

7 Asero R, Antonicelli L, Arena A, Bommarito L, Caruso B, Crivellaro M, De Carli M, Della Torre E, Della Torre F, Heffler E, Lodi Rizzini F, Longo R, Manzotti G, Marcotulli M, Melchiorre A, Minale P, Morandi P, Moreni B, Moschella A, Murzilli F, Nebiolo F, Poppa M, Randazzo S, Rossi G, Senna GE: EpidemAAITO: features of food allergy in Italian adults attending allergy clinics: a multi-centre study. Clin Exp Allergy 2009;39:547–555.

8 Blanco C: Latex-fruit syndrome. Curr Allergy Asthma Rep 2003;3:47–53.

9 Yagami T: Allergies to cross-reactive plant proteins. Latex-fruit syndrome is comparable with pollen-food allergy syndrome. Int Arch Allergy Immunol 2002;128:271–279.

10 Breiteneder H, Radauer C: A classification of plant food allergens. J Allergy Clin Immunol 2004;113:821–830.

11 Egger M, Mutschlechner S, Wopfner N, Gadermaier G, Briza P, Ferreira F: Pollen-food syndromes associated with weed pollinosis: an update from the molecular point of view. Allergy 2006;61: 461–476.

12 Andersen MB, Hall S, Dragsted LO: Identification of european allergy patterns to the allergen families PR-10, LTP, and profilin from Rosaceae fruits. Clin Rev Allergy Immunol 2011;41:4–19.

13 Kleine-Tebbe J, Vogel L, Crowell DN, Haustein UF, Vieths S: Severe oral allergy syndrome and anaphylactic reactions caused by a Bet v 1-related PR-10 protein in soybean, SAM22. J Allergy Clin Immunol 2002;110:797–804.

14 Fernández-Rivas M, Bolhaar S, González-Mancebo E, Asero R, van Leeuwen A,Bohle B, Ma Y, Ebner C, Rigby N, Sancho AI, Miles S, Zuidmeer L, Knulst A, Breiteneder H, Mills C, Hoffmann-Sommergruber K, van Ree R: Apple allergy across Europe: How allergen sensitization profiles determine the clinical expression of plant food allergies. J Allergy Clin Immunol 2006;118:481–488.

15 Fernández-Rivas M, González-Mancebo E, Rodríguez Pérez R, Benito C, Sánchez-Monge R, Salcedo G, Alonso MD, Rosado A, Tejedor MA, Vila C, Casas ML: Clinically relevant peach allergy is related to peach lipid transfer protein, Pru p 3, in the Spanish population. J Allergy Clin Immunol 2003;112:789–795.

16 Palacín A, Gómez-Casado C, Rivas LA, Aguirre J, Tordesillas L, Bartra J,Blanco C, Carrillo T, Cuesta-Herranz J, de Frutos C, Alvarez-Eire GG, Fernández FJ, Gamboa P, Muñoz R, Sánchez-Monge R, Sirvent S, Torres MJ, Varela-Losada S, Rodríguez R, Parro V, Blanca M, Salcedo G, Díaz-Perales A: Graph based study of allergen cross-reactivity of plant lipid transfer proteins (LTPs) using microarray in a multicenter study. PLoS One 2012;7:e50799.

17   Barber D, de la Torre F, Feo F, Florido F, Guardia P, Moreno C, Quiralte J, Lombardero M, Villalba M, Salcedo G, Rodríguez R: Understanding patient sensitization profiles in complex pollen areas: a molecular epidemiological study. Allergy 2008;63:1550–1558.

18   Barber D, de la Torre F, Lombardero M, Antépara I, Colas C, Dávila I, Tabar AI, Vidal C, Villalba M, Salcedo G, Rodríguez R: Component-resolved diagnosis of pollen allergy based on skin testing with profilin, polcalcin and lipid transfer protein pan-allergens. Clin Exp Allergy 2009;39:1764–1773.

19   Fernández Rivas M, van Ree R, Cuevas M: Allergy to *Rosaceae* fruits without related pollinosis. J Allergy Clin Immunol 1997;100:728–733.

20   Radauer C, Adhami F, Fürtler I, Wagner S, Allwardt D, Scala E, Ebner C, Hafner C, Hemmer W, Mari A, Breiteneder H: Latex-allergic patients sensitized to the major allergen hevein and hevein-like domains of class I chitinases show no increased frequency of latex-associated plant food allergy. Mol Immunol 2011; 48:600–609.

21   Le TM, Bublin M, Breiteneder H, Fernández-Rivas M, Asero R, Ballmer-Weber B, Barreales L, Bures P, Belohlavkova S, de Blay F, Clausen M, Dubakiene R, Gislason D, van Hoffen E, Jedrzejczak-Czechowicz M, Kowalski M, Kralimarkova T, Lidholm J, Marknell DeWitt A, Mills CEN, Papadopoulos NG, Popov T, Purohit A, van Ree R, Seneviratne S, Sinaniotis A, Summers C, Vázquez-Cortés S, Vieths S, Vogel L, Hoffmann-Sommergruber K, Knulst AC: Kiwifruit allergy across Europe: clinical manifestation and IgE recognition patterns to kiwifruit allergens. J Allergy Clin Immunol 2013;131:164–171.

22   Geroldinger-Simic M, Zelniker T, Aberer W, Ebner C, Egger C, Greiderer A, Prem N, Lidholm J, Ballmer-Weber BK, Vieths S, Bohle B: Birch pollen-related food allergy: clinical aspects and the role of allergen-specific IgE and IgG4 antibodies. J Allergy Clin Immunol 2011; 127:616–622.

23   Ballmer-Weber BK, Hoffmann A, Wüthrich B, Lüttkopf D, Pompei C, Wangorsch A, Kästner M, Vieths S: Influence of food processing on the allergenicity of celery: DBPCFC with celery spice and cooked celery in patients with celery allergy. Allergy 2002;57:228–235.

24   Pastorello EA, Farioli L, Pravettoni V, Scibilia J, Mascheri A, Borgonovo L, Piantanida M, Primavesi L, Stafylaraki C, Pasqualetti S, Schroeder J, Nichelatti M, Marocchi A: Pru p 3-sensitised Italian peach-allergic patients are less likely to develop severe symptoms when also presenting IgE antibodies to Pru p 1 and Pru p 4. Int Arch Allergy Immunol 2011; 156:362–372.

25   Cardona V, Luengo O, Garriga T, Labrador-Horrillo M, Sala-Cunill A, Izquierdo A, Soto L, Guilarte M: Co-factor-enhanced food allergy. Allergy 2012;67: 1316–1318.

26   Asero R, Antonicelli L, Arena A, Bommarito L, Caruso B, Colombo G, Crivellaro M, De Carli M, Della Torre E, Della Torre F, Heffler E, Lodi Rizzini F, Longo R, Manzotti G, Marcotulli M, Melchiorre A, Minale P, Morandi P, Moreni B, Moschella A, Murzilli F, Nebiolo F, Poppa M, Randazzo S, Rossi G, Senna GE: Causes of food-induced anaphylaxis in Italian adults: a multi-centre study. Int Arch Allergy Immunol 2009;150:271–277.

27   Asero R, Ballmer-Weber BK, Beyer K, Conti A, Dubakiene R, Fernandez-Rivas M, Hoffmann-Sommergruber K, Lidholm J, Mustakov T, Oude Elberink JN, Pumphrey RS, Stahl Skov P, van Ree R, Vlieg-Boerstra BJ, Hiller R, Hourihane JO, Kowalski M, Papadopoulos NG, Wal JM, Mills EN, Vieths S: IgE-mediated food allergy diagnosis: Current status and new perspectives. Mol Nutr Food Res 2007;51:135–147.

28   Crespo JF, Rodríguez J, James JM, Daroca P, Reaño M, Vives R: Reactivity to potential cross-reactive foods in fruit-allergic patients: implications for prescribing food avoidance. Allergy 2002; 57:946–949.

29   Reuter A, Lidholm J, Andersson K, Ostling J, Lundberg M, Scheurer S, Enrique E, Cistero-Bahima A, San Miguel-Moncin M, Ballmer-Weber BK, Vieths S: A critical assessment of allergen component-based in vitro diagnosis in cherry allergy across Europe. Clin Exp Allergy 2006;36:815–823.

30   Asero R, Jimeno L, Barber D: Component-resolved diagnosis of plant food allergy by SPT. Eur Ann Allergy Clin Immunol 2008;40:115–121.

31   Fernández-Rivas M, Garrido Fernández M, Nadal JA, Alonso Díaz de Durana MD, García BE, González-Mancebo E, Martín S, Barber D, Rico P, Tabar AI: Randomized double-blind, placebo-controlled trial of sublingual immunotherapy with a Pru p 3 quantified peach extract. Allergy 2009;64:876–883.

Montserrat Fernández-Rivas, MD, PhD
Allergy Department, Hospital Clínico San Carlos
IdISSC, c/ Prof. Martín Lagos s/n
ES–28040 Madrid (Spain)
E-Mail mariamontserrat.fernandez@salud.madrid.org

Ebisawa M, Ballmer-Weber BK, Vieths S, Wood RA (eds): Food Allergy: Molecular Basis and Clinical Practice.
Chem Immunol Allergy. Basel, Karger, 2015, vol 101, pp 171–180 (DOI: 10.1159/000371700)

Gastrointestinal Food Allergies

Ralf G. Heine

Department of Gastroenterology and Clinical Nutrition and Department of Allergy and Immunology,
The Royal Children's Hospital Melbourne, Melbourne, Vic., Murdoch Childrens Research Institute,
Melbourne, Vic., and Department of Paediatrics, The University of Melbourne, Melbourne, Vic., Australia

Abstract

Gastrointestinal food allergies present during early childhood with a diverse range of symptoms. Cow's milk, soy and wheat are the three most common gastrointestinal food allergens. Several clinical syndromes have been described, including food protein-induced enteropathy, proctocolitis and enterocolitis. In contrast with immediate, IgE-mediated food allergies, the onset of gastrointestinal symptoms is delayed for at least 1–2 hours after ingestion in non-IgE-mediated allergic disorders. The pathophysiology of these non-IgE-mediated allergic disorders is poorly understood, and useful *in vitro* markers are lacking. The results of the skin prick test or measurement of the food-specific serum IgE level is generally negative, although low-positive results may occur. Diagnosis therefore relies on the recognition of a particular clinical phenotype as well as the demonstration of clear clinical improvement after food allergen elimination and the re-emergence of symptoms upon challenge. There is a significant clinical overlap between non-IgE-mediated food allergy and several common paediatric gastroenterological conditions, which may lead to diagnostic confusion. The treatment of gastrointestinal food allergies requires the strict elimination of offending food allergens until tolerance has developed. In breast-fed infants, a maternal elimination diet is often sufficient to control symptoms. In formula-fed infants, treatment usually involves the use an extensively hydrolysed or amino acid-based formula. Apart from the use of hypoallergenic formulae, the solid diets of these children also need to be kept free of specific food allergens, as clinically indicated. The nutritional progress of infants and young children should be carefully monitored, and they should undergo ongoing, regular food protein elimination reassessments by cautious food challenges to monitor for possible tolerance development.

© 2015 S. Karger AG, Basel

Introduction

Food allergies are among the most common non-communicable diseases in young children [1]. While IgE-mediated food allergies are generally well understood, the management of children with non-IgE-mediated food allergies still poses significant diagnostic and therapeutic dilemmas.

There is significant clinical overlap between gastrointestinal food allergies and common non-allergic disorders that occur during infancy, such as gastro-oesophageal reflux disease (GORD) or carbohydrate malabsorption. The absence of clear diagnostic markers often delays the recognition of non-IgE-mediated gastrointestinal allergic manifestations and may lead to adverse nutritional outcomes, including protein-energy malnutrition, specific micronutrient deficiencies or feeding disorders.

Clinical Presentation

Food protein-induced enteropathy, enterocolitis syndrome (FPIES) and proctocolitis are the three main food allergic gastrointestinal disorders that occur during infancy. Symptoms include persistent regurgitation, vomiting, chronic diarrhoea, rectal bleeding, feeding difficulties and unsettled behaviour.

Food Protein-Induced Enteropathy

Infants and young children suffering from food protein-induced enteropathy typically present with chronic diarrhoea [2]. Cow's milk and soy milk proteins are considered to be the main offending food allergens. The prevalence of food protein-induced enteropathy appears to have decreased since the development of 'humanised' cow's milk and soy formula. However, current reliable prevalence figures are not available. Allergic inflammation in the small intestine causes mucosal damage with distortion of the villous architecture. The histological features share strong similarities with those of untreated coeliac disease (CD) [3]. Early studies of cow's milk-sensitive enteropathy have demonstrated that the mucosal damage is mediated by eosinophils in the presence of vascular cell adhesion molecule-1 [4]. More recently, cow's milk-specific T-helper 2 lymphocytes have been identified in biopsies of patients with duodenal eosinophilic gastroenteri-

tis or food protein-induced enteropathy [5]. Localised production of IgE in the mucosa of the small intestine in the absence of food-specific serum IgE may also be implicated in the pathogenesis of this condition [6].

The manifestations of cow's milk or soy enteropathy during infancy include chronic diarrhoea, vomiting, poor weight gain and associated micronutrient deficiencies (e.g. iron deficiency or rickets) [7]. Severe cases may also develop protein-losing enteropathy and present with peripheral oedema due to hypoalbuminaemia [2]. If treatment is delayed, infants may develop protein-energy malnutrition and growth impairment. Infants with cow's milk enteropathy often develop secondary lactose malabsorption due to reduced expression of brush border lactase in the shortened intestinal villi. Lactose therefore needs to be eliminated from the diets of these infants until the normal villus architecture has been restored. While lactose-free cow's milk-based formula reduces the severity of diarrhoea in cow's milk enteropathy, it is not suitable as a treatment formula due to its cow's milk protein content, which perpetuates allergic gut inflammation. Extensively hydrolysed formula is considered to be the first-line treatment for cow's milk or soy enteropathy in infants [8, 9]. Soy formula may be tolerated in infants from 6 months of age [10]. In severe cases, an amino acid-based formula (AAF) may be required [11]. Tolerance development needs to be assessed intermittently by cow's milk challenge. Strict cow's milk protein elimination needs to be continued until tolerance develops, which usually occurs between 12 and 24 months of age. In a subset of patients, residual gastrointestinal symptoms may persist to school age [12].

Food Protein-Induced Enterocolitis Syndrome

FPIES is characterised by profuse vomiting and dehydration, with onset at about 2 hours after allergen ingestion [13]. In a population-based study, FPIES reactions occurred in 0.34% of infants [14]. Similar to most cell-mediated food-allergic disorders, the pathological mechanisms causing FPIES are poorly understood. The term 'enterocolitis' may be misleading because direct evidence of allergic inflammation in the small intestine or colon is missing. Cow's milk and soy are considered to be the main causative allergens [13]. Solid foods, including rice, other cereals and poultry meats, may also cause FPIES reactions in infants [15, 16]. FPIES reactions to multiple food allergens are relatively common. Protracted vomiting may lead to hypovolaemic shock, which occurs in about 20% of patients with FPIES. These infants present with pallor, lethargy and floppiness. Cutaneous signs are absent, which, apart from the timing of reactions, is an important distinguishing clinical feature against anaphylaxis. No diagnostic test other than food challenge is currently available to confirm the diagnosis of this condition. Its diagnosis is therefore often not established at first presentation, and infants may develop further FPIES reactions before this type of food allergy is recognised [17]. This condition may be mistaken for gastroenteritis, sepsis or even intestinal obstruction [18]. Its treatment involves strict avoidance of the offending food allergens. FPIES does not appear to occur in breast-fed infants, and maternal elimination diets in these infants are therefore generally not required [8]. Tolerance is usually assessed by food challenge at around 2 years of age. Due to the risk of significant vomiting and dehydration during challenges, they are usually performed at a hospital.

Food Protein-Induced Proctocolitis
Food protein-induced proctocolitis is a relatively common and benign form of gastrointestinal food allergy that manifests with low-grade diarrhoea and bright rectal bleeding during the first weeks of life [19]. Infantile proctocolitis is the most common cause of low-grade rectal bleeding in infants less than 3 months of age [20]. Exact prevalence figures in infants are unavailable.

Symptoms usually develop between 3 and 6 weeks of age but may occasionally be seen in older infants. Infantile proctocolitis occurs in both breast- and formula-fed infants [21]. Its clinical presentation is generally limited to low-grade diarrhoea containing small amounts of fresh blood and mucus. These infants are otherwise healthy. Because the associated blood loss is usually minor, clinically significant anaemia is uncommon. Endoscopic biopsies typically demonstrate eosinophilic proctocolitis with the presence of more than 10 eosinophils per microscopic high-power field [21]. Numbers of intraepithelial lymphocytes, predominantly CD8[+] cells, are also increased [22]. The differential diagnosis of rectal bleeding in infancy includes colonic polyps, non-allergic colitis, bacterial gastroenteritis, duplication cysts or vascular malformations. Rectal suction biopsy may be indicated in infants with severe constipation to assess for the possible presence of Hirschsprung's disease. The treatment of infantile allergic proctocolitis involves the dietary elimination of the offending food proteins. In the majority of cases, the elimination of cow's milk protein is sufficient and can be achieved by a maternal elimination diet in breast-fed infants or by the use of an extensively hydrolysed hypoallergenic formula. The prognosis of infantile allergic proctocolitis is excellent, and most infants outgrow this condition between 9 and 12 months of age [21].

Multiple Food Protein Intolerance of Infancy
Multiple food protein intolerance (MFPI) is a severe form of gastrointestinal food allergy to cow's milk, soy milk, casein or whey hydrolysate formula and other common weaning foods [23, 24]. Infants with MFPI present with gastrointestinal manifestations, including persistent vomiting, diarrhoea, severe irritability, feeding difficulties and poor weight gain. AAF is the treatment of choice, and symptoms typically remit within 2 weeks of commencing the elemental diet. Most

infants tolerate a small range of solid foods, including potato, pumpkin, zucchini, apple, pear, rice cereal and chicken meat. The diet is gradually expanded as tolerated, while the infants remain on an AAF. The majority of infants with MFPI develop tolerance to solid foods between 18 and 24 months of age, and only 10% require AAF by 3 years of age [24].

Food Protein-Induced Gastrointestinal Motility Disorders in Infants and Young Children
GORD and constipation are among the most common disorders that occur during infancy and early childhood. In at least a subset of infants with these functional disorders, improvement after the dietary elimination of specific food proteins has been demonstrated. Gastrointestinal food allergy should therefore be considered in the differential diagnosis of infants presenting with persistent regurgitation or constipation, particularly if conventional treatment has not been beneficial. Gastrointestinal biopsies with evidence of tissue eosinophilia prior to the initiation of a hypoallergenic diet may provide important diagnostic clues. However, better diagnostic markers of paediatric allergic gastrointestinal motility disorders are required.

Gastro-Oesophageal Reflux Disease in Infancy
Gastro-oesophageal reflux (GOR) involves the involuntary, passive regurgitation of gastric contents into the oesophagus and occurs in about 20–25% of healthy young infants [25]. In the vast majority of cases, infantile GOR does not require treatment and resolves at around 12–18 months of age [26]. If it is associated with clinical complications (e.g. reflux oesophagitis, aspiration or failure to thrive), it represents GORD. The thickening of formula and acid suppression with a proton pump inhibitor may be required in severe cases with significant ongoing regurgitation. However, the effectiveness of the use of proton pump inhibitors during infancy has recently been questioned [27].

Several studies have linked reflux oesophagitis during infancy to non-IgE-mediated cow's milk allergy [28, 29]. In a study of infants with biopsy-proven oesophagitis, about 42% improved after treatment with an extensively hydrolysed formula and relapsed following subsequent blinded cow's milk challenges [29]. The mechanisms by which food allergens induce GOR and oesophagitis are poorly understood. In oesophageal tissue, the number of mucosal eosinophils in food protein-induced GORD is not increased (<5/high power field), distinguishing it from eosinophilic oesophagitis [30]. Typically, infants with cow's milk-induced GORD present with frequent regurgitation. Feeding refusal is a common problem and may lead to poor weight gain [31]. Infants with cow's milk protein-induced GORD typically respond to treatment with an extensively hydrolysed formula or an AAF if symptoms are severe [28]. If symptoms improve significantly following the initiation of a hypoallergenic diet, a diagnosis of cow's milk protein-induced GORD is assumed. This diagnosis should be confirmed by cautious cow's milk challenge to avoid unnecessary elimination diets. If challenges fail, they can be repeated every 3–6 months until tolerance has been demonstrated.

Constipation
Food protein-induced constipation is a poorly defined clinical entity, and its incidence during infancy is not known [32]. Only a small proportion of constipation in children less than 2 years of age is due to food allergies, and the vast majority of cases are functional in nature. Minor non-allergic constipation commonly occurs at the transition from breast to formula feeding. Cow's milk formula with a high casein:whey protein ratio and high levels of palmitic acid has been shown to negatively affect stool consistency [33]. Infants with cow's milk allergic constipation typically present with infrequent bowel movements from the first weeks of life or after the dietary introduction of cow's milk-based products. In severe cases,

this symptom may be associated with significant abdominal distension and should be distinguished from Hirschsprung's disease by rectal suction biopsy [34]. In some cases, eosinophilic proctocolitis can be demonstrated [32]. Anal sphincter tone may be increased in infants with eosinophilic proctocolitis and predispose them to faecal retention [35]. The treatment of cow's milk-induced constipation relies on a trial of a strict cow's milk-free diet, which often involves the use of an AAF for several weeks to months. In breast-fed infants, a strict maternal dairy-free elimination diet may also be effective. The assessment of treatment outcomes in patients with significant secondary megarectum may be difficult because the treatment response may be delayed. Stool softeners or laxatives should be continued during dietary trials and gradually weaned over weeks to months, as tolerated. The differential diagnosis of severe constipation includes Hirschsprung's disease, slow transit constipation and other gastrointestinal motility disorders. The prognosis of food allergic constipation appears to be generally good. Dietary restrictions need to be maintained until tolerance to cow's milk protein has been demonstrated. No formal longitudinal studies on the natural history of cow's milk-induced constipation are available.

Infantile Colic
Infantile colic presents with episodes of persistent and inconsolable crying during the first weeks of life. In the vast majority of infants with colic, no organic cause is found [36, 37]. However, colic symptoms may cause maternal exhaustion and significant family stress [38]. Only few randomised, placebo-controlled studies on the treatment of colic are available. Most treatments initiated at the peak of crying at around 6 weeks of age are no better than placebo because spontaneous improvement of colic symptoms usually occurs at between 3 and 4 months of age [39]. Recently, several randomised clinical trials have demonstrated that treatment or prophylaxis with probi-

otics (e.g. *Lactobacillus reuteri*) significantly reduces crying duration in infants with colic [40].

In a subset of infants, colic symptoms may be caused by a non-IgE-mediated cow's milk allergy. However, the vast majority of young infants with colic do not suffer from underlying food allergies, and the relationship between colic and cow's milk allergy remains controversial. Previous studies have had methodological limitations and have typically not been population-based. Cow's milk allergy should be suspected in infants with severe colic if the persistent crying is associated with gastrointestinal symptoms, feeding refusal or poor weight gain. Several clinical trials have assessed the effects of formula on colic and have demonstrated a significant treatment benefit of hypoallergenic formula [41–47]. A systematic review has demonstrated the benefit of extensively hydrolysed and soy-based formula for infants with colic [48]. Partially hydrolysed formula or lactose-free formula, however, is not suitable for the treatment of non-IgE-mediated cow's milk allergy. Maternal elimination diets may also be an effective treatment for a proportion of breast-fed infants with colic [41]. The diagnosis of cow's milk allergy needs to be confirmed by subsequent cow's milk challenge to avoid unnecessary dietary restrictions for the mother or infant. The exact role of cow's milk allergy in infants with colic requires further study.

Carbohydrate Malabsorption and Food Intolerance
Carbohydrate malabsorption during early childhood presents with intermittent, food-associated diarrhoea as well as abdominal bloating and pain. It is therefore one of the main differential diagnoses of gastrointestinal food allergy. The diagnostic overlap of non-IgE-mediated cow's milk allergy and lactose malabsorption is particularly close. Other forms of carbohydrate malabsorption, including congenital sucrase-isomaltase deficiency [49], may also masquerade as food allergies. Lactose and fructose malabsorption are often

implicated in children with recurrent abdominal pain. However, clinical trials have demonstrated that these conditions do not generally cause recurrent abdominal pain [50].

Lactose Intolerance/Malabsorption

Lactose is the main carbohydrate in human milk [51]. In breast-fed infants, low-grade lactose malabsorption is considered to be physiological [52]. Lactose requires enzymatic hydrolysis by lactase before its subunits D-glucose and D-galactose can be absorbed [53]. Lactase is expressed in the brush border by mature enterocytes and is the most highly expressed in the mid-jejunum. Maximal lactase expression occurs during the first months of life [54]. In 65–70% of the world's population, lactase activity significantly declines by adulthood ('non-persistence'). Lactase persistence is more common in people with Northern European, West African or Middle Eastern backgrounds [55]. Congenital (primary) lactose malabsorption is a rare genetic disorder that mainly occurs in Finland and Western Russia [56]. Secondary lactose malabsorption is relatively common during infancy and is the result of another underlying disorder, such as infective gastroenteritis, CD, cow's milk protein-induced enteropathy or rare epithelial dysplasia syndromes.

Lactose malabsorption in infancy presents with abdominal distension, diarrhoea and perianal excoriation due to acidic stools. Depending on the underlying pathology and duration of symptoms, weight gain may also be slow [57]. The treatment of formula-fed infants consists of lactose restriction, which involves a shift to a lactose-reduced, cow's milk-based formula. In breast-fed infants, it is more difficult to limit the intake of lactose. Expressed breast milk can be incubated with lactase drops if symptoms are severe. The need for long-term lactose restriction depends on the type of underlying process. In infants with infective gastroenteritis, adequate lactase activity is usually restored within 2–4 weeks. However, in very young infants, recovery may be delayed. If

cow's milk enteropathy is suspected, infants should be started on a hypoallergenic formula and avoid dietary cow's milk protein.

Coeliac Disease

CD is a gluten-sensitive enteropathy with a community prevalence of about 1% [58, 59]. The clinical presentation of CD and cow's milk allergic enteropathy are very similar and difficult to distinguish by histology. Over the past decade, there have been significant breakthroughs in the understanding of the pathophysiology of CD, particularly regarding the involvement of human leukocyte antigens (HLA-DQ2/DQ8) and tissue transglutaminase in the immune processing of gluten-derived peptides by antigen-presenting cells and T-lymphocytes [60, 61]. Highly sensitive and specific serological markers, such as serum IgA and IgG antibodies against tissue transglutaminase and deamidated gliadin peptides, have become available in recent years [62, 63]. From a diagnostic perspective, it is important to test for CD before wheat is eliminated from the diet. The combination of HLA-DQ2/DQ8 screening and antibody testing has significantly improved the diagnostic accuracy of the serological diagnosis of this disease. However, despite these recent advances, its diagnosis still requires confirmation by small bowel biopsy [64–66]. Conversely, the absence of HLA-DQ2/DQ8 in the setting of a negative serology practically rules out CD. The treatment of CD involves a life-long, strict, gluten-free diet.

Diagnostic Evaluation and Differential Diagnosis

The diagnosis of gastrointestinal food allergy generally relies on the demonstration of a significant clinical improvement within 2–4 weeks after food allergen elimination and a relapse of symptoms after re-challenge. The challenge phase is often deferred until nutritional rehabilitation has been achieved. Skin prick testing and measurement of the food-specific serum IgE antibody level are generally not diagnostic because gastrointestinal food allergies are not IgE-mediated. Atopy patch testing has been proposed as a useful diagnostic test for non-IgE-mediated food allergies [67]. However, its clinical application is hampered by its subjective interpretation and low sensitivity [68].

Endoscopic examination of the upper gastrointestinal tract may be valuable in patients with frequent regurgitation or vomiting. Oesophageal biopsies allow for the differentiation between GORD and eosinophilic oesophagitis [30]. In infants with bilious vomiting, an upper gastrointestinal barium study should be performed to rule out any anatomical anomalies, particularly intestinal malrotation. An increase in the number of eosinophils in gastric or duodenal biopsies may be a useful marker of gastrointestinal cow's milk allergy in infants [2]. Small bowel biopsies are important in the assessment for possible CD or other enteropathies. Patients need to maintain a wheat-containing diet for at least 2–3 months before biopsy to confidently assess for possible CD. In infants with persistent diarrhoea, measurements of duodenal disaccharidase levels (lactase, sucrase and maltase/isomaltase) are useful to test for carbohydrate malabsorption due to disaccharidase deficiency [69, 70]. Hydrogen breath testing after ingestion of specific sugars (lactose, fructose, and sucrose) can also be helpful in assessing for possible carbohydrate malabsorption, e.g. lactose or fructose intolerance.

Dietary Management

The treatment of gastrointestinal food allergies is based on the strict dietary avoidance of the offending food allergens. Because there are no clear diagnostic markers, dietary allergen elimination is often empirical. Cow's milk, soy and wheat are the main suspected gastrointestinal food allergens. However, other solid foods may also be of importance (e.g. rice, corn, and chicken). After making a presumed diagnosis of non-IgE-mediated food allergy, a dietary plan is implemented with the help of a paediatric dietician. After 2–4 weeks, the clinical response to the elimination diet is assessed. In patients with significantly improved gastrointestinal symptoms, the diet is continued. In patients with no response, the diet is either normalised, or a more broad-based elimination diet is trialled. In some cases, an elemental diet may be used. In breast-fed infants, a maternal cow's milk-free elimination diet (sometimes in combination with soy or wheat) can be attempted. The maternal diet should be assessed by a dietician for its nutritional adequacy, and a calcium supplement should be prescribed (1.2 g daily in several divided doses). In formula-fed infants, a trial of an extensively hydrolysed formula or a soy-based formula (in infants >6 months) should be attempted. Infants that experience ongoing symptoms while on an extensively hydrolysed formula may benefit from an AAF. Reintroduction of the eliminated food allergens by cautious challenge should be attempted every 3–6 months until tolerance develops. Prolonged elimination diets should be closely supervised by a dietician to minimise the risk of adverse nutritional outcomes, and growth parameters should be carefully monitored.

Conclusion

Gastrointestinal food allergy is a common clinical problem in infants and young children. Recognition may be delayed due to a lack of diagnostic markers and clinical overlaps with other non-allergic gastrointestinal problems that occur during infancy. The diagnosis of non-IgE-mediated food allergy requires a high degree of clinical suspicion and a careful dietary assessment. Involvement of a paediatric dietician in the management of elimination diets is recommended to reduce the risk of nutritional deficiencies or growth impairment.

References

1 Sicherer SH: Epidemiology of food allergy. J Allergy Clin Immunol 2011;127: 594–602.
2 Chehade M, Magid MS, Mofidi S, Nowak-Wegrzyn A, Sampson HA, Sicherer SH: Allergic eosinophilic gastroenteritis with protein-losing enteropathy: intestinal pathology, clinical course, and long-term follow-up. J Pediatr Gastroenterol Nutr 2006;42:516–521.
3 Iyngkaran N, Abdin Z, Davis K, Boey CG, Prathap K, Yadav M, Lam SK, Puthucheary SD: Acquired carbohydrate intolerance and cow milk protein-sensitive enteropathy in young infants. J Pediatr 1979;95:373–378.
4 Chung HL, Hwang JB, Kwon YD, Park MH, Shin WJ, Park JB: Deposition of eosinophil-granule major basic protein and expression of intercellular adhesion molecule-1 and vascular cell adhesion molecule-1 in the mucosa of the small intestine in infants with cow's milk-sensitive enteropathy. J Allergy Clin Immunol 1999;103:1195–1201.
5 Beyer K, Castro R, Birnbaum A, Benkov K, Pittman N, Sampson HA: Human milk-specific mucosal lymphocytes of the gastrointestinal tract display a TH2 cytokine profile. J Allergy Clin Immunol 2002;109:707–713.
6 Lin XP, Magnusson J, Ahlstedt S, Dahlman-Höglund A, Hanson LL, Magnusson O, Bengtsson U, Telemo E: Local allergic reaction in food-hypersensitive adults despite a lack of systemic food-specific IgE. J Allergy Clin Immunol 2002;109:879–887.
7 Iyngkaran N, Robinson MJ, Prathap K, Sumithran E, Yadav M: Cows' milk protein-sensitive enteropathy. Combined clinical and histological criteria for diagnosis. Arch Dis Child 1978;53:20–26.
8 Allen KJ, Davidson GP, Day AS, Hill DJ, Kemp AS, Peake JE, Prescott SL, Shugg A, Sinn JK, Heine RG: Management of cow's milk protein allergy in infants and young children: an expert panel perspective. J Paediatr Child Health 2009; 45:481–486.

9 Fiocchi A, Brozek J, Schunemann H, Bahna SL, von Berg A, Beyer K, Bozzola M, Bradsher J, Compalati E, Ebisawa M, Guzman MA, Li H, Heine RG, Keith P, Lack G, Landi M, Martelli A, Rancé F, Sampson H, Stein A, Terracciano L, Vieths S: World Allergy Organization (WAO) Diagnosis and Rationale for Action against Cow's Milk Allergy (DRACMA) Guidelines. World Allergy Organ J 2010; 3:57–161.
10 Klemola T, Vanto T, Juntunen-Bäckman K, Kalimo K, Korpela R, Varjonen E: Allergy to soy formula and to extensively hydrolyzed whey formula in infants with cow's milk allergy: a prospective, randomized study with a follow-up to the age of 2 years. J Pediatr 2002;140: 219–224.
11 Hill DJ, Murch SH, Rafferty K, Wallis P, Green CJ: The efficacy of amino acid-based formulas in relieving the symptoms of cow's milk allergy: a systematic review. Clin Exp Allergy 2007;37:808–822.
12 Kokkonen J, Haapalahti M, Laurila K, Karttunen TJ, Mäki M: Cow's milk protein-sensitive enteropathy at school age. J Pediatr 2001;139:797–803.
13 Leonard SA, Nowak-Wegrzyn A: Clinical diagnosis and management of food protein-induced enterocolitis syndrome. Curr Opin Pediatr 2012;24:739–745.
14 Katz Y, Goldberg MR, Rajuan N, Cohen A, Leshno M: The prevalence and natural course of food protein-induced enterocolitis syndrome to cow's milk: a large-scale, prospective population-based study. J Allergy Clin Immunol 2011;127:647–653.e1–e3.
15 Nowak-Wegrzyn A, Sampson HA, Wood RA, Sicherer SH: Food protein-induced enterocolitis syndrome caused by solid food proteins. Pediatrics 2003; 111:829–835.
16 Mehr SS, Kakakios AM, Kemp AS: Rice: a common and severe cause of food protein-induced enterocolitis syndrome. Arch Dis Child 2009;94:220–223.
17 Mehr S, Kakakios A, Frith K, Kemp AS: Food protein-induced enterocolitis syndrome: 16-year experience. Pediatrics 2009;123:e459–e464.
18 Jayasooriya S, Fox AT, Murch SH: Do not laparotomize food-protein-induced enterocolitis syndrome. Pediatr Emerg Care 2007;23:173–175.

19 Odze RD, Bines J, Leichtner AM, Goldman H, Antonioli DA: Allergic proctocolitis in infants: a prospective clinicopathologic biopsy study. Hum Pathol 1993;24:668–674.
20 Chang JW, Wu TC, Wang KS, Huang IF, Huang B, Yu IT: Colon mucosal pathology in infants under three months of age with diarrhea disorders. J Pediatr Gastroenterol Nutr 2002;35:387–390.
21 Lake AM: Food-induced eosinophilic proctocolitis. J Pediatr Gastroenterol Nutr 2000;30(suppl):S58–S60.
22 Örmala T, Rintala R, Savilahti E: T cells of the colonic mucosa in patients with infantile colitis. J Pediatr Gastroenterol Nutr 2001;33:133–138.
23 Hill DJ, Cameron DJ, Francis DE, Gonzalez-Andaya AM, Hosking CS: Challenge confirmation of late-onset reactions to extensively hydrolyzed formulas in infants with multiple food protein intolerance. J Allergy Clin Immunol 1995;96:386–394.
24 Hill DJ, Heine RG, Cameron DJ, Francis DE, Bines JE: The natural history of intolerance to soy and extensively hydrolyzed formula in infants with multiple food protein intolerance. J Pediatr 1999; 135:118–121.
25 Nelson SP, Chen EH, Syniar GM, Christoffel KK: Prevalence of symptoms of gastroesophageal reflux during infancy. A pediatric practice-based survey. Pediatric Practice Research Group. Arch Pediatr Adolesc Med 1997;151:569–572.
26 Vandenplas Y, Rudolph CD, Di Lorenzo C, Hassall E, Liptak G, Mazur L, Sondheimer J, Staiano A, Thomson M, Veereman-Wauters G, Wenzl TG, North American Society for Pediatric Gastroenterology Hepatology and Nutrition, European Society for Pediatric Gastroenterology Hepatology and Nutrition: Pediatric gastroesophageal reflux clinical practice guidelines: joint recommendations of the North American Society for Pediatric Gastroenterology, Hepatology, and Nutrition (NASPGHAN) and the European Society for Pediatric Gastroenterology, Hepatology, and Nutrition (ESPGHAN). J Pediatr Gastroenterol Nutr 2009;49:498–547.

27 Davidson G, Wenzl TG, Thomson M, Omari T, Barker P, Lundborg P, Illueca M: Efficacy and safety of once-daily esomeprazole for the treatment of gastroesophageal reflux disease in neonatal patients. J Pediatr 2013;163:692–698.e1–e2.

28 Hill DJ, Heine RG, Cameron DJ, Catto-Smith AG, Chow CW, Francis DE, Hosking CS: Role of food protein intolerance in infants with persistent distress attributed to reflux esophagitis. J Pediatr 2000;136:641–647.

29 Iacono G, Carroccio A, Cavataio F, Montalto G, Kazmierska I, Lorello D, Soresi M, Notarbartolo A: Gastroesophageal reflux and cow's milk allergy in infants: a prospective study. J Allergy Clin Immunol 1996;97:822–827.

30 Liacouras CA, Furuta GT, Hirano I, Atkins D, Attwood SE, Bonis PA, Burks AW, Chehade M, Collins MH, Dellon ES, Dohil R, Falk GW, Gonsalves N, Gupta SK, Katzka DA, Lucendo AJ, Markowitz JE, Noel RJ, Odze RD, Putnam PE, Richter JE, Romero Y, Ruchelli E, Sampson HA, Schoepfer A, Shaheen NJ, Sicherer SH, Spechler S, Spergel JM, Straumann A, Wershil BK, Rothenberg ME, Aceves SS: Eosinophilic esophagitis: updated consensus recommendations for children and adults. J Allergy Clin Immunol 2011;128:3–20.e6; quiz 21–22.

31 Wu YP, Franciosi JP, Rothenberg ME, Hommel KA: Behavioral feeding problems and parenting stress in eosinophilic gastrointestinal disorders in children. Pediatr Allergy Immunol 2012;23:730–735.

32 Iacono G, Cavataio F, Montalto G, Florena A, Tumminello M, Soresi M, Notarbartolo A, Carroccio A: Intolerance of cow's milk and chronic constipation in children. N Engl J Med 1998;339:1100–1104.

33 Quinlan PT, Lockton S, Irwin J, Lucas AL: The relationship between stool hardness and stool composition in breast- and formula-fed infants. J Pediatr Gastroenterol Nutr 1995;20:81–90.

34 Lee JH, Choe YH, Lee SK, Seo JM, Kim JH, Suh YL: Allergic proctitis and abdominal distention mimicking Hirschsprung's disease in infants. Acta Paediatr 2007;96:1784–1789.

35 Iacono G, Bonventre S, Scalici C, Maresi E, Di Prima L, Soresi M, Di Gesu G, Noto D, Carroccio A: Food intolerance and chronic constipation: manometry and histology study. Eur J Gastroenterol Hepatol 2006;18:143–150.

36 Barr RG: Colic and crying syndromes in infants. Pediatrics 1998;102:1282–1286.

37 Freedman SB, Al-Harthy N, Thull-Freedman J: The crying infant: diagnostic testing and frequency of serious underlying disease. Pediatrics 2009;123:841–848.

38 Clifford TJ, Campbell MK, Speechley KN, Gorodzinsky F: Sequelae of infant colic: evidence of transient infant distress and absence of lasting effects on maternal mental health. Arch Pediatr Adolesc Med 2002;156:1183–1188.

39 Hall B, Chesters J, Robinson A: Infantile colic: a systematic review of medical and conventional therapies. J Paediatr Child Health 2012;48:128–137.

40 Sung V, Collett S, de Gooyer T, Hiscock H, Tang M, Wake M: Probiotics to prevent or treat excessive infant crying: systematic review and meta-analysis. JAMA Pediatr 2013;167:1150–1157.

41 Hill DJ, Roy N, Heine RG, Hosking CS, Francis DE, Brown J, Speirs B, Sadowsky J, Carlin JB: Effect of a low-allergen maternal diet on colic among breastfed infants: a randomized, controlled trial. Pediatrics 2005;116:e709–e715.

42 Lucassen PL, Assendelft WJ, Gubbels JW, van Eijk JT, van Geldrop WJ, Neven AK: Effectiveness of treatments for infantile colic: systematic review. BMJ 1998;316:1563–1569.

43 Evans RW, Fergusson DM, Allardyce RA, Taylor B: Maternal diet and infantile colic in breast-fed infants. Lancet 1981;1:1340–1342.

44 Campbell JP: Dietary treatment of infant colic: a double-blind study. J R Coll Gen Pract 1989;39:11–14.

45 Lothe L, Lindberg T, Jakobsson I: Cow's milk formula as a cause of infantile colic: a double-blind study. Pediatrics 1982;70:7–10.

46 Hill DJ, Hudson IL, Sheffield LJ, Shelton MJ, Menahem S, Hosking CS: A low allergen diet is a significant intervention in infantile colic: results of a community-based study. J Allergy Clin Immunol 1995;96:886–892.

47 Forsyth BW: Colic and the effect of changing formulas: a double-blind, multiple-crossover study. J Pediatr 1989;115:521–526.

48 Lucassen PL, Assendelft WJ: Systematic review of treatments for infant colic. Pediatrics 2001;108:1047–1048.

49 McMeans AR: Congenital sucrase-isomaltase deficiency: diet assessment and education guidelines. J Pediatr Gastroenterol Nutr 2012;55(suppl 2):S37–S39.

50 Gijsbers CF, Kneepkens CM, Buller HA: Lactose and fructose malabsorption in children with recurrent abdominal pain: results of double-blinded testing. Acta Paediatr 2012;101:e411–e415.

51 Fusch G, Choi A, Rochow N, Fusch C: Quantification of lactose content in human and cow's milk using UPLC-tandem mass spectrometry. J Chromatogr B Analyt Technol Biomed Life Sci 2011;879:3759–3762.

52 Mobassaleh M, Montgomery RK, Biller JA, Grand RJ: Development of carbohydrate absorption in the fetus and neonate. Pediatrics 1985;75:160–166.

53 Gupta SK, Chong SK, Fitzgerald JF: Disaccharidase activities in children: normal values and comparison based on symptoms and histologic changes. J Pediatr Gastroenterol Nutr 1999;28:246–251.

54 Hamosh M: Digestion in the newborn. Clin Perinatol 1996;23:191–209.

55 Itan Y, Jones BL, Ingram CJ, Swallow DM, Thomas MG: A worldwide correlation of lactase persistence phenotype and genotypes. BMC Evol Biol 2010;10:36.

56 Savilahti E, Launiala K, Kuitunen P: Congenital lactase deficiency. A clinical study on 16 patients. Arch Dis Child 1983;58:246–252.

57 Northrop-Clewes CA, Lunn PG, Downes RM: Lactose maldigestion in breast-feeding Gambian infants. J Pediatr Gastroenterol Nutr 1997;24:257–263.

58 Mäki M, Mustalahti K, Kokkonen J, Kulmala P, Haapalahti M, Karttunen T, Ilonen J, Laurila K, Dahlbom I, Hansson T, Hopfl P, Knip M: Prevalence of Celiac disease among children in Finland. N Engl J Med 2003;348:2517–2524.

59 Mustalahti K, Catassi C, Reunanen A, Fabiani E, Heier M, McMillan S, Murray L, Metzger MH, Gasparin M, Bravi E, Mäki M: The prevalence of celiac disease in Europe: results of a centralized, international mass screening project. Ann Med 2010;42:587–595.

60 Sollid LM, Qiao SW, Anderson RP, Gianfrani C, Koning F: Nomenclature and listing of celiac disease relevant gluten T-cell epitopes restricted by HLA-DQ molecules. Immunogenetics 2012;64:455–460.

61 Karell K, Louka AS, Moodie SJ, Ascher H, Clot F, Greco L, Ciclitira PJ, Sollid LM, Partanen J, European Genetics Cluster on Celiac Disease: HLA types in celiac disease patients not carrying the DQA1*05-DQB1*02 (DQ2) heterodimer: results from the European Genetics Cluster on Celiac Disease. Hum Immunol 2003;64:469–477.

62 Alessio MG, Tonutti E, Brusca I, Radice A, Licini L, Sonzogni A, Florena A, Schiaffino E, Marus W, Sulfaro S, Villalta D, Study Group on Autoimmune Diseases of Italian Society of Laboratory Medicine: Correlation between IgA tissue transglutaminase antibody ratio and histological finding in celiac disease. J Pediatr Gastroenterol Nutr 2012;55: 44–49.

63 Zanini B, Magni A, Caselani F, Lanzarotto F, Carabellese N, Villanacci V, Ricci C, Lanzini A: High tissue-transglutaminase antibody level predicts small intestinal villous atrophy in adult patients at high risk of celiac disease. Dig Liver Dis 2012;44:280–285.

64 Kurppa K, Salminiemi J, Ukkola A, Saavalainen P, Loytynoja K, Laurila K, Collin P, Mäki M, Kaukinen K: Utility of the new ESPGHAN criteria for the diagnosis of celiac disease in at-risk groups. J Pediatr Gastroenterol Nutr 2012;54:387–391.

65 Marsh MN: Gluten, major histocompatibility complex, and the small intestine. A molecular and immunobiologic approach to the spectrum of gluten sensitivity ('celiac sprue'). Gastroenterology 1992;102:330–354.

66 Oberhuber G, Granditsch G, Vogelsang H: The histopathology of coeliac disease: time for a standardized report scheme for pathologists. Eur J Gastroenterol Hepatol 1999;11:1185–1194.

67 Niggemann B, Reibel S, Roehr CC, Felger D, Ziegert M, Sommerfeld C, Wahn U: Predictors of positive food challenge outcome in non-IgE-mediated reactions to food in children with atopic dermatitis. J Allergy Clin Immunol 2001;108: 1053–1058.

68 Heine RG, Verstege A, Mehl A, Staden U, Rolinck-Werninghaus C, Niggemann B: Proposal for a standardized interpretation of the atopy patch test in children with atopic dermatitis and suspected food allergy. Pediatr Allergy Immunol 2006;17:213–217.

69 Iyngkaran N, Davis K, Robinson MJ, Boey CG, Sumithran E, Yadav M, Lam SK, Puthucheary SD: Cows' milk protein-sensitive enteropathy: an important contributing cause of secondary sugar intolerance in young infants with acute infective enteritis. Arch Dis Child 1979; 54:39–43.

70 Heyman MB, Committee on Nutrition: Lactose intolerance in infants, children, and adolescents. Pediatrics 2006;118: 1279–1286.

Dr. Ralf G. Heine, MD, FRACP
Department of Gastroenterology and Clinical Nutrition
The Royal Children's Hospital Melbourne
50 Flemington Road
Parkville, VIC 3052 (Australia)
E-Mail ralf.heine@rch.org.au

Ebisawa M, Ballmer-Weber BK, Vieths S, Wood RA (eds): Food Allergy: Molecular Basis and Clinical Practice.
Chem Immunol Allergy. Basel, Karger, 2015, vol 101, pp 181–190 (DOI: 10.1159/000371701)

Atopic Eczema and Food Allergy

Anja Wassmann[a, b] · Thomas Werfel[a]

[a]Department of Dermatology and Allergy, Hannover Medical School, Hannover, and
[b]Dermatological Ambulatory, Hamburg, Germany

Abstract

Approximately one-third of children with severe atopic eczema suffer from a food allergy, whereas in adult patients, food allergies are rare. In child patients, three different clinical reaction patterns can be differentiated as follows: (1) immediate-type reactions, (2) isolated late eczematous reactions, and (3) combined immediate-type and late eczematous reactions. In childhood food allergies, food allergens, such as cow's milk or hen's egg, are primarily responsible for allergic reactions, while in adolescents and adults, food allergies often develop consecutively after primary sensitization to pollen allergens. Dysfunctions in the epidermal barrier seem to be vitally important in the development of food allergies in patients with atopic eczema by facilitating sensitization after epicutaneous allergen exposure. Further investigation is required to determine the role of intestinal epithelial barrier defects in the pathogenesis of these allergies as well as the genetic characteristics associated with an increased risk of food allergy. The diagnosis of eczematous reactions to food requires a careful diagnostic procedure, taking into account a patient's history and sensitization patterns. The clinical relevance of sensitization often has to be proven by an oral food challenge, with the rating of the skin condition by validated scores after 24 h and the later evaluation of the eczematous reaction. © 2015 S. Karger AG, Basel

Prevalence and Natural History of Food Allergies in Atopic Eczema

A large subset of child patients with atopic eczema suffers from a concurrent food allergy, whereas in adolescent and adult patients, food allergies are rare. Data from studies based on the outcomes of double-blind placebo-controlled food challenges (DBPCFCs) have indicated that approximately one-third of children with severe atopic eczema are affected by an IgE-mediated food allergy. In addition to immediate-type reactions, foods can also induce a worsening of the skin condition in affected children [1–3]. In contrast, in adult patients, atopic eczema is rarely associated with food allergy [4]; however, data from controlled clinical trials is lacking.

Childhood food allergies tend to show remission after temporary food avoidance. A total of 50–80% of children with a cow's milk, hen's egg or soy allergy develop a tolerance to the food allergen before reaching school age [5–9], while allergies to peanuts, tree nuts and fish persist for a longer duration [9, 10].

To date, the DBPCFC serves as the 'gold standard' for the diagnosis of food allergy, especially in atopic eczema. Because DBPCFCs are costly with regard to both time and personnel, it is desir-

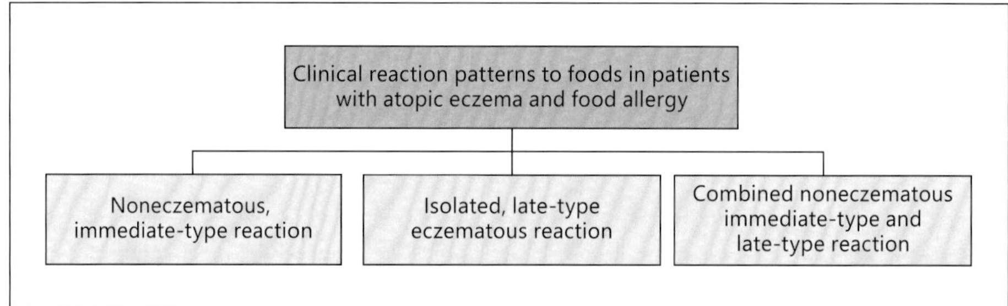

Fig. 1. Clinical reaction patterns to foods in patients with atopic eczema and a food allergy adapted from an EAACI position paper [1].

able to define decision points for the prediction of clinically relevant food allergies.

The Early Prevention of Asthma in Atopic Children study has proven that there is a correlation between sensitization against food allergens during early childhood and the manifestation of atopic eczema. In an international cohort of 2,184 children with atopic eczema, high-risk IgE titers were identified against cow's milk, hen's egg and peanuts, especially in infants who developed atopic eczema within the first 3 months of life as well as in those with the most severe eczema. In contrast, children who acquired atopic eczema after the age of twelve months showed the lowest high-risk IgE titer frequency [11]. Further investigations should be conducted to evaluate the clinical relevance of the defined IgE titers in this high-risk group to derive specific recommendations for clinical practice.

The early occurrence of sensitization against food allergens between the ages of 3–18 months is related to the manifestation of atopic eczema and bronchial asthma at the age of 6 years. The results of the Danish Allergy Research Center birth cohort study have illustrated the association between early sensitization patterns and subsequent allergic disease at the age of 6 years. In particular, early sensitization against food allergens has been identified as a risk marker for the later development of allergic diseases [12]. Data from this birth cohort based on the outcomes of oral food challenges showed a 6-year food allergy incidence of 3.7% (20/534). A total of 18 of these 20 children had also been diagnosed with atopic eczema at least once. The children who suffered from atopic eczema and food allergy showed higher food-specific IgE titers, while those children with atopic eczema without an accompanying food allergy did not differ significantly from the healthy control set concerning the frequency and level of food-specific IgE antibody detection [13].

Despite these recent results, which suggest that a score combining clinical signs and sensitization patterns may lead to the diagnosis of food allergy in the future, the DBPCFC remains the current 'gold standard' for the diagnosis of food allergy in patients with atopic eczema in routine clinical practice. Further research is needed to evaluate the scope of defining predictive markers for the diagnosis of clinically relevant food allergies in these patients.

Clinical Reaction Patterns to Foods in Patients with Atopic Eczema

In patients with atopic eczema and food allergies, three different clinical reaction patterns can be observed (fig. 1).

Immediate-type reactions are based on an IgE-mediated immune response and are characterized by the acute onset of symptoms within the first 2 h after allergen exposure. Delayed immediate type reactions can occur within 6 hours after food uptake. Immediate-type reactions can manifest as noneczematous cutaneous reactions, such as urticaria, angioedema or flush, as well as noncutaneous reactions in the forms of gastrointestinal symptoms, rhinitis and/or conjunctivitis, asthma or cardiovascular reactions up to anaphylactic shock [9]. Furthermore, in some patients with atopic eczema, a late T cell-mediated reaction with an exacerbation of eczema can be observed as early as 6 h and up to 48 h after food ingestion. A late-type eczematous reaction can occur in isolation or accompanied by a preceding immediate-type reaction [1].

Data from the DBPCFC performed on children with atopic eczema have indicated that 25% of all clinical reactions occur at 2 h or later after food ingestion [14, 15]. There is also evidence that birch pollen-related foods may act as triggers of the worsening of the skin condition in a subgroup of birch pollen-allergic patients with atopic eczema (Wassmann et al., unpublished data) [16, 17].

Allergens

In children, food allergies are predominantly caused by cow's milk, hen's egg, soy, wheat, fish, peanuts, or tree nuts. These foods cause about 90% of childhood food allergies [18, 19]. In contrast, data from oral provocation tests have confirmed that only a minority of adolescent and adults suffer from an allergy to 'classic' food allergens, such as wheat, cow's milk or hen's egg [20–22]. However, pollen-related food allergies increase in importance in adolescents and adults. In Northern and Central Europe, allergies to birch pollen-related foods (hazelnut, carrot, celery, and apple) are the most common. There is evidence that birch pollen-related foods can cause an exacerbation of eczema in adults [16] as well as in the subgroup of infantile patients with atopic eczema and birch pollen allergy [17]. Our recent

data obtained from larger patient cohorts have confirmed these previous results, showing that 49% out of 65 patients with atopic eczema and a proven birch pollen-related food allergy exhibit the exacerbation of eczema after oral food challenge with birch pollen-related foods (apple, carrot, celery, and/or hazelnut) (Wassmann et al., unpublished data).

Current research is focused on analyzing specific sensitization patterns, taking into account the roles of recombinant or native allergen components. Age-related and regional differences in sensitization patterns have already been described. Furthermore, risk markers for more severe allergic reactions have been characterized, such as lipid transfer proteins or storage proteins as well as pollen-related allergen components in foods, such as the homolog to the birch pollen major allergen Bet v 1, which is a member of the pathogenesis-related protein family 10 [23–27]. Further research needs to be conducted to evaluate whether the sensitization patterns of patients with atopic eczema and a food allergy differ from those with a suspected food allergy without atopic eczema.

Pathogenesis of Food Allergy in Atopic Eczema

Epidermal Barrier Dysfunction

Atopic eczema is characterized by a defective skin barrier function, which may also play an important role in the development of accompanying food allergies [28, 29]. In children with atopic eczema, food-specific sensitization is detectable even before the specific food has been introduced into the diet. This observation points to the involvement of skin barrier defects in the pathogenesis of food allergies. In animal models, it has been demonstrated that sensitization towards food allergens is enhanced after epidermal allergen exposure compared with other routes of sensitization. This effect is particularly observed after the removal of the stratum corneum or if a genetically determined impairment of the epidermal barrier exists [30–32]. The epidermal sensitization route enhances the T-helper type 2 immune response, which is typical of acute lesions in atopic eczema and is characterized by the production of interleukin-4 and IgE [33]. To date, several genes associated with atopic eczema have been identified. Of them, the gene encoding filaggrin (FLG) has been the most consistently replicated. FLG is an important protein that is involved in the maintenance of the skin barrier function and skin hydration [34]. Mutations in FLG or in the epidermal differentiation complex located on chromosome 1q21 [35] and variations in FLG expression due to the cytokine milieu could be of pathogenic importance in epidermal dysfunction in atopic eczema [36]. These findings support the theory of the outside-inside-outside pathogenic mechanisms in atopic eczema, which proposes that skin barrier defects are among the initiating pathogenic factors in this disease. Facilitated allergen penetration through the skin can enhance allergic skin inflammation [33].

Data from a recent case-control study of patients with a peanut allergy and non-peanut-sensitized population controls have shown that FLG-null mutations represent significant risk factors for IgE-mediated peanut allergies – even in the absence of clinical evidence of atopic eczema. These results point to a role of epithelial barrier dysfunction in the pathogenesis of food allergies [28].

Gut Barrier Dysfunction
The manifestation of food allergies is a result of a failure to develop oral tolerance or of a loss of pre-existing tolerance. Therefore, an impairment of the gut barrier is of vital importance in the pathogenesis of food allergies [37]. The gastrointestinal tract represents the largest immunologic organ of the human body. The gastrointestinal surface is lined with a single layer of epithelium that acts as a barrier between the abluminal side and luminal factors, such as food antigens [38]. Epithelial layer cells are joined by 'tight junctions,' which control antigen uptake from the intestinal lumen. Additionally, the immunogenicities of pathogens and food antigens are reduced by luminal and brush border enzymes, bile salts, and extreme pH values in the gastrointestinal tract. In addition to these functional barrier mechanisms, defense against foreign antigens involves components of intestinal innate immunity (polymorphonuclear neutrophils, macrophages, natural killer cells, epithelial cells, and Toll-like receptors) and the adaptive immune response (intraepithelial and lamina propria lymphocytes, Peyer's plaques, secretory IgA, and cytokines) [39]. A loss of tolerance can result from defects in immune or non-immune barrier factors (e.g. an increase in the gastric pH caused by antacid medicine [40], abnormalities in the development of regulatory T cells, soluble IgA, Peyer's plaques, and associated dendritic cells [41]). Therefore, the immaturity of various components of the gut barrier and gastrointestinal immunity might explain the high rate of food allergies in infants and young children [42]. In addition, it has been demonstrated that children with food allergies show a higher intestinal permeability than nonallergic children, which may contribute to the increased intestinal absorption of intact food proteins [43]. Likewise, the impairment of the intestinal barrier through physiological stress or bacterial infections enhances the risk of food sensitization [44].

There is evidence that a low diversity of gut microbiota during the first month of life is associated with an increased risk of the subsequent development of atopic eczema [45]. Further investigation is needed to determine whether the bacterial colonization of the gut influences the development of atopic eczema and food sensitization [46].

Immune Response
In addition to specific IgE antibodies, allergen-specific T cells can play an important role in the pathogenesis of food allergies in patients with atopic eczema [47]. While specific IgE antibodies are characteristic of immediate-type reactions to

food, specific T cells have been shown to be involved in the development of late eczematous reactions after food ingestion. Allergen-specific T cell clones and cutaneous lymphocyte-associated antigen-positive lymphocytes generated from children and adults with the food-induced worsening of atopic eczema show higher proliferative responses than those generated from nonresponders [48–50]. Furthermore, T cells generated from food-responsive patients show a distinct cytokine pattern, with a significantly higher release of the proinflammatory cytokines tumor necrosis factor-α and interleukin-1 [51].

Likewise, the outstanding role of birch pollen-specific T cells has been demonstrated in patients with atopic eczema and birch pollen-related food-induced eczematous reactions [16]. It has been shown that even cooked birch pollen-related food allergens can induce an immune response in Bet v 1-specific T cells *in vitro*, whereas the IgE-binding capacity of food allergens is abrogated by thermal processing [52]. Data form murine models have confirmed the role of T cells in food-sensitive atopic eczema [53].

Diagnosis of Food Allergy in Atopic Eczema

The identification of immediate-type reactions to food is relatively well achieved by the assessment of patient history, the testing of skin and the detection of specific IgE antibodies towards the suspected food. In contrast, in view of the occurrence of delayed eczema flare-ups after food ingestion, elucidation of a cause in patients with atopic eczema is difficult. In these cases, a patient's history is of reduced value [15].

There is no single parameter for the diagnosis of late-type allergic reactions to foods. Thus, a stepwise procedure referring to the diagnostic algorithm for immediate-type reactions is recommended. However, particularities in the diagnosis of late eczematous reactions to food and individual factors should be carefully taken into consid-

Table 1. Diagnostic algorithm in patients with persistent moderate-to-severe atopic eczema and a suspected food allergy (modified according to Werfel et al. [1, 2])

History of food allergy
History of suspected food allergy
Daily food-symptom diary (including the status of atopic eczema, intensity of itch and sleep loss) over a period of at least 2 weeks

***In vitro* diagnostics**
Specific IgE (together with total IgE)

***In vivo* diagnostics**
Skin tests
SPT (APT)
Diagnostic elimination diet
Specific diagnostic elimination diet over a period of at least 4 weeks
If there is no obvious association between food intake and allergic reaction, a diagnostic oligoallergenic diet should be introduced over a period of about 2 weeks. In adult patients this approach is only needed in exceptional cases.
Oral food challenge
First step of oral food challenge
– During a stable phase of the disease, oral food challenge should be conducted after the evaluation of the eczema score; ideally, a DBPCFC should be performed.*
– Titrated oral food challenge on the first challenge day:
    Evaluation of non-eczematous symptoms over the titration phase and the following 2 h
    Evaluation of the eczema score for at least 16–24 h after oral food challenge
– In the case of a negative reaction: the oral food challenge should be continued for a second consecutive day, with the cumulative dose corresponding to the average daily intake of the food.
– In the case of a negative reaction, if applicable: the oral food challenge should be continued over a period of several days with an average daily intake of food. The eczema score should be evaluated on every day during the challenge for up to 1 week.
Observation
– At least 1 challenge-free day
Second step of oral food challenge
– The next step of the oral food challenge is performed following the procedure described above.

SPT = Skin prick test; APT = atopy patch test.
* In the case of a DBPCFC, the first or second step of the oral food challenge should be performed with the suspected food or placebo.

eration (table 1) [1, 2]. If the role of a food as a trigger in persistent moderate-to-severe atopic eczema is uncertain, a daily food-symptom diary (including the status of atopic eczema, intensity of itch and sleep loss) over a period of 2–4 weeks should be recorded by patients or their parents [2].

In vitro Diagnostics

If a food allergy is suspected based on the history and/or the food-symptom diary, specific *in vivo* (e.g. the skin prick test, SPT) and *in vitro* tests (e.g. specific IgE) should follow [2]. However, it should be considered that in patients with atopic eczema and a suspected food allergy, the validity of specific IgE detection is limited. On the one hand, some patients with atopic eczema and late-type reactions to food have no detectable specific IgE antibodies [15]. On the other hand, these patients often show multiple IgE-mediated sensitizations that are not correlated with the occurrence of clinical symptoms (Wassmann et al., unpublished data) [54].

A multitude of research has been conducted to analyze the relationship between the degree of sensitization and the occurrence of clinically relevant childhood food allergies [14, 55, 56]; however, no cut-off levels for specific IgE have been established for routine clinical practice [1, 14]. Likewise, no cut-off levels have been identified for birch pollen- and food-specific IgE in patients with atopic eczema and a suspected late-type eczematous reaction to birch pollen-related foods (Wassmann et al., unpublished data). Thus, the clinical relevance of sensitization should be evaluated carefully. The detection of food-specific serum IgE antibodies alone is insufficient for the elimination of food from the diet [54].

Recently, semi-quantitative allergen microarrays have become available for component-resolved diagnostics. This relatively new *in vitro* diagnostic tool allows for the identification of specific sensitizations toward a multitude of veg-etable and animal allergen components in patients with atopic eczema (Wassmann et al., unpublished data) [57, 58]. However, current investigations of patients with atopic eczema and a verified birch pollen-related food allergy have suggested that microarray diagnostics cannot be used for distinguishing patients with a clinically relevant allergy from those with irrelevant sensitization against birch pollen-related food allergen (Wassmann et al., unpublished data). Further investigations of select cohorts of patients with atopic eczema and a suspected late-type food allergy are necessary to validate allergen microarrays for the diagnosis of food allergies in these patients. However, because of their capacities for broad and comprehensive negative IgE testing, allergen microarrays are reliable in the identification of the nonallergic form of atopic eczema [58].

In vivo Diagnostics
Skin Tests
For IgE-mediated disorders, the SPT provides a high negative predictive value of >90% [59]. Thus, a negative SPT response basically confirms the absence of an IgE-mediated allergic response. However, a positive skin prick response does not necessarily imply the presence of a clinically relevant allergy [18, 39]. In addition, the SPT has a low specificity for detecting food allergies to cow's milk, hen's egg, wheat and soy in children with atopic eczema, as confirmed by controlled oral food challenges [60]. Hence, the clinical relevance of a positive SPT reaction should be evaluated carefully [18, 39].

In comparison to the SPT, the atopy patch test (APT) with cow's milk, hen's egg, wheat and soy has shown a higher specificity but a lower sensitivity in children with atopic eczema [60]. Likewise, recent data from retrospective analysis of APT and oral food challenges conducted at the Hannover Medical School on infantile and adult patients with atopic eczema and a suspected birch pollen-related food allergy have confirmed that

Table 2. Example of an oligoallergenic diet for children older than one year of age and adults (Werfel et al. [2])

Food group and examples	
Grains	white rice
Meats	lamb, turkey and hen
Vegetables	cauliflower, broccoli, and cucumber
Fats	refined vegetable oil and dairy-free margarine
Beverages	mineral water and black tea
Spices	salt and sugar

for the diagnosis of a late-type eczematous reaction after the ingestion of birch pollen-related food, APTs with birch pollen extract and birch pollen-related food allergens show higher specificities compared with the detection of specific IgE antibodies (Wassmann et al., unpublished data).

Considering the fact that the APT is a time-consuming diagnostic procedure with limited diagnostic value, this test cannot be generally recommended for clinical routine use (Wassmann et al., unpublished data) [1, 60].

Oral Food Challenge

The results of specific IgE detection, the SPT and a patient's history often do not correlate with clinical findings [2, 15]. Hence, the DBPCFC should be regarded as the 'gold standard' for the diagnosis of a food-induced worsening of the skin condition in patients with atopic eczema [9].

A specific elimination diet over a period of at least 4 weeks conducted by a dietician should precede the oral food challenge [2]. The introduction of a diagnostic oligoallergenic diet over a period of about 2 weeks can be helpful in patients with severe atopic eczema, if (i) there is no obvious association between food intake and the allergic reaction and (ii) the diagnostic procedure does not provide clear indications concerning suspected foods. For infants, the oligoallergenic diet consists of an extensively hydrolyzed or amino acid formula [1]. In older children and adults, the composition of the diet should be determined individually based on the available allergological diagnostics and the patient's needs (table 2) [2].

In the case of the improvement of the skin condition, the elimination diet should be followed by an oral food challenge. After an oligoallergenic diet, the order of the re-introduction of food items should be chosen according to the patient's history, diagnostic results, individual habits, and nutritional physiological necessity [2].

If the skin condition does not improve during the elimination diet, no oral food challenge is indicated. However, if its condition worsens after the re-introduction of any of the eliminated food items, other triggers (e.g. stress, pollen season, or pet contact) should be considered that could bias the results of an elimination diet.

The oral food challenge should be carried out during a symptom-poor interval. If a stable skin condition cannot be achieved by the elimination diet alone, topical therapy must be intensified before the provocation and continued in the same fashion over the entire period of the oral food challenge. Antihistamine administration and UV therapy should be interrupted for an adequate period of time before the oral food challenge is conducted, as recommended in the guidelines [1].

Ideally, foods should be consumed on an empty stomach following the described procedure (fig. 2).

In routine practice, clinicians should aspire to achieve a 1:1 or 1:2 ratio for placebo to verum challenges. Provocation doses should be raised in 30 (to 60) minute intervals up to the highest dose or until a clinical reaction occurs. The highest dose should be based on the amount of the daily average intake of the food (e.g. 150 ml of cow's milk) [1].

If the oral food challenge is positive, a therapeutic elimination diet should be recommended that should be assisted by a nutritionist to ensure

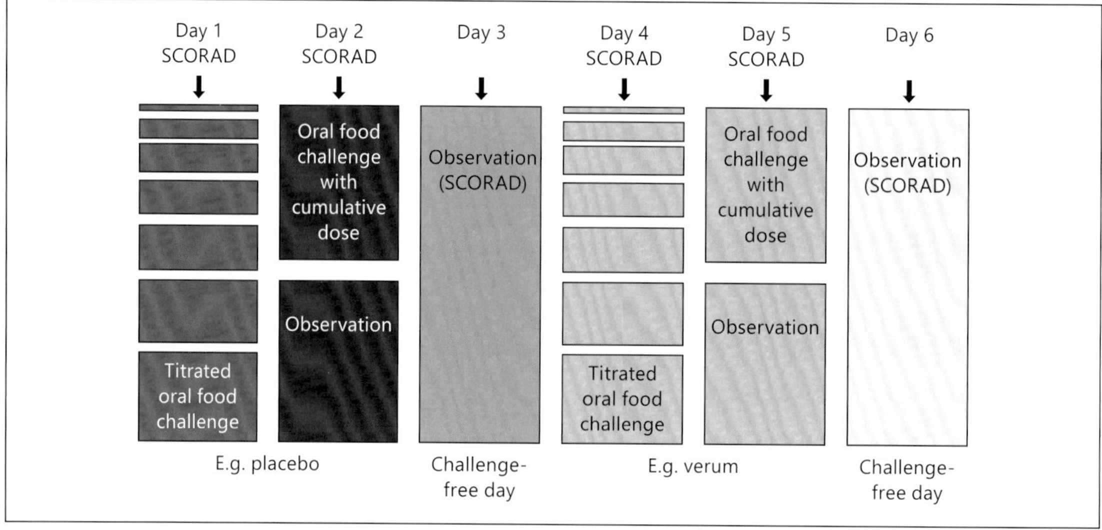

Fig. 2. Example of a DBPCFC procedure with food in patients with atopic eczema. Placebo and verum should be given on at least 2 consecutive days in a random order. On the first day, a titrated challenge test should be performed, and on the second day, the full dose can be given. The skin condition should be rated using an established score (e.g. the SCORing Atopic Dermatitis (SCORAD) and eczema area and severity index) on each day before the DBPCFC and at least 24 h after the last provocation dose has been given (adapted from [2]).

for the safe elimination of the allergenic food from the diet and the simultaneous provision of an adequate nutrient supply. In the case of a negative food challenge, no nutritional interventions are necessary.

In children, therapeutic diets should be recommended for a period of 12–24 months. Afterwards, clinical relevance should be re-evaluated by the determination of food-specific IgE antibodies and – when indicated – oral food challenges [9].

References

1 Werfel T, Ballmer-Weber B, Eigenmann PA, Niggemann B, Rancé F, Turjanmaa K, Worm M: Eczematous reactions to food in atopic eczema: position paper of the EAACI and GA2LEN. Allergy 2007; 62:723–728.

2 Werfel T, Erdmann S, Fuchs T, Henzgen M, Kleine-Tebbe J, Lepp U, Niggemann B, Raithel M, Reese I, Saloga J, Vieths S, Zuberbier T: Approach to suspected food allergy in atopic dermatitis. Guideline of the Task Force on Food Allergy of the German Society of Allergology and Clinical Immunology (DGAKI) and the Medical Association of German Allergologists (AeDA) and the German Society of Pediatric Allergology (GPA). JDDG 2009;7:265–271.

3 Greenhawt M: The role of food allergy in atopic dermatitis. Allergy Asthma Proc 2010;31:392–397.

4 Worm M, Forschner K, Lee H, Roehr CC, Edenharter G, Niggemann B, Zuberbier T: Frequency of atopic dermatitis and relevance of food allergy in adults in Germany. Acta Derm Venereol 2006;86: 119–122.

5 Savage JH, Matsui EC, Skripak JM, Wood RA: The natural history of egg allergy. J Allergy Clin Immunol 2007; 120:1413–1417.

6 Savage JH, Kaeding AJ, Matsui EC, Wood RA: The natural history of soy allergy. J Allergy Clin Immunol 2010; 125:683–686.

7 Heratizadeh A, Wichmann K, Werfel T: Food allergy and atopic dermatitis: how are they connected? Curr Allergy Asthma Rep 2011;11:284–291.

8 Wood RA, Sicherer SH, Vickery BP, Jones SM, Liu AH, Fleischer DM, Henning AK, Mayer L, Burks AW, Grishin A, Stablein D, Sampson HA: The natural history of milk allergy in an observational cohort. J Allergy Clin Immunol 2013;131:805–812.

9 Burks AW, Tang M, Sicherer S, Muraro A, Eigenmann PA, Ebisawa M, Fiocchi A, Chiang W, Beyer K, Wood R, Hourihane J, Jones SM, Lack G, Sampson HA: ICON: food allergy. J Allergy Clin Immunol 2012;129:906–920.

10 Fleischer DM, Conover-Walker MK, Matsui EC, Wood RA: The natural history of tree nut allergy. J Allergy Clin Immunol 2005;116:1087–1093.

11 Hill DJ, Hosking CS, Benedictis FM de, Oranje AP, Diepgen TL, Bauchau V: Confirmation of the association between high levels of immunoglobulin E food sensitization and eczema in infancy: an international study. Clin Exp Allergy 2008;38:161–168.

12 Kjaer HF, Eller E, Andersen KE, Høst A, Bindslev-Jensen C: The association between early sensitization patterns and subsequent allergic disease. The DARC birth cohort study. Pediatr Allergy Immunol 2009;20:726–734.

13 Eller E, Kjaer HF, Høst A, Andersen KE, Bindslev-Jensen C: Food allergy and food sensitization in early childhood: results from the DARC cohort. Allergy 2009:64:1023–1029.

14 Celik-Bilgili S, Mehl A, Verstege A, Staden U, Nocon M, Beyer K, Niggemann B: The predictive value of specific immunoglobulin E levels in serum for the outcome of oral food challenges. Clin Exp Allergy 2005;35:268–273.

15 Breuer K, Heratizadeh A, Wulf A, Baumann U, Constien A, Tetau D, Kapp A, Werfel T: Late eczematous reactions to food in children with atopic dermatitis. Clin Exp Allergy 2004;34:817–824.

16 Reekers R, Busche M, Wittmann M, Kapp A, Werfel T: Birch pollen-related foods trigger atopic dermatitis in patients with specific cutaneous T-cell responses to birch pollen antigens. J Allergy Clin Immunol 1999;104:466–472.

17 Breuer K, Wulf A, Constien A, Tetau D, Kapp A, Werfel T: Birch pollen-related food as a provocation factor of allergic symptoms in children with atopic eczema/dermatitis syndrome. Allergy 2004;59:988–994.

18 Suh K: Food allergy and atopic dermatitis: separating fact from fiction. Semin Cutan Med Surg 2010;29:72–78.

19 Ho MH, Wong WH, Chang C: Clinical spectrum of food allergies: a comprehensive review. Clin Rev Allergy Immunol 2014;46:225–240.

20 Celakovská J, Ettlerová K, Ettler K, Vanecková J, Bukac J: The effect of wheat allergy on the course of atopic eczema in patients over 14 years of age. Acta Medica (Hradec Kralove) 2011;54:157–162.

21 Celakovská J, Ettlerová K, Ettler K, Vaněčková J: Egg allergy in patients over 14 years old suffering from atopic eczema. Int J Dermatol 2011;50:811–818.

22 Celakovská J, Ettlerová K, Ettler K, Vanecková J, Bukac J: Evaluation of cow's milk allergy in a large group of adolescent and adult patients with atopic dermatitis. Acta Medica (Hradec Kralove) 2012;55:125–129.

23 Ballmer-Weber BK, Skamstrup Hansen K, Sastre J, Andersson K, Bätscher I, Ostling J, Dahl L, Hanschmann K, Holzhauser T, Poulsen LK, Lidholm J, Vieths S: Component-resolved in vitro diagnosis of carrot allergy in three different regions of Europe. Allergy 2012;67:758–766.

24 de Knop KJ, Verweij MM, Grimmelikhuijsen M, Philipse E, Hagendorens MM, Bridts CH, Clerck LS de, Stevens WJ, Ebo DG: Age-related sensitization profiles for hazelnut (Corylus avellana) in a birch-endemic region. Pediatr Allergy Immunol 2011;22:e139–e149.

25 Fernández-Rivas M, Bolhaar S, González-Mancebo E, Asero R, van Leeuwen A, Bohle B, Ma Y, Ebner C, Rigby N, Sancho AI, Miles S, Zuidmeer L, Knulst A, Breiteneder H, Mills C, Hoffmann-Sommergruber K, van Ree R: Apple allergy across Europe: how allergen sensitization profiles determine the clinical expression of allergies to plant foods. J Allergy Clin Immunol 2006;118:481–488.

26 Reuter A, Lidholm J, Andersson K, Ostling J, Lundberg M, Scheurer S, Enrique E, Cistero-Bahima A, San Miguel-Moncin M, Ballmer-Weber BK, Vieths S: A critical assessment of allergen component-based in vitro diagnosis in cherry allergy across Europe. Clin Exp Allergy 2006;36:815–823.

27 Skamstrup Hansen K, Ballmer-Weber BK, Sastre J, Lidholm J, Andersson K, Oberhofer H, Lluch-Bernal M, Ostling J, Mattsson L, Schocker F, Vieths S, Poulsen LK: Component-resolved in vitro diagnosis of hazelnut allergy in Europe. J Allergy Clin Immunol 2009;123:1134–1141.

28 Brown SJ, Asai Y, Cordell HJ, Campbell LE, Zhao Y, Liao H, Northstone K, Henderson J, Alizadehfar R, Ben-Shoshan M, Morgan K, Roberts G, Masthoff LJN, Pasmans SGMA, van den Akker PC, Wijmenga C, Hourihane JO, Palmer CNA, Lack G, Clarke A, Hull PR, Irvine AD, McLean WHI: Loss-of-function variants in the filaggrin gene are a significant risk factor for peanut allergy. J Allergy Clin Immunol 2011;127:661–667.

29 Irvine AD, McLean WHI, Leung DYM: Filaggrin mutations associated with skin and allergic diseases. N Engl J Med 2011;365:1315–1327.

30 Hsieh K, Tsai C, Wu CHH, Lin R: Epicutaneous exposure to protein antigen and food allergy. Clin Exp Allergy 2003;33:1067–1075.

31 Strid J, Hourihane J, Kimber I, Callard R, Strobel S: Disruption of the stratum corneum allows potent epicutaneous immunization with protein antigens resulting in a dominant systemic Th2 response. Eur J Immunol 2004;34:2100–2109.

32 Fallon PG, Sasaki T, Sandilands A, Campbell LE, Saunders SP, Mangan NE, Callanan JJ, Kawasaki H, Shiohama A, Kubo A, Sundberg JP, Presland RB, Fleckman P, Shimizu N, Kudoh J, Irvine AD, Amagai M, McLean WHI: A homozygous frameshift mutation in the mouse Flg gene facilitates enhanced percutaneous allergen priming. Nat Genet 2009;41:602–608.

33 Elias PM, Hatano Y, Williams ML: Basis for the barrier abnormality in atopic dermatitis: outside-inside-outside pathogenic mechanisms. J Allergy Clin Immunol 2008;121:1337–1343.

34 McAleer MA, Irvine AD: The multifunctional role of filaggrin in allergic skin disease. J Allergy Clin Immunol 2013;131:280–291.

35 Barnes KC: An update on the genetics of atopic dermatitis: scratching the surface in 2009. J Allergy Clin Immunol 2010;125:16–29.

36 Howell MD, Kim BE, Gao P, Grant AV, Boguniewicz M, DeBenedetto A, Schneider L, Beck LA, Barnes KC, Leung DYM: Cytokine modulation of atopic dermatitis filaggrin skin expression. J Allergy Clin Immunol 2007;120:150–155.

37 Chahine BG, Bahna SL: The role of the gut mucosal immunity in the development of tolerance versus development of allergy to food. Curr Opin Allergy Clin Immunol 2010;10:394–399.

38 Groschwitz KR, Hogan SP: Intestinal barrier function: Molecular regulation and disease pathogenesis. J Allergy Clin Immunol 2009;124:3–20.

39 Sicherer SH, Sampson HA: Food allergy. J Allergy Clin Immunol 2010;125:116–125.

40 Untersmayr E, Jensen-Jarolim E: The role of protein digestibility and antacids on food allergy outcomes. J Allergy Clin Immunol 2008;121:1301–1308.

41 Brandtzaeg P: Food allergy: separating the science from the mythology. Nat Rev Gastroenterol Hepatol 2010;7:380–400.

42 Chehade M, Mayer L: Oral tolerance and its relation to food hypersensitivities. J Allergy Clin Immunol 2005;115:3–12.

43 Ventura M, Polimeno L, Amoruso A, Gatti F, Annoscia E, Marinaro M, Di Leo E, Matino M, Buquicchio R, Bonini S, Tursi A, Francavilla A: Intestinal permeability in patients with adverse reactions to food. Dig Liver Dis 2006;38:732–736.

44 Kunisawa J, Kiyono H: Aberrant interaction of the gut immune system with environmental factors in the development of food allergies. Curr Allergy Asthma Rep 2010;10:215–221.

45 Abrahamsson TR, Jakobsson HE, Andersson AF, Björkstén B, Engstrand L, Jenmalm MC: Low diversity of the gut microbiota in infants with atopic eczema. J Allergy Clin Immunol 2012;129:434–440.e1–e2.

46 Adlerberth I, Strachan DP, Matricardi PM, Ahrné S, Orfei L, Aberg N, Perkin MR, Tripodi S, Hesselmar B, Saalman R, Coates AR, Bonanno CL, Panetta V, Wold AE: Gut microbiota and development of atopic eczema in 3 European birth cohorts. J Allergy Clin Immunol 2007;120:343–350.

47 Werfel T, Breuer K: Role of food allergy in atopic dermatitis. Curr Opin Allergy Clin Immunol 2004;4:379–385.

48 Reekers R, Beyer K, Niggemann B, Wahn U, Freihorst J, Kapp A, Werfel T: The role of circulating food antigen-specific lymphocytes in food allergic children with atopic dermatitis. Br J Dermatol 1996;135:935–941.

49 Werfel T, Morita A, Grewe M, Renz H, Wahn U, Krutmann J, Kapp A: Allergen specificity of skin-infiltrating T cells is not restricted to a type-2 cytokine pattern in chronic skin lesions of atopic dermatitis. J Invest Dermatol 1996;107:871–876.

50 Werfel T, Ahlers G, Schmidt P, Boeker M, Kapp A, Neumann C: Milk-responsive atopic dermatitis is associated with a casein-specific lymphocyte response in adolescent and adult patients. J Allergy Clin Immunol 1997;99:124–133.

51 Bordignon V, Sinagra JL, Trento E, Pietravalle M, Capitanio B, Cordiali Fei P: Antigen specific cytokine response in pediatric patients with atopic dermatitis. Pediatr Allergy Immunol 2005;16:113–120.

52 Bohle B, Zwölfer B, Heratizadeh A, Jahn-Schmid B, Antonia YD, Alter M, Keller W, Zuidmeer L, van Ree R, Werfel T, Ebner C: Cooking birch pollen-related food: divergent consequences for IgE- and T cell-mediated reactivity in vitro and in vivo. J Allergy Clin Immunol 2006;118:242–249.

53 Li X, Kleiner G, Huang C, Lee SY, Schofield B, Soter NA, Sampson HA: Murine model of atopic dermatitis associated with food hypersensitivity. J Allergy Clin Immunol 2001;107:693–702.

54 Fleischer DM, Bock SA, Spears GC, Wilson CG, Miyazawa NK, Gleason MC, Gyorkos EA, Murphy JR, Atkins D, Leung DYM: Oral food challenges in children with a diagnosis of food allergy. J Pediatr 2011;158:578–583.e1.

55 Sampson HA: Utility of food-specific IgE concentrations in predicting symptomatic food allergy. J Allergy Clin Immunol 2001;107:891–896.

56 Perry TT, Matsui EC, Kay Conover-Walker M, Wood RA: The relationship of allergen-specific IgE levels and oral food challenge outcome. J Allergy Clin Immunol 2004;114:144–149.

57 Ott H, Fölster-Holst R, Merk HF, Baron JM: Allergen microarrays: a novel tool for high-resolution IgE profiling in adults with atopic dermatitis. Eur J Dermatol 2010;20:54–61.

58 Mari A, Scala E, Alessandri C: The IgE-microarray testing in atopic dermatitis: a suitable modern tool for the immunological and clinical phenotyping of the disease. Curr Opin Allergy Clin Immunol 2011;11:438–444.

59 Chapman JA, Bernstein IL, Lee RE, Oppenheimer J: Food allergy: a practice parameter. Ann Allergy Asthma Immunol 2006;96:1–68.

60 Mehl A, Rolinck-Werninghaus C, Staden U, Verstege A, Wahn U, Beyer K, Niggemann B: The atopy patch test in the diagnostic workup of suspected food-related symptoms in children. J Allergy Clin Immunol 2006;118:923–929.

Thomas Werfel, MD
Department of Dermatology and Allergy
Hannover Medical School
Carl Neuberg Strasse 1
DE–30449 Hannover (Germany)
E-Mail werfel.thomas@mh-hannover.de

Ebisawa M, Ballmer-Weber BK, Vieths S, Wood RA (eds): Food Allergy: Molecular Basis and Clinical Practice.
Chem Immunol Allergy. Basel, Karger, 2015, vol 101, pp 191–198 (DOI: 10.1159/000371702)

Anaphylaxis in Food Allergy

Robbie D. Pesek[a, b] · Stacie M. Jones[a, b]

[a]Division of Allergy and Immunology, University of Arkansas for Medical Sciences and [b]Arkansas Children's
Hospital, Little Rock, Ark., USA

Abstract

Food allergy is a known trigger of anaphylaxis. Although the awareness of food allergies has improved, food-related allergic reactions and anaphylaxis still commonly occur. The recognition of anaphylaxis, its prompt treatment, and patient education are important for the prevention of future food reactions. Patients and health care providers should also recognize the importance of epinephrine as the primary treatment of anaphylaxis. When food-related anaphylaxis occurs, patients should receive education regarding their food allergies, an epinephrine auto-injector, and follow-up with a food allergy specialist to reduce the risk of future food-related reactions.   © 2015 S. Karger AG, Basel

Introduction

Anaphylaxis is defined as a 'serious allergic reaction that is rapid in onset and might cause death' [1]. The overall prevalence of anaphylaxis due to all causes is estimated to be 0.05–2% and is increasing. Over the last decade alone, there has been an 18% increase in the number of cases. Of all causes of anaphylaxis, food accounts for up to 50% of cases that present to emergency departments [2, 3]. In children, food allergy is the most common cause of anaphylaxis outside of the hospital setting, with most reactions occurring inside of the home and affecting patients who are aware of their allergies [4]. The most commonly implicated foods in children include milk, eggs, wheat, soy, peanuts, tree nuts, fish and shellfish, while peanuts, tree nuts, fish, and shellfish are the most common in adults [5]. Approximately 150–200 people die each year from food-induced anaphylaxis, and 300–500 million US dollars in health care costs are spent for food-induced allergic reactions and anaphylaxis in the USA [6, 7]. It is also believed that many cases of anaphylaxis are miscoded or underreported. The prompt recognition of symptoms of anaphylaxis, the correct identification of offending foods, and early treatment are vitally important for managing anaphylaxis and preventing future food reactions.

Table 1. Diagnostic criteria for anaphylaxis

Anaphylaxis is highly likely when any one of the following 3 criteria are fulfilled:
(1) Acute onset of an illness (within minutes to several hours) with involvement of the skin, mucosal tissue, or both (e.g. generalized hives, pruritis, flushing, or swollen lips-tongue-uvula)
And at least one of the following:
  a) Respiratory compromise (e.g. dyspnea, wheeze-bronchospasm, stridor, reduced peak expiratory flow, or hypoxemia)
  b) Reduced blood pressure (BP) or associated symptoms of end-organ dysfunction (e.g. hypotonia (collapse), syncope, or incontinence)

(2) Two or more of the following, occurring rapidly after the exposure of a patient to a likely allergen (within minutes to several hours):
  a) Involvement of the skin-mucosal tissue (e.g. generalized hives, itch-flush, or swollen lips-tongue-uvula)
  b) Respiratory compromise (e.g. dyspnea, wheeze-bronchospasm, stridor, reduced peak expiratory flow, or hypoxemia)
  c) Reduced BP or associated symptoms of end-organ dysfunction (e.g. hypotonia (collapse), syncope, or incontinence)
  d) Persistent gastrointestinal symptoms (e.g. crampy abdominal pain or vomiting)

(3) Reduced BP after the exposure of a patient to a known allergen (within minutes to several hours)
  a) Infants and children: low systolic BP (age-specific) or a greater than 30% decrease in systolic BP*
  b) Adults: systolic BP <90 mm Hg or a greater than 30% decrease from a patient's baseline

* Low systolic BP for children: 1 month to 1 year <70 mm Hg; 1–10 years < (70 mm Hg + (2 × age)); 11–17 years <90 mm Hg.

Diagnosis

Anaphylaxis is a multi-organ system reaction, and although the skin, gastrointestinal, and respiratory tracts are most commonly affected, any organ system can be involved. There is debate regarding what defines anaphylaxis and thus, some cases go unrecognized, which can lead to delays in providing appropriate treatment, with increases in morbidity and even in mortality. In 2006, a consensus guideline was published by the National Institute of Allergy and Infectious Diseases in conjunction with the Food Allergy and Anaphylaxis Network to help improve the recognition of anaphylaxis by health care providers [1] (table 1).

These criteria are useful in most patients presenting with cutaneous manifestations, as is the case for nearly 80% of patients. Thus, the remaining 20% do not have skin findings, which is particularly common in children with peanut- or tree nut-related anaphylaxis, and many of these children present with gastrointestinal manifestations alone [8]. Cardiovascular compromise is uncommon in food-related anaphylaxis, but clinical suspicion should remain high because it can result in significant morbidity.

Although death related to anaphylaxis is rare, there are multiple risk factors that can put patients at an increased risk of a fatal or near fatal reaction [6, 9] (table 2). In a study of 202 cases of fatal anaphylaxis, food allergens were shown to account for nearly 30% of the cases, with nuts causing the majority of the reactions [10]. In this same cohort, a history of a previous reaction was not predictive of the severity of future reactions; however, age (especially adolescents and young adults), comorbidities such as asthma, and concomitant medications all increased the risks of anaphylaxis and anaphylaxis-related death. In addition, the delayed administration of epi-

Table 2. Risk factors for anaphylaxis and anaphylaxis-related death

---

Peanut and/or tree nut allergies
Asthma (adolescents and young adults)
Cardiovascular disease
Severe atopic diseases (atopic dermatitis and allergic rhinitis)
Other disorders
    Systemic mastocytosis or clonal mast cell disorders
    Chronic lung diseases (other than asthma)
    Anatomic airway obstructions (airway hemangiomas or laryngotracheomalacia)
Medications
    Angiotensin-converting enzyme inhibitors/angiotensin receptor blockers
    Beta-adrenergic blockers
    Alpha-blockers
Delayed administration of epinephrine
Elevated serum PAF/decreased serum PAF-acetylhydrolase

---

nephrine and a low level of platelet-activating factor (PAF)-acetylhydrolase are associated with an increased risk of severe, life-threatening anaphylaxis [9].

Symptoms of food reactions typically begin within seconds to hours after the ingestion of the offending food, and most occur within the first hour. There are three possible phases of IgE-mediated food reactions: uniphasic, biphasic, and protracted [11]. Uniphasic reactions begin immediately after the ingestion of the offending food but resolve within minutes to hours with or without treatment and do not recur within the same reaction. Biphasic reactions include an initial reaction that begins within hours of the ingestion of the offending food and recurs after the initial symptoms have resolved. Biphasic reactions are highly variable, ranging from 1 to 78 hours, with most occurring within 8 hours of the initial presentation [11]. Symptoms may be less or more severe than those seen during the initial reaction. Biphasic reactions occur in only 3–20% of adult food reactions but account for nearly 25% of fatal or near-fatal cases. Delayed administration, inadequate dosing, or the need for larger doses of epinephrine during the initial reaction increases the risk of a bi-phasic reaction [11]. A protracted reaction involves symptoms that may last for hours to days after the initial presentation.

Laboratory Evaluation

While there are no laboratory tests that are specific for food-related anaphylaxis, several tests can be used to confirm the clinical diagnosis. Food-specific IgE and skin prick testing can be helpful in confirming a diagnosis of IgE-mediated food allergy based upon clinical history and will be covered elsewhere. Serum histamine, urine histamine metabolites, and serum tryptase have been the most frequently studied. Serum histamine has a very short half-life, with levels rising within 5–10 minutes of an allergic reaction but remaining elevated for only 60–90 minutes [12]. Serum used for histamine analysis is also labile and must be kept on ice, which, combined with its short half-life, limits its usefulness for many patients. The levels of urinary histamine metabolites, including N-methylhistamine, can be measured, but samples must be collected over a period of 24 hours. When they are elevated, the diagnosis of anaphylaxis is confirmed; however, normal levels do not rule out this condition. The serum tryptase level peaks at 60–90 minutes following the onset of anaphylaxis and does not return to a normal level for 12–24 hours. In food-induced anaphylaxis, tryptase is not typically elevated, limiting the usefulness of its measurement [8]. Another marker that has been studied is CD63, which is localized to the surfaces of basophils and is upregulated during anaphylaxis [13]. Prostaglandin D2, carboxypeptidase A3, leukotriene C4, and PAF levels are also elevated during episodes of anaphylaxis, while the level of PAF-acetylhydrolase is decreased [14–16]. Not all of these tests are commercially available, limiting their clinical utility.

Management of Anaphylaxis

Acute Management
The management of anaphylaxis is focused on making a prompt diagnosis followed by the rapid administration of adrenaline (epinephrine), which is the drug of choice [1, 5, 17] (table 3). Epinephrine is a direct-acting alpha and beta-adrenergic agent that rapidly reverses symptoms associated with anaphylaxis and can be life-saving. Epinephrine should be administered as quickly as possible because delays in administration increase the risk of a fatal reaction [8]. Intramuscular (IM) injection into the vastus lateralis muscle of the leg is the preferred method of delivery because it leads to a faster onset of action with more sustained plasma and tissue levels. Inhaled and sublingual routes are available but do not result in consistent efficacies. For children, a dose of 0.01 mg/kg up to 0.3 mg is recommended, while 0.2–0.5 mg is recommended for adults. Doses can be repeated every 5–15 minutes as needed. Intravenous administration may be required in patients who do not respond to repeated IM doses, and a slow, continuous infusion is superior to bolus administration [17]. Although there are no prospective, randomized trials evaluating the use

of epinephrine in the treatment of anaphylaxis, it is recommended as the first-line therapy based upon its effectiveness in treating life-threatening reactions [17].

The use of epinephrine is associated with anxiety, restlessness, headache, presyncope, palpitations, tremor, and pallor. Rarely, ventricular arrhythmias, angina, myocardial infarction, hypertensive emergency, pulmonary edema, and intracranial bleeding occur, and these symptoms are more frequently associated with intravenous administration. There are no absolute contraindications for the use of epinephrine to treat anaphylaxis, but pre-existing cardiovascular or central nervous system disorders, pregnancy, or the use of monoamine oxidase inhibitors, beta-blockers, tricyclic antidepressants, stimulants, or illegal drugs, such as cocaine, increase the risk of side effects and are relative contraindications [1, 5, 17].

In addition to the administration of epinephrine, other adjunctive treatments can be employed. These treatments are routinely recommended but do not have an evidence base for their use. Patients may require aggressive fluid resuscitation because vasodilation caused by anaphylaxis can lead to a decrease of up to 35% in the circulating blood volume and cardiac arrest. Patients should be placed in the supine position with their legs elevated, and fluids and even vasopressors may be required to maintain adequate tissue perfusion and normal blood pressure [9]. Respiratory compromise may also occur, requiring the uses of inhaled beta-agonists as well as supplemental oxygen and other airway support measures. Antihistamines, including both H1 and H2 antihistamines, may also be used. The use of their combination may be more effective than that of either alone, but due to their slower onset of action (1–2 hours) and ineffectiveness in reversing respiratory and cardiovascular symptoms, antihistamines cannot take the place of epinephrine in the treatment of anaphylaxis [18]. While corticosteroids are not recommended for the treatment of the immediate phase of anaphylaxis, they

Table 3. Pharmacologic management of anaphylaxis (modified from the National Institute of Allergy and Infectious Diseases-Sponsored Guidelines, 2010) [5]

With the exception of adrenaline as the first-line treatment, these treatments often occur concomitantly and are not meant to be sequential

Outpatient setting
First-line treatment
    Adrenaline, IM; auto-injector or 1:1,000 solution
        Weight = 10–25 kg: 0.15 mg adrenaline auto-injector, IM (anterior-lateral thigh)
        Weight >25 kg: 0.3 mg adrenaline auto-injector, IM (anterior-lateral thigh)
        Adrenaline (1:1,000 solution) (IM), 0.01 mg/kg per dose; maximum = 0.5 mg per dose (anterior-lateral thigh)
    Adrenaline doses may need to be repeated every 5–15 minutes
Adjunctive treatment
    Place the patient in the recumbent position if tolerated, with the lower extremities elevated
    Bronchodilator (β2-agonist): albuterol
        MDI (child: 4–8 puffs; adult: 8 puffs) or
        Nebulized solution (child: 1.5 ml; adult: 3 ml) every 20 minutes or continuously as needed
    H_1 antihistamine: less-sedating, second-generation antihistamines are recommended

Hospital setting
First-line treatment
    Adrenaline IM as above, consider continuous adrenaline infusion for persistent hypotension (ideally with the continuous non-invasive monitoring of the blood pressure and heart rate); an alternative is endotracheal or intra-osseous adrenaline
Adjunctive treatment
    Place the patient in the recumbent position if tolerated, with the lower extremities elevated
    Bronchodilator (β2-agonist): albuterol
        MDI (child: 4–8 puffs; adult: 8 puffs) or
        Nebulized solution (child: 1.5 ml; adult: 3 ml) every 20 minutes or continuously as needed
    H_1 antihistamine: less-sedating, second-generation antihistamines are suggested
    Corticosteroids
        Prednisone at 1 mg/kg with a maximum dose of 60–80 mg oral or
        Methylprednisolone at 1 mg/kg with a maximum dose of 60–80 mg IV
    Supplemental oxygen therapy
    IV fluids in large volumes for patients presenting with orthostasis, hypotension, or an incomplete response to IM adrenaline
    Vasopressors (other than adrenaline) for refractory hypotension, titrate to effect
    Glucagon for refractory hypotension, titrate to effect
        Child: 20–30 µg/kg
        Adult: 1–5 mg
        Dose may be repeated or followed by the infusion of 5–15 µg/minute atropine for bradycardia, titrate to effect

At time of discharge
First-line treatment
    Adrenaline auto-injector prescription (2 doses) and instructions
    Education on avoidance of allergen and emergency action plan
    Follow-up with primary care physician
    Consider referral to an allergist if first presentation or cause is unknown
    H_1 antihistamine: diphenhydramine every 6 hours for 2–3 days; alternative dosing with a non-sedating second-generation antihistamine
    H_2 antihistamine: ranitidine twice daily for 2–3 days
    Corticosteroid: prednisone daily for 2–3 days

IV = Intravenous; MDI = metered-dose inhaler.

may be useful for preventing biphasic reactions, although their efficacy has not been proven [19]. Glucagon may also be required in patients taking beta-blockers who do not respond to other treatments. It is important to note that all of these therapies are adjunctive treatments and should not be used in place of epinephrine in patients presenting with anaphylaxis [1, 5, 17].

Long-Term Management and Prevention
Depending on the severity of the reaction, patients should be monitored for up to 4–6 hours following the successful treatment of anaphylaxis in the case of relapse or the occurrence of a biphasic reaction. During this time, patients should be educated regarding their food allergy and anaphylaxis, and the acronym 'SAFE' can be used by health care professionals in providing instructions [20] (table 4).

Patients should be told that they have experienced anaphylaxis, a potentially life-threatening reaction, and that symptoms may recur for up to 3 days following the initial presentation. Patients should also be educated regarding the signs and symptoms of anaphylaxis and that if symptoms recur, they should initiate treatment with self-injectable epinephrine and seek medical attention. Health care providers should make efforts to correctly identify the offending food trigger and to provide instructions for proper food avoidance. A follow-up for additional testing and consultation with a food allergy specialist should also be arranged. All patients should be given a twin-pack epinephrine auto-injector or a prescription for one prior to discharge, with instructions to regularly check the expiration date, and they should be made aware of the importance of carrying it at all times [17]. Limitations to epinephrine auto-injectors include the lack of a dose range because only 2 doses are commercially available: 0.15 mg for patients weighing less than 25 kg or 0.3 mg for patients weighing more than 25 kg. Also, the needle length of these injectors may not be ideal for overweight or obese patients, preventing the delivery of epinephrine into the IM space. The shelf life varies depending on the manufacturer but ranges from 12 to 18 months. All family members should also be educated regarding the proper use of an epinephrine auto-injector, and the patient should receive a written anaphylaxis action plan. Medical alert jewelry with the identification of allergic foods is also available and can be helpful in preventing future allergic reactions [5].

Food-Dependent Exercise-Induced Anaphylaxis

There are many triggers of anaphylaxis, including foods, drugs, insects, and even exercise. An uncommon cause that should be considered in patients presenting with anaphylaxis due to an uncertain trigger is food-dependent exercise-induced anaphylaxis (FDEIA). This syndrome was initially described in 1979 by Maulitz et al. in a patient with exercise-induced anaphylaxis following ingestion of shellfish [21]. In these patients, anaphylaxis is triggered by the combination of ingestion of an offending food followed by exercise [22]. If the patient exercises independently of ingesting the offending food, anaphylaxis will not occur. The patient also may not have had an allergic reaction to ingestion of the offending food without subsequent exercise.

FDEIA is more common in adolescent or young adult males following prolonged endurance exercise [23]. Symptoms may be delayed for 60 minutes up to 3 hours following ingestion of the offending food but typically occur within 10–15 minutes of starting to exercise. There may be premonitory symptoms, including pruritis of the hands, paresthesia, sneezing, cough, dyspnea, flushing, and/or abdominal pain, prior to the onset of anaphylaxis. Common offending foods include wheat and shellfish, while less common trigger foods include celery, egg, milk, tomatoes, peanuts, and tree nuts [24, 25]. Regional variations in diets may result in other foods acting as potential triggers. Many of these patients will have positive skin prick or specific IgE tests that may help with the identification of the offending food [23]. Patients may also require a food challenge, which involves the ingestion of the suspected food followed by a period of exercise; however, a negative challenge does not necessarily rule out FDEIA. Patients should be counseled to avoid the offending food for at least 4 hours prior to exercise or to avoid exercise for at least 4 hours after eating the offending food [5].

Summary

Foods are an important trigger of anaphylaxis. Although the awareness of food allergies continues to increase, a significant number of cases of anaphylaxis occur each year. Improvements in the recognition, diagnosis, and treatment of anaphylaxis have been made in an attempt to prevent fatal episodes. In addition to promptly identifying cases of food-related anaphylaxis, patients and health care providers should understand the importance of the rapid administration of epinephrine, which can be life saving. All patients who present with anaphylaxis should receive education regarding their food allergies, an epinephrine auto-injector, and follow-up with a food allergy specialist to reduce the risk of future food-related reactions.

References

1 Sampson HA, Munoz-Furlong A, Campbell RL, et al: Second symposium on the definition and management of anaphylaxis – summary report – Second National Institute of Allergy and Infectious Disease/Food allergy and anaphylaxis network symposium. J Allergy Clin Immunol 2006;117:391–397.

2 Brown AF, McKinnon D, Chu K: Emergency department anaphylaxis: a review of 142 patients in a single year. J Allergy Clin Immunol 2001;108:861–866.

3 Clark S, Espinola J, Rudders SA, et al: Frequency of US emergency department visits for food-related acute allergic reactions. J Allergy Clin Immunol 2011; 127:682–683.

4 Fleischer DM, Perry TT, Atkins D, et al: Allergic reactions to foods in preschool-aged children in a prospective observational food allergy study. Pediatrics 2012;130:e25–e32.

5 Boyce JA, Assa'ad A, Burks AW, et al: Guidelines for the Diagnosis and Management of Food Allergy in the United States: Summary of the NIAID-Sponsored Expert Panel Report. J Allergy Clin Immunol 2010;126:1105–1118.

6 Bock SA, Munoz-Furlong A, Sampson HA: Further fatalities caused by anaphylactic reactions to food, 2001–2006. J Allergy Clin Immunol 2007;119:1016–1018.

7 Patel DA, Holdford DA, Edward E, et al: Estimating the economic burden of food-induced allergic reactions and anaphylaxis in the United States. J Allergy Clin Immunol 2011;128:110–115.

8 Sampson HA, Mendelson L, Rosen JP: Fatal and near-fatal anaphylactic reactions to food in children and adolescents. N Engl J Med 1992;327:380–384.

9 Simons FER: Anaphylaxis. J Allergy Clin Immunol 2010;125:S161–S181.

10 Pumphrey R: Anaphylaxis: can we tell who is at risk of a fatal reaction? Curr Opin Allergy Clin Immunol 2004;4:285–290.

11 Lieberman P: Biphasic anaphylactic reactions. Ann Allergy Asthma Immunol 2005;95:217–226.

12 Lieberman P: Anaphylaxis and anaphylactoid reactions; in Middleton E, Ellis EF, Yunginger JW, et al (eds): Allergy: Principles and Practice, ed 5. St. Louis, MO, Mosby-Year Book, 1998, vol II, section E, chapter 77, pp 1079–1092.

13 Ebo DG, Hagendorens MM, Bridts CH, et al: In vitro allergy diagnosis: should we follow the flow? Clin Exp Allergy 2004;34:332–339.

14 Zhou X, Buckley MG, Lau LC, et al: Mast cell carboxypeptidase as a new clinical marker for anaphylaxis. J Allergy Clin Immunol 2006;117:S85.

15 Zhou X, Lau L, Eren E, et al: Mast cell carboxypeptidase as a confirmatory and predictive marker in allergic reactions to drugs. J Allergy Clin Immunol 2011;127: 143.

16 Vadas P, Gold M, Perelman B, et al: Platelet-activating factor, PAF acetylhydrolase, and severe anaphylaxis. N Engl J Med 2008;358:28–35.

17 Simons FER, Ardusso LRF, Bilo MB, et al: World Allergy Organization anaphylaxis guidelines: summary. J Allergy Clin Immunol 2011;127:587–593.

18 Kaliner M, Shelhamer JH, Ottesen EA: Effects of infused histamine: correlation of plasma histamine levels and symptoms. J Allergy Clin Immunol 1982;69: 283–289.

19 Choo KJ, Simons E, Sheikh A: Glucocorticoids for the treatment of anaphylaxis: Cochrane systematic review. Allergy 2010;10:1205–1211.

20 Lieberman P, Decker W, Camargo CA Jr, et al: SAFE: a multidisciplinary approach to anaphylaxis education in the emergency department. Ann Allergy Asthma Immunol 2007;98:519–523.

21 Maulitz RM, Pratt DS, Schocket AL: Exercise-induced anaphylactic reaction to shellfish. J Allergy Clin Immunol 1979; 63:433–434.

22 Du Toit G: Food-dependent exercise-induced anaphylaxis in childhood. Pediatr Allergy Immu 2007;18:455–463.

23 Dutau G, Micheau P, Juchet A, et al: Exercise and food-induced anaphylaxis. Pediatr Pulmonol 2001;S23:48–51.

24 Romano A, DiFonso M, Giuffreda F, et al: Food dependent exercise-induced anaphylaxis: clinical and laboratory findings in 54 subjects. Int Arch Allergy Immunol 2011;125:264–272.

25 Beaudouin E, Renaudin JM, Morisset M, et al: Food-dependent exercise-induced anaphylaxis-update and current data. Eur Ann Allergy Clin Immunol 2006;38: 45–51.

Robbie D. Pesek, MD
Arkansas Children's Hospital
13 Children's Way, Slot 512–13
Little Rock, AR 72202 (USA)
E-Mail rdpesek@uams.edu

Ebisawa M, Ballmer-Weber BK, Vieths S, Wood RA (eds): Food Allergy: Molecular Basis and Clinical Practice.
Chem Immunol Allergy. Basel, Karger, 2015, vol 101, pp 199–208 (DOI: 10.1159/000371703)

Eosinophilic Oesophagitis

Ralf G. Heine[a–c] · Katrina J. Allen[a–c]

[a]Department of Gastroenterology and Clinical Nutrition and Department of Allergy and Immunology,
The Royal Children's Hospital Melbourne, Melbourne, Vic., [b]Murdoch Childrens Research Institute,
Melbourne, Vic., and [c]Department of Paediatrics, The University of Melbourne, Melbourne, Vic., Australia

Abstract

Eosinophilic oesophagitis (EoE) is an antigen-driven pan-oesophagitis that is defined by the presence of at least 15 eosinophils per high power field on oesophageal histology in conjunction with upper gastrointestinal symptoms. EoE is closely associated with atopic disorders, in particular with food allergy, and as for other atopic diseases in childhood, there is a strong preponderance of male patients who have this disorder. The mechanisms leading to EoE have been characterised at the molecular level. Eotaxin-3, interleukin-5 and interleukin-13 are the key effector molecules in EoE pathogenesis. EoE presents with a diverse range of gastrointestinal symptoms, including regurgitation, vomiting, feeding difficulties or feeding refusal in infancy, as well as heartburn, dysphagia and food bolus impaction in older children and adults. The diagnosis may also be ascertained as an incidental finding in patients undergoing gastroscopy for other suspected conditions, including coeliac disease. EoE is different from gastro-oesophageal reflux disease and does not improve in response to proton pump inhibitors. Therefore, EoE needs to be distinguished from so-called PPI-responsive oesophageal eosinophilia. The long-term prognosis of EoE remains poorly defined, and complications mainly relate to subepithelial remodelling and fibrosis that may result in dysmotility, dysphagia and oesophageal strictures. The treatment of EoE involves elimination diets and topical swallowed aerosolised corticosteroids, while biological therapies targeting molecular mechanisms have so far been unsuccessful. In children, elemental diets have proved highly effective, but multiple food elimination diets are more sustainable in the long term. Further randomised, controlled trials on dietary or pharmacological interventions are needed to inform the optimal long-term management of EoE.

© 2015 S. Karger AG, Basel

Introduction

Eosinophilic oesophagitis (EoE) is a recently recognised form of pan-oesophagitis in children and adults that is closely associated with food allergy and atopic disorders [1]. The oesophagus is typically devoid of eosinophils, and the presence of any eosinophils in oesophageal tissue was previously thought to be due to gastro-oesophageal reflux disease [2]. However, Kelly et al. [3] recognised that patients with high numbers of oesophageal mucosal eosinophils, i.e. EoE, represented a separate disease entity that was resistant to proton pump inhibitor (PPI) treatment but improved clinically and histologically after treatment with an amino-acid-based (elemental) diet.

Patients with EoE present to both gastroenterologists and allergists with a diverse range of symptoms, including vomiting, feeding difficulties, heartburn, failure to thrive, dysphagia or food bolus impaction. Clinicians still face complex issues with regard to the optimal diagnosis and management of these difficult-to-treat patients. EoE may be under-recognised since its diagnosis requires gastroscopic examination and oesophageal biopsy [1]. To date, there are no guidelines for clinicians as to which patient should undergo gastroscopy for possible EoE. This is particularly problematic as non-specific upper gastrointestinal tract symptoms have a high prevalence in the general population.

Despite recent advances in understanding the pathophysiology of EoE, major knowledge deficits remain in the optimal management of EoE. Although population-based data on the long-term consequences of poorly managed or untreated EoE are not available, there is strong evidence that some patients will develop oesophageal strictures or dysphagia, particularly if the diagnosis is delayed [4]. To date, there are few randomised, controlled trials (RCTs) investigating the optimal long-term management of EoE, including trials on dietary interventions, topical corticosteroids or biological agents. Prospective studies are urgently needed to define the natural history of the disease and to develop an evidence base to inform optimal management strategies [5, 6].

Epidemiology

Since its initial recognition in 1995, the prevalence of EoE appears to be rapidly rising – although increased ascertainment is likely to have contributed to a degree [7]. Previous studies have found a preponderance of males in both adults (76%) and children (66%) with EoE [8]. Familial clusters of EoE have also been described [9]. However, reliable population-based data are not available. The reported incidence of EoE in American children in 2003 was 1.28 in 10,000 children, which is similar to recent incidence figures for ulcerative colitis (1.74 in 10,000) [10, 11]. In our retrospective review of consecutive EoE patients in Australia, the rate of new diagnoses appears to have reached a plateau over the past decade [12].

Clinical Presentation in Children and Adults

EoE can present at any age with a diverse range of symptoms, including regurgitation, vomiting, heartburn, abdominal pain, food refusal, weight loss, dysphagia or food bolus impaction [1]. Irritability, feeding refusal and failure to thrive are classic presenting features in infancy [10], while dysphagia and food bolus impaction are the most characteristic symptoms in school-aged children and young adults. Patients frequently, but not always, have co-existent food allergies, eczema, allergic rhinitis, asthma or at least a family history of atopy. In 89 children with EoE from a tertiary referral centre, 75–79% of patients had a history of atopic disorders or were sensitised to food or inhalant allergens [13]. A large population-based study in Swedish adults showed that asymptomatic EoE was relatively common [14]. In that study, about 1% of patients had evidence of likely EoE, but only half of them were symptomatic.

Distinguishing Eosinophilic Oesophagitis from Gastro-Oesophageal Reflux Disease
EoE commonly presents with gastro-oesophageal reflux disease-like symptoms, including vomiting, heartburn and regurgitation. By definition, EoE does not respond to treatment with PPIs, and failure to respond to a trial of high-dose PPIs is part of the diagnostic criteria [1, 8]. Acid suppression alone may reduce oesophageal mucosal eosinophilia in some patients [5, 15]. This condition, which is different from EoE, has been labelled 'PPI-responsive oesophageal eosinophilia' (PPI-ROE). The exact mechanism by which PPIs reduce mucosal eosinophil counts is not clear. Apart

from acid suppression, a direct anti-inflammatory effect is also possible. Zhang et al. [16] showed that PPIs suppress IL-13-induced eotaxin-3 expression by squamous epithelial cells via an acid-independent mechanism. Untersmayr et al. have suggested that acid-suppressive medications may also increase the risk of allergies and EoE, as reduced gastric acid may increase the protein degradation of the upper gastrointestinal tract and increase the allergenicity of food proteins [17]. However, the role of PPIs in the development of EoE has never been formally investigated.

Eosinophilic Oesophagitis in Patients with Coeliac Disease

EoE and coeliac disease (CD) commonly co-exist [18], and it has been speculated that these two disorders are causally related [19]. However, a recent population-based study from Sweden failed to demonstrate a significant association between EoE and CD [20]. From a pathophysiological perspective, this is plausible, as there are striking differences between both conditions [21]. CD is a T helper (Th)1-mediated and HLA DQ2/DQ8 restricted disorder that aligns with autoimmunity. By contrast, EoE is a Th2-mediated disorder that is closely associated with food allergy and atopic disorders. HLA DQ2/DQ8 is not overrepresented in adult patients with EoE, making a true association unlikely [22]. An Italian study suggested that there was at least a partial treatment response in EoE severity after patients with concomitant CD began a gluten-free diet [23]. However, a more recent case series found no such treatment effect [20].

Mechanisms of Disease

Our understanding of the mechanisms involved in the pathophysiology of EoE has evolved rapidly [24] due to sophisticated animal experiments, as well as human gene array studies [25]. Similar to eczema and asthma, EoE is predominantly a Th2 lymphocyte-driven disorder, with upregulation of interleukins (IL) 5 and 13 [26, 27]. Furthermore, the number of mucosal mast cells is increased [28]. The migration of eosinophils into the oesophagus is under the control of three critical effector molecules: IL-5, IL-13 and eotaxin-3. Human gene array studies have demonstrated that the eotaxin-3 gene is markedly upregulated in EoE, and it has been speculated that susceptibility to EoE may, in part, be explained by polymorphisms in the eotaxin-3 gene [25]. IL-13 plays a central role in initiating the cascade of mediators leading to increased eotaxin-3 expression and chemo-attraction of tissue eosinophils [29]. Variants of the thymic stromal lymphopoietin located on chromosome 5q22 have been shown to be associated with an increased predisposition to EoE [30]. Thymic stromal lymphopoietin is believed to be a key regulatory molecule in the initiation of Th2-mediated inflammation and plays a role in other atopic conditions, such as asthma and eczema.

Basal cell proliferation is a key histological feature in patients with EoE. Subepithelial remodelling and mucosal deposition of collagen has been demonstrated in patients with EoE and may contribute to dysphagia [31, 32]. Oesophageal dysmotility even occurs in children with EoE, which suggests that the development of peristaltic dysfunction occurs early in the disease course [25, 26]. Eosinophils may also directly disrupt the integrity of submucosal neuronal networks and promote lower oesophageal sphincter dysfunction and peristaltic dysfunction [33].

In experimental models, intratracheal egg challenge in ovalbumin-sensitised mice has been shown to elicit oesophageal eosinophilia, suggesting that EoE is a food antigen-driven process [34]. This observation aligns with a high prevalence of both IgE- and non-IgE-mediated food allergy in patients with EoE [15, 35]. Inhalant allergens, e.g. grass pollen, appear to play a greater aetiological role in adults than in children [36], and sensitisation to grass and tree pollen may explain some seasonal variability in symptom severity, mucosal eosinophilia and incidence of EoE [37]. In a significant proportion of patients, EoE does not appear to be associated with other atopic disorders [38]. The pathophysiology of non-atopic EoE is poorly understood.

Diagnostic Evaluation

The diagnosis of EoE requires gastroscopic evaluation and oesophageal biopsy [1, 8], and EoE diagnosis is assumed if more than 15 eosinophils per high power field (HPF) are demonstrated in oesophageal biopsies (at 400-times magnification) in conjunction with clinical symptoms attributable to upper gastrointestinal inflammation [1]. Recently, PPI-ROE has been described as a separate diagnostic entity [1, 5, 39]. Patients with PPI-ROE respond to acid-suppressive medication alone and do not follow the clinical course of EoE. EoE diagnosis therefore needs to be made in the context of a non-response to PPI treatment.

The endoscopic appearance of EoE is often characteristic, including longitudinal furrowing and thickening of the mucosa [40]. White mucosal plaques are also common, reflecting fibrinous exudate due to epithelial eosinophilic inflammation [41]; these plaques may be mistaken for candidiasis. Other features include concentric rings (trachealisation), strictures or a narrow oesophageal calibre [40]. Importantly, a macroscopically normal oesophageal appearance does not rule out EoE. The consensus guidelines therefore recommend taking several biopsies from several levels along the oesophagus, regardless of its macroscopic appearance [1, 8]. Repeat gastroscopy is required to assess the effectiveness of any therapeutic intervention.

Allergic evaluation of patients with EoE relies on skin prick testing (SPT), as the use of food-specific serum IgE has not been standardised for this condition. Atopic patch testing (APT) is also used to screen for possible trigger foods; however, evidence for its clinical usefulness is limited [42]. Spergel et al. [43] have defined the diagnostic accuracy of SPT and APT for food allergens in children with EoE. Apart from food allergens, aeroallergens are thought to be of importance in the pathogenesis of EoE, but it is often difficult to ascertain to what extent inhalants specifically contribute to the aetiology. SPT and APT findings may form the basis for targeted elimination diets, particularly if patients are only sensitised to a small number of food allergens. In recent years, empiric elimination diets have been increasingly used, as they seem to achieve a similar efficacy compared to targeted elimination diets [44]. The role of allergy testing in the management of EoE has therefore been questioned [45].

Natural History and Complications

There are few longitudinal studies that have prospectively followed treated and untreated patients with EoE, and population-based data on the natural history of EoE are not available. In general, EoE appears to follow a chronic or relapsing course, and complete resolution of the disease is thought to be uncommon [46, 47]. A longitudinal study suggests that even the persistence of small numbers of oesophageal eosinophils (>5/HPF) may have prognostic significance for EoE [46], and observational studies found a progression of symptoms in untreated EoE [4]. Strictures in the paediatric population are relatively uncommon [12, 15]. By contrast, adolescent and adult patients may develop long-term sequelae, including dysphagia, strictures, crêpe-paper mucosa or even oesophageal perforation [1]. However, it is not clear whether all patients with poorly managed or undiagnosed EoE are at increased risk of strictures. There is currently a debate as to whether stricturing disease is a marker of a more aggressive phenotype of EoE or, alternatively, a result of long-standing untreated disease. As such, there is little evidence to guide gastroenterologists and allergists as to whether aggressive treatment should aim for complete eradication of eosinophils from oesophageal biopsies or whether a symptom-free outcome is a sufficient clinical end-point. Well-designed, longitudinal studies on the natural history of untreated EoE are needed to identify markers of progressive EoE that would warrant dietary, corticosteroid or other immune-modulating therapy.

Treatment

The treatment of EoE relies on three main pillars: diets, drugs and oesophageal dilatation – often referred to as DDD. Treatments aim to improve symptoms, prevent long-term sequelae and relieve oesophageal obstruction. Both corticosteroids and elimination diets can reverse or ameliorate subepithelial fibrosis and may therefore reduce the risk of dysphagia and stricturing disease [32, 48]. In children, and more recently in adults, various types of elimination diets have been shown to be effective in reducing eosinophilic inflammation. In older children and adults, topical swallowed corticosteroid preparations are also commonly used. Finally, endoscopic food bolus disimpaction and oesophageal dilatation may be required in patients with dysphagia and oesophageal strictures.

Proton Pump Inhibitors
A significant proportion of patients with oesophageal eosinophilia respond to treatment with proton pump inhibitors (PPIs). These patients do not suffer from EoE and have instead been labelled as 'PPI-responsive eosinophilia (PPI-ROE)'. A high-dose trial of a PPI for 4–8 weeks followed by repeat gastroscopy is therefore an integral part in the diagnostic assessment for EoE [1, 5]. Two studies assessed the effect of esomeprazole (a potent PPI) against swallowed fluticasone aerosol for oesophageal eosinophilia [49, 50]. Both studies found a similar effect for both treatments in terms of tissue eosinophilia and oesophageal symptoms, highlighting the importance of PPI in delineating EoE against PPI-ROE.

Elimination Diets
Three types of elimination diets are currently available for the treatment of EoE: amino acid-based (elemental) diets, individualised targeted elimination diets that are based on allergy testing, and empiric elimination diets that avoid the most common food allergens. In recent years, the trend has been towards an increased use of empiric elimination diets, which are easier to establish and achieve a similar efficacy compared to skin test-directed elimination diets [51].

Elemental Diet
The initial recognition of EoE as a new disease entity was based on the observation that EoE resolved after treatment with an amino acid-based formula [3]. In children, amino acid-based diets are highly effective. Markowitz et al. [52] reported that after treatment with an amino acid-based formula for 4 weeks, 96% of children with EoE achieved mucosal remission, with a drop in eosinophils from 33.7/HPF to 2.1/HPF. Symptoms also resolved within 7–10 days. Recently, a small case series in adults also confirmed that elemental diets induced histological remission in 72% of patients after 4 weeks [53]. However, symptomatic improvement was incomplete, and compliance with the diet was poor. These studies demonstrate that elemental diets are highly effective in treating paediatric EoE but often are not tolerated in the long term, mainly due to poor palatability.

Targeted Elimination Diets
Targeted elimination diets that are based on allergy testing are often attempted. Spergel et al. [35] reported resolution of EoE in 75% of patients after removing foods that were positive on SPT or APT. The investigation of underlying food allergies in patients is often complex, as patients may present with multiple IgE-mediated and non-IgE-mediated food allergies. In a retrospective review, the overall response rate after removal of foods identified on SPT/APT was 53%, which was the same as for an empiric 6-food-elimination diet

[42]. The remission rate increased to 77% when empiric cow's milk elimination was added to the SPT/APT-guided elimination diet [42]. By contrast, in a study of 22 adults with EoE, the efficacy of targeted elimination diets was much lower, with remission in only 26% of patients [54].

Empiric Elimination Diet
As the long-term use of elemental diets is impractical, many gastroenterologists have moved to the empiric elimination of the most commonly implicated food allergens in patients with EoE. Initially, Kagalwalla et al. [44] compared the clinical response between a 6-food-elimination diet in children (i.e. avoidance of cow's milk, soy, egg, wheat, fish/shellfish and peanut/nuts) and an elemental diet using a retrospective, non-randomised study design. In that study, remission was achieved in 88% of subjects on the elemental diet, compared to 74% subjects on the 6-food elimination diet. The 6-food elimination diet thereby offered a less cumbersome treatment modality with reasonable efficacy. Gonsalves et al. [55] found a remission rate of 70% in adults with EoE (defined as less than 10 eosinophils/HPF), and after step-wise re-introduction of foods, wheat (60%) and cow's milk (50%) were the most common trigger foods in the adults. Another adult study on a 6-food elimination diet by Lucenda et al. [56] found a response rate of 73%. In that study, the most common trigger foods were cow's milk (61.9%), wheat (28.6%), egg (26.2%) and legumes (23.8%). The single elimination of cow's milk has also recently been proposed as an empiric diet in children with EoE, with a histological response rate of 65%, in an uncontrolled, retrospective study [57].

Integrating the results of these studies, the four foods cow's milk, soy, egg and wheat appear to be the predominant trigger foods in children with EoE. The reduced number of avoided food allergens and better palatability, compared to an elemental diet, make the 4-food elimination diet a promising candidate for a sustainable dietary intervention that will be effective in a significant proportion of children with EoE. We have recently initiated the first RCT on this novel 4-food elimination diet (the 4-FEED RCT). Because it is ethically difficult to randomise children with newly identified EoE to 'no treatment', this study aims to assess the effect of a 4-food elimination diet (plus PPIs) versus PPI alone. Apart from assessing the overall clinical response rate to the elimination diet, the study will allow for estimating the rate of PPI-ROE in the control group.

Corticosteroids
While prednisolone is effective in the treatment of EoE, topical corticosteroids are more commonly used because of their fewer adverse effects [58]. Dose and delivery regimens for steroid medications in EoE are largely empirical, and only few RCTs (including only one head-to-head trial) of topical corticosteroids are available to inform best treatment [59]. In a comparative trial, prednisolone was superior to topical steroids in suppressing eosinophilic inflammation in the oesophagus [60]. However, the use of systemic corticosteroids is now mainly limited to short courses for severe EoE or after food impaction [58].

Several clinical trials have assessed the clinical efficacy of swallowed topical corticosteroids, including aerosolised fluticasone [38, 60–63], viscous budesonide [64–67], and more recently, aerosolised ciclesonide [68]. While generally effective, topical steroids are limited by a high relapse rate after discontinuation [59] as well as by a blunted response in patients with atopic disorders or food allergy [38, 63]. Konikoff et al. [38] found that fluticasone (440 μg twice daily) was effective in only 50% of paediatric patients with EoE, and non-response was more common in patients with underlying atopic disorders or food allergy. Aceves et al. [64] first described the use of viscous budesonide (suspended in sucralose powder; Splenda™, McNeil Nutritionals) as an alternative to fluticasone. An RCT in children showed that after 3 months of treatment with oral viscous budesonide, 68% of patients had <6 eosinophils/

HPF on repeat biopsy [66]. A recent RCT also confirmed that aerosolised budesonide is effective in adolescents and adults with EoE [67]. Long-term administration of budesonide appeared to be well tolerated and to adequately maintain clinical and histological remission [69]. In another RCT in adults, swallowed fluticasone aerosol appeared to improve histology but was not effective in terms of a symptomatic response when compared to placebo [70]. The role of fluticasone in adults is therefore uncertain.

Other Immune-Modulating Agents
Montelukast, a leukotriene inhibitor used in asthma prevention, has been studied in an uncontrolled adult trial, but its use is limited because of side effects and is therefore no longer recommended [71]. Several other novel medications have been trialled for the treatment of EoE, many of which were developed based on our emerging understanding of the basic biology of EoE. Mepolizumab, a humanised monoclonal antibody against IL-5, has been shown to effectively reduce oesophageal eosinophil counts, but its effect on symptoms was disappointing [72, 73]. Therefore, given its cost and limited clinical efficacy, the role of this medication requires further evaluation. Reslizumab, another humanised neutralising antibody against IL-5, was assessed in patients with EoE. Both the reslizumab and placebo-treated groups showed improvements in eosinophil counts, without significant differences [74]. Finally, the CRTH2 antagonist OC000459 achieved a modest reduction in eosinophil counts in adults with EoE when compared to placebo [75]. The role of these monoclonal antibodies in the treatment of EoE requires further study.

Endoscopic Oesophageal Food Disimpaction and Dilatation of Strictures
EoE is one of the most common reasons for dysphagia and food bolus impaction in children and young adults [76]. Despite this, the diagnosis may not be recognised at the time of endoscopic disimpaction unless biopsies are obtained. In patients who have failed to respond to topical steroid treatment, endoscopic dilatation is an effective way of relieving oesophageal obstruction due to strictures [77]. However, endoscopic dilatation is associated with a significant risk of oesophageal perforation, particularly after rigid oesophagoscopy [76]. Endoscopic balloon dilatation can generally be safely achieved [77–79].

Conclusion and Future Directions

EoE remains a complex disorder that still poses clinical challenges in children and adults. The development of consensus guidelines in the Unites States [1, 8] and Europe [6] have been helpful in standardising the care for patients with EoE and in identifying gaps in the evidence base. The treatment of EoE requires a team approach between gastroenterologists, allergists, dieticians, and even speech pathologists to optimise management. We urgently require high-quality evidence from RCTs to assess both the efficacy of dietary interventions and to find the optimal dose/delivery mode of topical steroid treatments. Head-to-head trials of diet versus corticosteroid management would also be beneficial. Finally, further mechanistic studies that unravel the biology of EoE may lead to the development of novel therapies in the future.

References

1 Liacouras CA, Furuta GT, Hirano I, Atkins D, Attwood SE, Bonis PA, Burks AW, Chehade M, Collins MH, Dellon ES, Dohil R, Falk GW, Gonsalves N, Gupta SK, Katzka DA, Lucendo AJ, Markowitz JE, Noel RJ, Odze RD, Putnam PE, Richter JE, Romero Y, Ruchelli E, Sampson HA, Schoepfer A, Shaheen NJ, Sicherer SH, Spechler S, Spergel JM, Straumann A, Wershil BK, Rothenberg ME, Aceves SS: Eosinophilic esophagitis: updated consensus recommendations for children and adults. J Allergy Clin Immunol 2011;128:3–20.e6.

2 Winter HS, Madara JL, Stafford RJ, Grand RJ, Quinlan JE, Goldman H: Intraepithelial eosinophils: a new diagnostic criterion for reflux esophagitis. Gastroenterology 1982;83:818–823.

3 Kelly KJ, Lazenby AJ, Rowe PC, Yardley JH, Perman JA, Sampson HA: Eosinophilic esophagitis attributed to gastroesophageal reflux: improvement with an amino acid-based formula. Gastroenterology 1995;109:1503–1512.

4 Schoepfer AM, Safroneeva E, Bussmann C, Kuchen T, Portmann S, Simon HU, Straumann A: Delay in diagnosis of eosinophilic esophagitis increases risk for stricture formation in a time-dependent manner. Gastroenterology 2013;145: 1230–1236.e1–e2.

5 Dellon ES, Gonsalves N, Hirano I, Furuta GT, Liacouras CA, Katzka DA: ACG clinical guideline: evidenced based approach to the diagnosis and management of esophageal eosinophilia and eosinophilic esophagitis (EoE). Am J Gastroenterol 2013;108:679–692.

6 Papadopoulou A, Koletzko S, Heuschkel R, Dias JA, Allen KJ, Murch SH, Chong S, Gottrand F, Husby S, Lionetti P, Mearin ML, Ruemmele FM, Schappi MG, Staiano A, Wilschanski M, Vandenplas Y, ESPGHAN Eosinophilic Esophagitis Working Group and the Gastroenterology Committee: Management guidelines of eosinophilic esophagitis in childhood. J Pediatr Gastroenterol Nutr 2014;58: 107–118.

7 Dellon ES: Epidemiology of eosinophilic esophagitis. Gastroenterol Clin North Am 2014;43:201–218.

8 Furuta GT, Liacouras CA, Collins MH, Gupta SK, Justinich C, Putnam PE, Bonis P, Hassall E, Straumann A, Rothenberg ME: Eosinophilic esophagitis in children and adults: a systematic review and consensus recommendations for diagnosis and treatment. Gastroenterology 2007;133:1342–1363.

9 Collins MH, Blanchard C, Abonia JP, Kirby C, Akers R, Wang N, Putnam PE, Jameson SC, Assa'ad AH, Konikoff MR, Stringer KF, Rothenberg ME: Clinical, pathologic, and molecular characterization of familial eosinophilic esophagitis compared with sporadic cases. Clin Gastroenterol Hepatol 2008;6:621–629.

10 Noel RJ, Putnam PE, Rothenberg ME: Eosinophilic esophagitis. N Engl J Med 2004;351:940–941.

11 Cherian S, Smith NM, Forbes DA: Rapidly increasing prevalence of eosinophilic oesophagitis in Western Australia. Arch Dis Child 2006;91:1000–1004.

12 Nethercote M, Heine RG, Kansal S, Ho SSC, Chow CW, Cameron D, Alex G, Erbas B, Osborne N, Stevens L, Davidson D, Allen KJ: Clinical features of eosinophilic esophagitis in a consecutive series of pediatric patients in an Australian tertiary referral center. J Food Allergy 2012;1:160–169.

13 Assa'ad AH, Putnam PE, Collins MH, Akers RM, Jameson SC, Kirby CL, Buckmeier BK, Bullock JZ, Collier AR, Konikoff MR, Noel RJ, Guajardo JR, Rothenberg ME: Pediatric patients with eosinophilic esophagitis: an 8-year follow-up. J Allergy Clin Immunol 2007; 119:731–738.

14 Ronkainen J, Talley NJ, Aro P, Storskrubb T, Johansson SE, Lind T, Bolling-Sternevald E, Vieth M, Stolte M, Walker MM, Agreus L: Prevalence of oesophageal eosinophils and eosinophilic oesophagitis in adults: the population-based Kalixanda study. Gut 2007;56: 615–620.

15 Liacouras CA, Spergel JM, Ruchelli E, Verma R, Mascarenhas M, Semeao E, Flick J, Kelly J, Brown-Whitehorn T, Mamula P, Markowitz JE: Eosinophilic esophagitis: a 10-year experience in 381 children. Clin Gastroenterol Hepatol 2005;3:1198–1206.

16 Zhang X, Cheng E, Huo X, Yu C, Hormi-Carver KK, Anderson J, Spechler SJ, Souza RF: 877 in esophageal squamous epithelial cell lines from patients with eosinophilic esophagitis (EoE), omeprazole blocks the stimulated secretion of eotaxin-3: a potential anti-inflammatory effect of omeprazole in EoE that is independent of acid inhibition. Gastroenterology 2010;138(suppl 1):S-122.

17 Untersmayr E, Scholl I, Swoboda I, Beil WJ, Forster-Waldl E, Walter F, Riemer A, Kraml G, Kinaciyan T, Spitzauer S, Boltz-Nitulescu G, Scheiner O, Jensen-Jarolim E: Antacid medication inhibits digestion of dietary proteins and causes food allergy: a fish allergy model in BALB/c mice. J Allergy Clin Immunol 2003;112:616–623.

18 Ooi CY, Day AS, Jackson R, Bohane TD, Tobias V, Lemberg DA: Eosinophilic esophagitis in children with celiac disease. J Gastroenterol Hepatol 2008;23: 1144–1148.

19 Leslie C, Mews C, Charles A, Ravikumara M: Celiac disease and eosinophilic esophagitis: a true association. J Pediatr Gastroenterol Nutr 2010;50:397–399.

20 Ludvigsson JF, Aro P, Walker MM, Vieth M, Agreus L, Talley NJ, Murray JA, Ronkainen J: Celiac disease, eosinophilic esophagitis and gastroesophageal reflux disease, an adult population-based study. Scand J Gastroenterol 2013; 48:808–814.

21 Heine RG: Eosinophilic esophagitis in children with celiac disease: new diagnostic and therapeutic dilemmas. J Gastroenterol Hepatol 2008;23:993–994.

22 Lucendo AJ, Arias A, Perez-Martinez I, Lopez-Vazquez A, Ontanon-Rodriguez J, Gonzalez-Castillo S, De Rezende LC, Rodrigo L: Adult patients with eosinophilic esophagitis do not show an increased frequency of the HLA-DQ2/DQ8 genotypes predisposing to celiac disease. Dig Dis Sci 2011;56:1107–1111.

23 Quaglietta L, Coccorullo P, Miele E, Pascarella F, Troncone R, Staiano A: Eosinophilic oesophagitis and coeliac disease: is there an association? Aliment Pharmacol Ther 2007;26:487–493.

24 Mishra A: Mechanism of eosinophilic esophagitis. Immunol Allergy Clin North Am 2009;29:29–40, viii.

25 Blanchard C, Wang N, Stringer KF, Mishra A, Fulkerson PC, Abonia JP, Jameson SC, Kirby C, Konikoff MR, Collins MH, Cohen MB, Akers R, Hogan SP, Assa'ad AH, Putnam PE, Aronow BJ, Rothenberg ME: Eotaxin-3 and a uniquely conserved gene-expression profile in eosinophilic esophagitis. J Clin Invest 2006;116:536–547.

26 Blanchard C, Mingler MK, Vicario M, Abonia JP, Wu YY, Lu TX, Collins MH, Putnam PE, Wells SI, Rothenberg ME: IL-13 involvement in eosinophilic esophagitis: transcriptome analysis and reversibility with glucocorticoids. J Allergy Clin Immunol 2007;120:1292–1300.

27 Bullock JZ, Villanueva JM, Blanchard C, Filipovich AH, Putnam PE, Collins MH, Risma KA, Akers RM, Kirby CL, Buckmeier BK, Assa'ad AH, Hogan SP, Rothenberg ME: Interplay of adaptive th2 immunity with eotaxin-3/c-C chemokine receptor 3 in eosinophilic esophagitis. J Pediatr Gastroenterol Nutr 2007;45:22–31.

28 Lucendo AJ, Bellon T, Lucendo B: The role of mast cells in eosinophilic esophagitis. Pediatr Allergy Immunol 2009;20: 512–518.

29 Blanchard C, Stucke EM, Burwinkel K, Caldwell JM, Collins MH, Ahrens A, Buckmeier BK, Jameson SC, Greenberg A, Kaul A, Franciosi JP, Kushner JP, Martin LJ, Putnam PE, Abonia JP, Wells SI, Rothenberg ME: Coordinate interaction between IL-13 and epithelial differentiation cluster genes in eosinophilic esophagitis. J Immunol 2010;184:4033–4041.

30 Rothenberg ME, Spergel JM, Sherrill JD, Annaiah K, Martin LJ, Cianferoni A, Gober L, Kim C, Glessner J, Frackelton E, Thomas K, Blanchard C, Liacouras C, Verma R, Aceves S, Collins MH, Brown-Whitehorn T, Putnam PE, Franciosi JP, Chiavacci RM, Grant SF, Abonia JP, Sleiman PM, Hakonarson H: Common variants at 5q22 associate with pediatric eosinophilic esophagitis. Nat Genet 2010;42:289–291.

31 Chehade M, Sampson HA, Morotti RA, Magid MS: Esophageal subepithelial fibrosis in children with eosinophilic esophagitis. J Pediatr Gastroenterol Nutr 2007;45:319–328.

32 Aceves SS, Ackerman SJ: Relationships between eosinophilic inflammation, tissue remodeling, and fibrosis in eosinophilic esophagitis. Immunol Allergy Clin North Am 2009;29:197–211, xiii–xiv.

33 Lucendo AJ: Motor disturbances participate in the pathogenesis of eosinophilic oesophagitis, beyond the fibrous remodelling of the oesophagus. Aliment Pharmacol Ther 2006;24:1264–1267.

34 Hogan SP, Mishra A, Brandt EB, Foster PS, Rothenberg ME: A critical role for eotaxin in experimental oral antigen-induced eosinophilic gastrointestinal allergy. Proc Natl Acad Sci U S A 2000; 97:6681–6686.

35 Spergel JM, Andrews T, Brown-Whitehorn TF, Beausoleil JL, Liacouras CA: Treatment of eosinophilic esophagitis with specific food elimination diet directed by a combination of skin prick and patch tests. Ann Allergy Asthma Immunol 2005;95:336–343.

36 Almansa C, Krishna M, Buchner AM, Ghabril MS, Talley N, DeVault KR, Wolfsen H, Raimondo M, Guarderas JC, Achem SR: Seasonal distribution in newly diagnosed cases of eosinophilic esophagitis in adults. Am J Gastroenterol 2009;104:828–833.

37 Wang FY, Gupta SK, Fitzgerald JF: Is there a seasonal variation in the incidence or intensity of allergic eosinophilic esophagitis in newly diagnosed children? J Clin Gastroenterol 2007;41:451–453.

38 Konikoff MR, Noel RJ, Blanchard C, Kirby C, Jameson SC, Buckmeier BK, Akers R, Cohen MB, Collins MH, Assa'ad AH, Aceves SS, Putnam PE, Rothenberg ME: A randomized, double-blind, placebo-controlled trial of fluticasone propionate for pediatric eosinophilic esophagitis. Gastroenterology 2006;131:1381–1391.

39 Schroeder S, Capocelli KE, Masterson JC, Harris R, Protheroe C, Lee JJ, Furuta GT: Effect of proton pump inhibitor on esophageal eosinophilia. J Pediatr Gastroenterol Nutr 2013;56:166–172.

40 Croese J, Fairley SK, Masson JW, Chong AK, Whitaker DA, Kanowski PA, Walker NI: Clinical and endoscopic features of eosinophilic esophagitis in adults. Gastrointest Endosc 2003;58:516–522.

41 Sundaram S, Sunku B, Nelson SP, Sentongo T, Melin-Aldana H, Kumar R, Li BU: Adherent white plaques: an endoscopic finding in eosinophilic esophagitis. J Pediatr Gastroenterol Nutr 2004; 38:208–212.

42 Spergel JM, Brown-Whitehorn TF, Cianferoni A, Shuker M, Wang ML, Verma R, Liacouras CA: Identification of causative foods in children with eosinophilic esophagitis treated with an elimination diet. J Allergy Clin Immunol 2012;130: 461–467.e5.

43 Spergel JM, Brown-Whitchorn T, Beausoleil JL, Shuker M, Liacouras CA: Predictive values for skin prick test and atopy patch test for eosinophilic esophagitis. J Allergy Clin Immunol 2007;119: 509–511.

44 Kagalwalla AF, Sentongo TA, Ritz S, Hess T, Nelson SP, Emerick KM, Melin-Aldana H, Li BU: Effect of six-food elimination diet on clinical and histologic outcomes in eosinophilic esophagitis. Clin Gastroenterol Hepatol 2006;4: 1097–1102.

45 Greenhawt M, Rubenstein JH: Tailored versus empiric dietary therapy for eosinophilic esophagitis: is there a superior option? Gastroenterology 2013;144: 1560–1561.

46 DeBrosse CW, Collins MH, Buckmeier Butz BK, Allen CL, King EC, Assa'ad AH, Abonia JP, Putnam PE, Rothenberg ME, Franciosi JP: Identification, epidemiology, and chronicity of pediatric esophageal eosinophilia, 1982–1999. J Allergy Clin Immunol 2010;126:112–119.

47 Spergel JM, Brown-Whitehorn TF, Beausoleil JL, Franciosi J, Shuker M, Verma R, Liacouras CA: 14 years of eosinophilic esophagitis: clinical features and prognosis. J Pediatr Gastroenterol Nutr 2009;48:30–36.

48 Lieberman JA, Morotti RA, Konstantinou GN, Yershov O, Chehade M: Dietary therapy can reverse esophageal subepithelial fibrosis in patients with eosinophilic esophagitis: a historical cohort. Allergy 2012;67:1299–1307.

49 Moawad FJ, Veerappan GR, Dias JA, Baker TP, Maydonovitch CL, Wong RK: Randomized controlled trial comparing aerosolized swallowed fluticasone to esomeprazole for esophageal eosinophilia. Am J Gastroenterol 2013;108:366–372.

50 Peterson KA, Thomas KL, Hilden K, Emerson LL, Wills JC, Fang JC: Comparison of esomeprazole to aerosolized, swallowed fluticasone for eosinophilic esophagitis. Dig Dis Sci 2010;55:1313–1319.

51 Henderson CJ, Abonia JP, King EC, Putnam PE, Collins MH, Franciosi JP, Rothenberg ME: Comparative dietary therapy effectiveness in remission of pediatric eosinophilic esophagitis. J Allergy Clin Immunol 2012;129:1570–1578.

52 Markowitz JE, Spergel JM, Ruchelli E, Liacouras CA: Elemental diet is an effective treatment for eosinophilic esophagitis in children and adolescents. Am J Gastroenterol 2003;98:777–782.

53 Peterson KA, Byrne KR, Vinson LA, Ying J, Boynton KK, Fang JC, Gleich GJ, Adler DG, Clayton F: Elemental diet induces histologic response in adult eosinophilic esophagitis. Am J Gastroenterol 2013;108:759–766.

54 Molina-Infante J, Martin-Noguerol E, Alvarado-Arenas M, Porcel-Carreno SL, Jimenez-Timon S, Hernandez-Arbeiza FJ: Selective elimination diet based on skin testing has suboptimal efficacy for adult eosinophilic esophagitis. J Allergy Clin Immunol 2012;130:1200–1202.

55 Gonsalves N, Yang GY, Doerfler B, Ritz S, Ditto AM, Hirano I: Elimination diet effectively treats eosinophilic esophagitis in adults; food reintroduction identifies causative factors. Gastroenterology 2012;142:1451–1459.e1.

56 Lucendo AJ, Arias A, Gonzalez-Cervera J, Yague-Compadre JL, Guagnozzi D, Angueira T, Jimenez-Contreras S, Gonzalez-Castillo S, Rodriguez-Domingez B, De Rezende LC, Tenias JM: Empiric 6-food elimination diet induced and maintained prolonged remission in patients with adult eosinophilic esophagitis: a prospective study on the food cause of the disease. J Allergy Clin Immunol 2013;131:797–804.

57 Kagalwalla AF, Amsden K, Shah A, Ritz S, Manuel-Rubio M, Dunne K, Nelson SP, Wershil BK, Melin-Aldana H: Cow's milk elimination: a novel dietary approach to treat eosinophilic esophagitis. J Pediatr Gastroenterol Nutr 2012;55: 711–716.

58 Liacouras CA, Wenner WJ, Brown K, Ruchelli E: Primary eosinophilic esophagitis in children: successful treatment with oral corticosteroids. J Pediatr Gastroenterol Nutr 1998;26:380–385.

59 Elliott EJ, Thomas D, Markowitz JE: Non-surgical interventions for eosinophilic esophagitis. Cochrane Database Syst Rev 2010;3:CD004065.

60 Schaefer ET, Fitzgerald JF, Molleston JP, Croffie JM, Pfefferkorn MD, Corkins MR, Lim JD, Steiner SJ, Gupta SK: Comparison of oral prednisone and topical fluticasone in the treatment of eosinophilic esophagitis: a randomized trial in children. Clin Gastroenterol Hepatol 2008;6:165–173.

61 Helou EF, Simonson J, Arora AS: 3-yr-follow-up of topical corticosteroid treatment for eosinophilic esophagitis in adults. Am J Gastroenterol 2008;103: 2194–2199.

62 Teitelbaum JE, Fox VL, Twarog FJ, Nurko S, Antonioli D, Gleich G, Badizadegan K, Furuta GT: Eosinophilic esophagitis in children: immunopathological analysis and response to fluticasone propionate. Gastroenterology 2002; 122:1216–1225.

63 Noel RJ, Putnam PE, Collins MH, Assa'ad AH, Guajardo JR, Jameson SC, Rothenberg ME: Clinical and immunopathologic effects of swallowed fluticasone for eosinophilic esophagitis. Clin Gastroenterol Hepatol 2004;2:568–575.

64 Aceves SS, Dohil R, Newbury RO, Bastian JF: Topical viscous budesonide suspension for treatment of eosinophilic esophagitis. J Allergy Clin Immunol 2005;116:705–706.

65 Aceves SS, Newbury RO, Chen D, Mueller J, Dohil R, Hoffman H, Bastian JF, Broide DH: Resolution of remodeling in eosinophilic esophagitis correlates with epithelial response to topical corticosteroids. Allergy 2010;65:109–116.

66 Dohil R, Newbury R, Fox L, Bastian J, Aceves S: Oral viscous budesonide is effective in children with eosinophilic esophagitis in a randomized, placebo-controlled trial. Gastroenterology 2010; 139:418–429.

67 Straumann A, Conus S, Degen L, Felder S, Kummer M, Engel H, Bussmann C, Beglinger C, Schoepfer A, Simon H-U: Budesonide is effective in adolescent and adult patients with active eosinophilic esophagitis. Gastroenterology 2010;139:1526–1537.e1.

68 Lee JJ, Fried AJ, Hait E, Yen EH, Perkins JM, Rubinstein E: Topical inhaled ciclesonide for treatment of eosinophilic esophagitis. J Allergy Clin Immunol 2012;130:1011.

69 Straumann A, Conus S, Degen L, Frei C, Bussmann C, Beglinger C, Schoepfer A, Simon HU: Long-term budesonide maintenance treatment is partially effective for patients with eosinophilic esophagitis. Clin Gastroenterol Hepatol 2011;9:400–409.e1.

70 Alexander JA, Jung KW, Arora AS, Enders F, Katzka DA, Kephardt GM, Kita H, Kryzer LA, Romero Y, Smyrk TC, Talley NJ: Swallowed fluticasone improves histologic but not symptomatic response of adults with eosinophilic esophagitis. Clin Gastroenterol Hepatol 2012;10:742–749.e1.

71 Attwood SE, Lewis CJ, Bronder CS, Morris CD, Armstrong GR, Whittam J: Eosinophilic oesophagitis: a novel treatment using Montelukast. Gut 2003;52: 181–185.

72 Stein ML, Collins MH, Villanueva JM, Kushner JP, Putnam PE, Buckmeier BK, Filipovich AH, Assa'ad AH, Rothenberg ME: Anti-IL-5 (mepolizumab) therapy for eosinophilic esophagitis. J Allergy Clin Immunol 2006;118:1312–1319.

73 Straumann A, Conus S, Grzonka P, Kita H, Kephart G, Bussmann C, Beglinger C, Smith DA, Patel J, Byrne M, Simon HU: Anti-interleukin-5 antibody treatment (mepolizumab) in active eosinophilic oesophagitis: a randomised, placebo-controlled, double-blind trial. Gut 2010; 59:21–30.

74 Spergel JM, Rothenberg ME, Collins MH, Furuta GT, Markowitz JE, Fuchs G, 3rd, O'Gorman MA, Abonia JP, Young J, Henkel T, Wilkins HJ, Liacouras CA: Reslizumab in children and adolescents with eosinophilic esophagitis: results of a double-blind, randomized, placebo-controlled trial. J Allergy Clin Immunol 2012;129:456–463.e1–e3.

75 Straumann A, Hoesli S, Bussmann C, Stuck M, Perkins M, Collins LP, Payton M, Pettipher R, Hunter M, Steiner J, Simon HU: Anti-eosinophil activity and clinical efficacy of the CRTH2 antagonist OC000459 in eosinophilic esophagitis. Allergy 2013;68:375–385.

76 Straumann A, Bussmann C, Zuber M, Vannini S, Simon HU, Schoepfer A: Eosinophilic esophagitis: analysis of food impaction and perforation in 251 adolescent and adult patients. Clin Gastroenterol Hepatol 2008;6:598–600.

77 Schoepfer AM, Gschossmann J, Scheurer U, Seibold F, Straumann A: Esophageal strictures in adult eosinophilic esophagitis: dilation is an effective and safe alternative after failure of topical corticosteroids. Endoscopy 2008;40:161–164.

78 Dellon ES, Gibbs WB, Rubinas TC, Fritchie KJ, Madanick RD, Woosley JT, Shaheen NJ: Esophageal dilation in eosinophilic esophagitis: safety and predictors of clinical response and complications. Gastrointest Endosc 2010;71:706–712.

79 Jacobs JW Jr, Spechler SJ: A systematic review of the risk of perforation during esophageal dilation for patients with eosinophilic esophagitis. Dig Dis Sci 2010;55:1512–1515.

Prof. Katrina J. Allen, PhD, FRACP
Department of Allergy and Immunology
The Royal Children's Hospital Melbourne
50 Flemington Road, Parkville, VIC 3052 (Australia)
E-Mail katrina.allen@rch.org.au

Ebisawa M, Ballmer-Weber BK, Vieths S, Wood RA (eds): Food Allergy: Molecular Basis and Clinical Practice.
Chem Immunol Allergy. Basel, Karger, 2015, vol 101, pp 209–220 (DOI: 10.1159/000373904)

Nutritional Aspects and Diets in Food Allergy

Anna Nowak-Węgrzyn · Marion Groetch

Jaffe Food Allergy Institute, Icahn School of Medicine at Mount Sinai, New York, N.Y., USA

Abstract

Dietary intervention is a crucial component of food allergy management but can negatively impact nutrient intake. A comprehensive nutrition assessment with appropriate intervention is warranted in all children with food allergies to meet nutrient needs and optimize growth. Nutrition assessment may also be indicated in adults with food allergy. Frequently, an elimination diet is absolutely necessary to prevent potentially life-threatening anaphylaxis. Allergen elimination can also improve chronic symptoms, such as atopic dermatitis, when a food is proven to trigger symptoms. Allergen elimination goals are to prevent acute and chronic food-allergic reactions in the safest and least restrictive environment to supply a balanced diet that promotes health in children and adults.
© 2015 S. Karger AG, Basel

Food allergy management is focused on food allergen avoidance, which can have profound consequences on nutritional status. Recent food allergy guidelines recommend nutrition therapy or consultation with a dietitian [1, 2]. Dietary assessment and guidance are necessary for successful diagnosis and management of all types of food-allergic disorders [3]. Elimination of a food or

food group from the pediatric diet is associated with nutritional risk, so it is therefore important that elimination diets be prescribed only for the treatment of a diagnosed food allergy or for diagnostic purposes for a limited period of time. As many food allergies of early childhood resolve over time, regular reassessment by an allergist is also important to avoid extended, unnecessary elimination diets.

Elimination Diet in Food Allergy Diagnosis

A short-term elimination diet, e.g., 2–3 weeks for atopic dermatitis (AD) or 6–8 weeks for eosinophilic gastroenteropathies, can be used for diagnostic purposes [1]. Following symptom resolution, the food(s) may be slowly re-introduced to determine if symptoms recur. After more extended elimination, a physician-supervised oral food challenge should be performed since, in some instances, acute reactions may occur after a period of avoidance, even in patients who previously manifested only chronic eczema when food was in their diet on a regular basis [4]. In cases of gastrointestinal food allergy (e.g., eosinophilic

Box 1. Clinical vignette: pitfalls with label reading

A 7-year-old boy with wheat allergy developed severe anaphylaxis with pharyngeal edema (stridor), cough, wheezing, generalized urticaria and emesis within 45 minutes of ingesting a small piece of cornbread that was baked at home from a store-bought mix. The inspection of the package revealed that the mix contained wheat flour as the second ingredient on the list. The boy's father recalled reading labels on two cornbread mixes in the store: one that was wheat-free and one that contained wheat. He thought he had purchased the wheat-free cornbread mix.

Key message: Label reading is challenging, and mistakes are common. Furthermore, the ingredients may change at any time, and constant vigilance is imperative. Reading product labels once at the point of purchase and then again prior to ingestion will help patients catch errors in label reading before a reaction occurs.

Reprinted with permission from Groetch and Nowak-Węgrzyn [3].

esophagitis, allergic proctocolitis), food may be slowly reintroduced at home over the course of days or weeks, with the exception of food protein-induced enterocolitis syndrome, where supervised challenge is recommended [5].

Elimination Diet in Food Allergy Management

Following the confirmation of food allergy diagnosis by appropriate testing, the standard of care for food allergy management is strict avoidance of the offending food(s). Avoidance of food allergens is not simple and may have far-reaching nutritional consequences that impact the quality of life for the patient and the family. Mistakes in avoidance are common and may have grave consequences for individuals with the most severe phenotype of food allergy and who develop anaphylactic reactions from ingestion of trace

amounts of foods [6] [see Box 1, Clinical vignette: pitfalls with label reading]. Avoidance of food allergens limits the selection of store-bought food choices, imposes additional costs associated with purchasing specialty foods, and affects participation in social events, which typically revolve around food [7]. The commercial food industry is ever expanding, adding thousands of new food items each year. Additionally, ingredients in these commercial products can change frequently, so consumers must learn to read product labels each and every time an item is purchased [8]. Food allergen labelling laws begin by identifying foods that are considered the 'common allergens' or 'major allergens'. These common allergens must be listed on the product label using the common name (e.g., milk, egg, wheat) rather than a scientific name (e.g., casein, albumin, starch). Additionally, major allergens may be hidden in a vague ingredient term such as 'natural flavoring'. Laws that guide the labelling of food allergens vary from country to country, and each country or region identifies those foods that are considered common food allergens (see table 1). However, many countries do not yet have specific food allergen labelling laws; therefore, any allergen may remain hidden on product labels in these countries. Health care practitioners and patients should know their country's food allergen labelling laws. Furthermore, when travelling abroad, patients with food allergies should familiarize themselves with labelling laws of their destination country prior to purchasing and consuming packaged foods [9].

Loopholes in the Labeling Laws

Food allergen labelling laws simplified the identification of allergenic ingredients but did not address the potential presence of allergens due to cross contact. The presence of allergenic ingredients due to cross contact confers a small but real risk of allergen exposure to consumers with food

Table 1. Major food allergens based on country-specific labeling laws

Country or Countries	EU	USA, Mexico, Hong Kong, China	Australia and New Zealand	Canada	Japan	Korea
Identified allergens requiring full disclosure on product labels	Milk Egg Soy Gluten-containing grains Peanut Tree nuts Fish Shellfish-Crustacean and Mollusks Mustard Celery Lupine Sesame	Milk Egg Soy Wheat Peanut Tree nut Fish Shellfish-Crustacean	Milk Egg Soy Wheat Peanut Tree nut Fish Shellfish-Crustacean Sesame	Milk Egg Soy Wheat Peanut Tree nut Fish Shellfish-Crustacean and Mollusks Sesame	Milk Egg Wheat Buckwheat Peanut Shrimp Crab	Milk Egg Wheat Buckwheat Soy Peanut Mackerel Crab Shrimp Pork Peach Tomato

Table 1 lists the foods that are considered allergens, by country. Ingredients derived from the listed foods require full disclosure on product labels.
Reprinted with permission from Groetch and Nowak-Węgrzyn [3].

allergies. Manufacturers may address this risk with a precautionary label such as 'may contain milk' or 'manufactured in a facility that manufactures milk products', but these labels are not mandatory, and they are unregulated, leaving consumers feeling unsure about the safety of manufactured products [10]. The National Institute of Allergy and Infectious Diseases food allergy guidelines suggest that consumers avoid products with precautionary labels for their allergens [1].

The labelling laws only apply to foods considered major allergens. While the vast majority of allergic reactions occur to 8 foods – milk, egg, wheat, soy, peanut, tree nut, fish, shellfish – consumers who are allergic to other ingredients may have a more difficult time interpreting product labels. For those allergic to an ingredient not considered a major allergen, additional precautions are necessary. These ingredients may be denoted by a vague labelling term such as 'natural flavoring' or 'spice'. These vague ingredient terms will alert the consumer with allergies that they should either avoid the product or call the manufacturer to determine if their specific allergen is an ingredient in the product.

Changing Paradigms in the Management of Milk and Egg Allergy: Baked Milk and Egg Diet

As many as 70% of children with milk or egg allergy tolerate extensively heated milk or egg ingredients in baked goods [11, 12]. Extensive heating of milk and egg ingredients decreases protein allergenicity by destroying conformational epitopes and enhancing gastrointestinal digestion [13, 14]. The consumption of extensively heated milk and egg protein in the diet of children with milk or egg allergy who can tolerate the baked form appears to accelerate the resolution of milk and egg allergy [15, 16]. Children who incorporated baked milk into the diet were 16 times more likely to become tolerant to un-

Box 2. Clinical vignette: baked-milk diet

A 5-year old child with milk allergy passed an oral food challenge, under physician supervision, to a muffin baked with 1.3 g of milk protein. She added baked milk products to her diet and reported several episodes of itchy mouth and abdominal pain with baked products such as cakes and breads. The inspection of the baked products revealed that they were not baked through and were too moist and soggy in the middle. After thorough baking was enforced, the child had no subsequent complaints.

Key message: Under-baking may result in allergic symptoms.

Reprinted with permission from Groetch and Nowak-Węgrzyn [3].

baked milk compared to a group of children who continued strict avoidance of milk ingredients [15]. Children who incorporated baked egg into the diet were 14.6 times more likely to develop regular egg tolerance than children in the comparison group (p < 0.0001), and they developed tolerance earlier (median 50.0 vs. 78.7 months; p < 0.0001) [16]. In patient populations at large, the adherence to the principles of the baked milk/egg diet may be less stringent than that in clinical trials [see Box 2, Clinical vignette: baked milk diet]. Monitoring is necessary; physicians, dietitians, and nurses must understand how to provide guidance on incorporating baked foods with milk and eggs. For instance, it is not always obvious from a product label how an ingredient was processed [17]. For example, a frosted cookie or cake may contain baked milk in the cake and unbaked milk in the frosting, or a flavored cracker may have a baked milk ingredient or it may have a milk ingredient in the flavoring that is topically applied after the cracker is baked. So, while introducing baked milk or baked egg ingredients into the diet may greatly improve the quality and diversity of the diet, it also introduc-

es additional nuances to avoidance that must be conveyed to the consumer with allergies. In such situations, dietary education is necessary. Table 2 provides examples of foods tolerated by patients who pass a baked milk or baked egg challenge. A physician may choose to advise the family to add additional baked milk or egg items or may even limit some of these items or the serving sizes of these items based on the patient's clinical history [17].

The Effects of Allergen Avoidance on Nutrition in Children

Children with food allergies are at nutritional risk because they are likely to avoid foods of important nutritional value, such as cow's milk, and their nutritional needs for growth and development are substantial. The younger the child and the greater the number of food allergens avoided, the higher the risk of nutritional deficiencies. An avoidance diet must fulfill the nutrient needs of an individual child within the context of the allergen-restricted diet. Therefore, comprehensive dietary education entails the avoidance of specific allergens and guidance on how to properly substitute for the nutrients provided by the avoided food(s).

Children with food allergy on elimination diets are at risk for poor energy intake [18, 19], and children with food allergies tend to be smaller than children without food allergies, even when nutrient intake is similar. Suppressed growth may result from higher protein and energy requirements in children with moderate to severe AD, which is common in many children with food allergies [20]. Children with cow's milk protein allergy and AD had lower albumin levels than healthy controls, despite similar protein intake [21]. Loss of nutrients may occur through abnormal intestinal permeability and absorption caused by poor adherence to the avoidance diet, additional undiagnosed food allergen, residual

Table 2. Guidelines for incorporating baked milk and baked egg in the diet

Types of foods	Allowed	Not allowed
Baked milk diet	– Store-bought baked goods such as rolls, muffins, cupcakes, cookies, crackers and bread, with milk or milk protein ingredients listed as the third ingredient or further down the list of ingredients. – Home-baked goods (such as rolls, muffins, cupcakes or cookies) that have 240 ml of milk per batch of a recipe (yield of 6 servings per batch or approximately 40 ml of baked milk per serving). – Home-baked items with center that is thoroughly cooked through (not moist or soft). Products should be baked in individual serving size: cupcakes, not cakes; brownie muffins, not brownies; rolls, not bread. – Baked milk containing baked goods with milk-free chocolate chips. – Remember to check store-bought products and ingredients based on the patient's other food allergies in order to avoid a reaction to other allergens. – Servings are specified in the nutritional information section of the food label or determined by the yield of the recipe.	– Store-bought baked goods such as rolls, muffins, cupcakes, cookies, crackers and bread, with milk or milk protein ingredients listed as the first or second ingredient. – Home-baked goods with more than 40 ml of baked milk per serving. – Full-sized, home-baked products such as cakes, brownies and breads (commercial breads are safe) that may not be fully cooked in the middle. – Baked milk-containing baked goods with milk chocolate chips. – Continue to avoid milk products that are not fully baked, such as milk-based frostings, icings, and milk-containing flavorings that are topically applied after the product is baked.
Baked egg diet	– Store-bought baked products with egg listed as the third ingredient or further down the list of ingredients. – Home-baked products that have no more than 2 eggs per batch of a recipe (yield of 6 servings) or 1/3 of a large egg. – Home-baked items with center that is thoroughly cooked through (not moist or soft). Products should be baked in individual serving size: cupcakes, not cakes; brownie muffins, not brownies; rolls, not bread. – Remember to check store-bought products and ingredients based on your child's food allergies in order to avoid a reaction to other allergens.	– Store-bought baked products with egg listed as the first or second ingredient. – Home-baked products that have more than 2 eggs per batch of a recipe (yield of 6 servings) or 1/3 of a large egg. – Full-sized, home-baked products such as cakes, brownies and breads (commercial breads are safe) that may not be fully cooked in the middle. – Continue to avoid: Caesar salad dressing; custard; eggs in the form of hard boiled, scrambled or poached, etc.; French toast; frosting; ice cream; mayonnaise; quiche.

Reprinted with permission from Groetch and Nowak-Węgrzyn [3].

reactivity to the substitute formula, or intrinsic factors that predispose the individual to food allergy [21]. Optimal nutrition is of paramount importance because suboptimal nutrient intake may exacerbate the risk of lower growth rates in children with food allergies.

Cow's Milk Allergy

Cow's milk and cow's milk products are major sources of calcium, riboflavin, phosphorus, pantothenic acid, vitamin B12 and vitamin D (in countries with vitamin D-fortified milk), protein and fat. Avoidance of cow's milk compared to

Table 3. Alternative sources for nutrients in cow's milk

Nutrient	Alternative dietary sources
Calcium	Fortified alternative beverages (soy, rice, oat, almond, coconut, hemp, potato), calcium-fortified tofu, calcium-fortified juice
Vitamin D*	Fortified alternative beverages, fortified margarine, fortified alternative yogurts, fish oils, salmon and other fatty fish
Vitamin B12	Meat, fish, poultry, eggs, enriched alternative 'milk' beverages
Vitamin A	Liver, egg yolk, fortified margarine, dark green leafy vegetables, deep orange fruits and vegetables, fortified alternative beverages
Pantothenic acid	Meat, vegetables, eggs, whole grains, legumes, fish
Riboflavin	Dark green leafy vegetables, enriched and whole grain products
Protein	Meat, fish, poultry, eggs, soy products, peanut, other legumes, tree nuts and seeds
Fat	Vegetable oils, margarine, avocado, meats, fish, poultry, peanut, tree nuts, seeds

* In countries where milk is fortified, read labels of alternative 'milk' products for degree of fortification. Fortified alternative beverages are not appropriate for infants and may not be safe and appropriate as a substitute for fluid milk for toddlers and young children. Please consider the overall nutrient intake and potential risks.
Reprinted with permission from Groetch and Nowak-Węgrzyn [3].

avoidance of other food allergens is more likely to result in inadequate nutrient intake and decreased growth [18, 19] (see table 3).

Exclusive breastfeeding is recommended for infants up to 4–6 months of age, at which time the gradual introduction of complementary solid foods should begin. Some infants with cow's milk allergy may require elimination of cow's milk from the maternal diet due to allergic symptoms. In this case, the maternal diet should be evaluated for adequate nutrient intact, most specifically calcium and vitamin D, and supplementing the maternal diet might be necessary. The World Allergy Organization's Diagnosis and Rationale for Action against Cow's Milk Allergy guidelines recommend continuing either breastfeeding (with maternal milk avoidance) or a substitute formula for all infants and toddlers up to 2 years of age with milk allergy [2] (see table 4). After 2 years of age, a dietary assessment and guidance to ensure adequate intake of all es-

sential micro- and macronutrients is recommended. In a population-based survey, children (age 31–37 months old) on milk-free diets had significantly lower intakes of energy, fat, protein, calcium, riboflavin and niacin [18]. When a milk substitute (either a soy formula or hydrolyzed formula) was included in the diet, the nutritional content improved significantly, although calcium and riboflavin intakes remained below the recommended levels. Micronutrient supplementation may be necessary to meet nutrient needs in this population.

Enriched alternative beverages are often used as milk substitutes for toddlers and older children. If tolerated, an enriched soy beverage can be a good substitute because it contains appropriate amounts of protein and adequate fats [3]. Other plant-based beverages such as rice, almond and potato 'milk' are very low in protein and fat and are not appropriate as a primary substitute for cow milk. In addition, an enriched rice

Table 4. Substitute formula recommendations for infants and toddlers with cow's milk allergy, as per the Diagnosis and Rationale for Action against Cow's Milk Allergy guidelines*

Food allergy disorder	First formula recommendation	Second formula recommendation	Third formula recommendation
Low risk of anaphylaxis	eHF-C	AAF	Soy
High risk of anaphylaxis	AAF	eHF-C	Soy
Non-IgE (FPIES or Proctocolitis)	eHF-C	AAF	–
Eosinophilic esophagitis	AAF	–	–

* Diagnosis and Rationale for Action against Cow's Milk Allergy guidelines should be interpreted with consideration for patient preference, individual clinical circumstance and cost.
FPIES = Food protein-induced enterocolitis syndrome; eHF-C = Hypoallergenic, extensively hydrolysed casein-based formula; AAF = Hypoallergenic amino acid-based formula; Soy = Soy-based formula.
Reprinted with permission from Groetch and Nowak-Węgrzyn [3].

beverage, when consumed in quantities similar to the average consumption of cow's milk (approximately 280 ml), presents the additional concern of increased exposure to daily dietary inorganic arsenic. The European Food Standards Agency advises against the substitution of breast milk, infant formula or cow's milk by rice beverages for toddlers and young children (up to 4.5 years of age) based on the poor nutritional quality and the concern for increased exposure to inorganic arsenic.

Young toddlers require 30–40% of their daily energy intake from fat. However, children on milk avoidance diets must eliminate common sources of fat such as full-fat yogurts, butter and cheeses as well as many manufactured and processed foods that contain milk as an ingredient. If dietary fats are not intentionally added, the resulting diet may be too low in fat, essential fatty acids and energy. Adding sufficient oil (e.g., milk-free margarine or vegetable oils such as olive, canola, soy, corn, safflower) to meet fat, essential fatty acid and energy needs is a practical suggestion. Adequate protein is another area of concern for individuals on a pediatric milk elimination diet. Young toddlers may be unable to eat or may not accept meat, fish, poultry, eggs, nuts, legumes and seeds, which are additional sources of protein in the diet. Protein intake in children should comprise 10–30% of the daily energy intake (5–20% in infants). In addition to an appropriate milk substitute, protein intake can be improved by incorporating a variety of small amounts of protein-rich foods in each meal and snack.

Grains

Whole and enriched grains are excellent sources of complex carbohydrates, vitamins (thiamin, niacin, riboflavin, vitamin B6), dietary fiber, iron and magnesium. In some countries, grains are also enriched with folic acid. Wheat is the most common grain allergy, with major allergens contained in the gluten fraction. Gluten is also found in rye, barley, spelt and their hybridized varieties. When wheat is eliminated, nutrient-dense alternative grains should be provided to substitute for the nutrients normally provided by wheat in the diet (see table 5 for suggestions). Gluten-free products are also wheat-free and may be useful on a wheat elimination diet when other wheat-free grains are tolerated. These products are more expensive, however, and may not be universally available, so the wheat-allergic population may benefit from advice and re-

Table 5. Alternative sources for nutrients in wheat

Nutrient	Alternative dietary sources
Niacin	Meat, poultry, tuna, salmon, liver, peanuts, seeds, legumes, enriched and whole grain alternative grain products
Thiamin	Liver, pork, other meats, sunflower seeds, enriched and whole grain alternative grain products, nuts and legumes
Riboflavin	Milk, dark green leafy vegetables, enriched and whole grain alternative grain products
Iron	Heme iron: Meat, fish, shellfish, poultry Non-heme irons*: Enriched and whole grain alternative grain products, legumes and dried fruits
Folic acid	Enriched and whole grain alternative grain products**, beef liver, spinach, legumes (especially lentils), avocado, orange juice
Carbohydrates	Fruits, vegetables, legumes and products made with alternative grains or flours such as rice, oat, corn, buckwheat, potato, tapioca, amaranth, millet, quinoa
Fiber	Fruits, vegetables, alternative whole grains

* Non-heme iron sources are better absorbed if consumed with a food that provides vitamin C. ** Product labels must be read, as policies regarding enrichment vary based on country of origin.
Reprinted with permission from Groetch and Nowak-Węgrzyn [3].

sources for on-line ordering or education regarding how to prepare wheat or gluten-free meals and snacks from 'scratch,' which would be less expensive.

Soy, Egg, Peanut, Tree Nut, Fish and Shellfish Allergies

Although these common food allergens in children are all nutrient-dense, they typically do not supply a large percentage of daily energy intakes. If the diet is diverse, the nutrients in these foods can easily be provided by other foods in the diet. Additional dietary constraints, such as a vegetarian diet, a picky or faddy eater or a diet restricted for religious reasons may make meeting nutritional needs more challenging. Avoidance of peanut and tree nuts is more challenging due to the ubiquitous presence of these foods in candy, chocolates and baked goods as well as the high allergenic potential for inducing severe reactions upon exposure to trace amounts of the foods.

Nutritional Impact of Specific Food-Allergic Disorders

In addition to the type of food that is avoided, the type of food-allergic disorder may influence the potential for nutritional risk. Table 6 highlights nutritional issues in AD, eosinophilic esophagitis, food protein-induced enterocolitis syndrome and allergic proctocolitis.

Feeding and Developmental Needs

Infants with food allergies have the same developmental needs associated with eating as all other infants. A healthy baby is born with the ability to coordinate sucking, breathing and swallowing and so can instinctively nurse or take a bottle. Other feeding skills are learned, and infants master foods of varying flavors and textures through practice. Thus, the gradual

Table 6. Nutritional issues of selected food allergy disorders

Disorder	Food allergy relevance	Nutritional risks	Management
Atopic dermatitis (AD)	About 35% of children with moderate-severe persistent AD have symptoms upon food ingestion. Elimination of the offending food can improve the AD symptoms.	Due to the chronic waxing/waning nature of AD, multiple foods may be unnecessarily eliminated by caregivers.	National Institute of Allergy and Infectious Diseases guidelines support the removal of suspected foods to identify potential triggers, followed by physician-supervised oral food challenge. Following a period of food avoidance (as soon as 2 weeks), acute symptoms may be elicited by foods that previously caused chronic eczema.
Eosinophilic esophagitis (EoE)	A subset of children and adults with EoE has food allergies.	Chronic emesis, abdominal pain, poor appetite, food refusal or other maladaptive feeding behaviors.	Whether and which foods are implicated in EoE are determined by documenting the resolution of EoE with specific food removal followed by a recurrence of disease when the specific food is reintroduced. As such, dietary management of EoE requires an elimination diet to determine trigger foods.
Food protein-induced proctocolitis	Typically begins in early infancy in response to milk or soy proteins either in the breast milk or infant formula.	Blood and mucous in the stool and possibly diarrhea appear benign without an accompanying growth delay or overt nutritional risk. These symptoms typically resolve within 48–72 hours after removal of the suspected antigen.	Nutritional risk is minimal because tolerance is typically acquired by 1 year of age and nutritional substitution in infancy is easily achieved. Infants can continue breastfeeding with maternal dietary elimination of the trigger food(s) or can be fed a hypoallergenic formula with maternal elimination of cow's milk. The maternal diet should be evaluated, and a safe alternative milk substitute or supplementation of calcium and vitamin D in the maternal diet may be required.
Food protein-induced enterocolitis syndrome (FPIES)	FPIES is often associated with milk proteins in infant formulas, with a potential risk of concomitant soy protein allergy reported in the U.S. FPIES to solid food proteins may also occur and has been reported most commonly in response to grains such as rice, oats, barley but also to chicken, turkey, egg white, green pea, peanut, sweet potato, white potato, fruit protein, fish, and mollusks (in adults).	FPIES usually begins prior to 6 months of age and is resolved by 3 years of age; children may be affected throughout the toddler years or longer. Children with FPIES exhibit gastrointestinal symptoms that include delayed, recurrent vomiting (100%) and diarrhea (25%). In infants with reactions to multiple foods, feeding refusal and difficulties are common.	FPIES differs from proctocolitis and IgE-mediated allergies in that the breastfed infant can typically continue nursing without maternal dietary avoidance of the allergen. Only rare cases of FPIES in exclusively breastfed infants have been reported. Infants with milk or soy FPIES have a greater chance of developing solid food FPIES, most commonly to rice and other grains. Introduction of fruits and vegetables is often recommended prior to grains, and these fruits and vegetables may not provide the iron and zinc needed in this age group (30). If supplemental substitute formulas are not in the diet, micronutrient supplementation may be required until the diet has greater diversity. In infants with reactions to multiple foods, feeding difficulties are common.

Box 3. Clinical vignette: feeding refusal

A 10-month-old infant had been breast-fed since birth without any formula or micronutrient supplementation. At the age of 5 months, he had two episodes of repetitive, forceful emesis within 2 hours following ingestion of rice cereal that was treated with intravenous rehydration in the emergency department. He had milder emesis episodes followed by diarrhea with the ingestion of oatmeal and sweet potato. He was given a presumptive diagnosis of food protein-induced enterocolitis syndrome and was referred for diagnostic oral food challenges. Following a negative skin prick test, his parents were advised to gradually add apples and butternut squash to his diet at home. His mother was reluctant to try these foods at home, so an office oral food challenge was done. During the challenge, he consistently refused the foods, pushing away the spoon and spitting up the contents. He also refused additional solids such as banana and pear. He was referred to a feeding specialist for evaluation, and elemental semi-solid food was recommended as an alternative to improve feeding skills and to provide an additional source of energy and micronutrients, specifically zinc. A multivitamin supplement was added to meet his vitamin D and iron needs.

Key message: Young, breast-fed infants with a history of reactions to solid foods and delayed introduction of solid foods to their diet may develop feeding difficulties. The food refusal may be related to past unpleasant experiences with solid food, and the problem can be compounded by parental apprehension about trying new foods because of past traumatic experiences. Counseling parents about strategies for enhancing feeding and oral skills is critical in these infants.

Reprinted with permission from Groetch and Nowak-Węgrzyn [3].

presentation of foods of various flavors and appropriate textures is required. It is best if feeding opportunities can be presented when developmentally appropriate, and there appear to be critical periods in infant development when chewing and taste acceptance are more easily learned. For instance, when textured foods are introduced after 10 months of age, children are more likely to refuse solid foods [22] [see Box 3, Clinical vignette: feeding refusal]. If necessary, a commercial, semi-solid, hypoallergenic food may be provided.

Feeding age-appropriate textures is more challenging for a child with food allergies due to food avoidance, and families will benefit from specific guidance regarding food introduction. An infant with milk or soy allergy may be introduced to a variety of flavors and textures through grains, fruits, vegetables, and meats in a skill-appropriate manner. Even an infant with a very limited diet can be provided a variety of textures with safe ingredients with a little creativity. For instance, a diet of only butternut squash can provide multi-

ple textures. It can be mixed with breast milk (or a safe substitute formula) into a smooth, thin or thick puree, mashed so that it is lumpy, or soft cooked and chopped so it provides an appropriate finger food texture.

Nutritional Issues in Adults with Food Allergy

Although we are more often concerned about the nutritional needs of children with food allergies, adults with food allergies would benefit from nutritional guidance as well. The most common allergens of adult IgE-mediated food allergy are peanut, tree nuts, fish, shellfish, fruits and vegetables [23]. Although peanuts, tree nuts and seafood contain concentrated nutrients, they can be omitted without nutritional consequence from an otherwise healthy diet. Systemic allergy to multiple fruits and vegetables is uncommon; it is more common for adults with hay fever to have pollen food allergy syndrome (PFAS), resulting in oropharyngeal symptoms to specific raw plant proteins. PFAS occurs in about 5–50% of patients with pollen allergies and is caused by structural homologies between raw plant proteins and pollen allergens. As these proteins are heat-labile and easily denatured upon exposure to initial digestion, symptoms are most commonly limited to the mouth and pharynx. Therefore, cooked versions of the fruits and vegetables are typically well tolerated, so it is not necessary to eliminate all raw fruits and vegetables. Of course, primary allergy to fruits and vegetables may also occur. Fruits and vegetables are important sources of beta-carotene, fiber, and phytonutrients and are the sole sources of vitamin C in the diet. There is one reported case of scurvy caused by vitamin C deficiency in an adult male patient who removed all fruits and vegetables due to PFAS [24].

Wheat allergy, although less common in adults, may manifest as food-dependent, exercise-induced anaphylaxis in adults [25, 26]. Avoidance of wheat will present the same nutritional consequences in adults, so instructions on when wheat should be avoided and when it can be safely included can be helpful. Safe alternative grain options should be discussed.

Milk avoidance in adults may result in calcium deficiency, so ensuring an appropriate calcium-fortified milk substitute or calcium supplementation is essential.

Adults are also not immune to poor dietary intake, picky eating or fad diets that limit nutrient intake or even specific foods such as wheat or casein in the belief that these foods are harmful. The nutritional content of any one diet is multifactorial, so an assessment is warranted to ensure that any elimination diet continues to provide adequate nutrition.

Summary

Dietary intervention is a crucial component of food allergy management but can negatively impact nutrient intake. A comprehensive nutrition assessment with appropriate intervention is warranted in all children with food allergies to meet nutrient needs and optimize growth. Nutrition assessment may also be indicated in food-allergic adults. Frequently, an elimination diet is absolutely necessary to prevent potentially life-threatening anaphylaxis, and allergen elimination can improve chronic symptoms, such as AD, when a food is proven to trigger symptoms. Allergen elimination goals are to prevent acute and chronic food-allergic reactions in the safest and least restrictive environment to supply a balanced diet that promotes health in children and adults.

References

1 Boyce JA, Assa'ad A, Burks AW, Jones SM, Sampson HA, Wood RA, Plaut M, Cooper SF, Fenton MJ, Arshad SH, et al: Guidelines for the diagnosis and management of food allergy in the United States: summary of the NIAID-sponsored expert panel report. Nutr Res 2011;31:61–75.

2 Fiocchi A, Schunemann HJ, Brozek J, Restani P, Beyer K, Troncone R, Martelli A, Terracciano L, Bahna SL, Rance F, et al: Diagnosis and Rationale for Action Against Cow's Milk Allergy (DRACMA): a summary report. J Allergy Clin Immunol 2010; 126:1119–1128.e12.

3 Groetch M, Nowak-Węgrzyn A: Practical approach to nutrition and dietary intervention in pediatric food allergy. Pediatr Allergy Immunol 2013;24:212–221.

4 Flinterman AE, Knulst AC, Meijer Y, Bruijnzeel-Koomen CA, Pasmans SG: Acute allergic reactions in children with AEDS after prolonged cow's milk elimination diets. Allergy 2006;61:370–374.

5 Leonard SA, Nowak-Węgrzyn A: Clinical diagnosis and management of food protein-induced enterocolitis syndrome. Curr Opin Pediatr 2012; 24:739–745.

6 Bock SA, Munoz-Furlong A, Sampson HA: Fatalities due to anaphylactic reactions to foods. J Allergy Clin Immunol 2001;107:191–193.
7 Ravid NL, Annunziato RA, Ambrose MA, Chuang K, Mullarkey C, Sicherer SH, Shemesh E, Cox AL: Mental health and quality-of-life concerns related to the burden of food allergy. Immunol Allergy Clin North Am 2012;32:83–95.
8 Pieretti MM, Chung D, Pacenza R, Slotkin T, Sicherer SH: Audit of manufactured products: use of allergen advisory labels and identification of labeling ambiguities. J Allergy Clin Immunol 2009;124:337–341.
9 Gendel SM: Comparison of international food allergen labeling regulations. Regul Toxicol Pharmacol 2012; 63:279–285.
10 National guidelines on management and labeling of allergens. http://www. foodallergens.info/Manufac? Guidelines (accessed May 2013).
11 Nowak-Węgrzyn A, Bloom KA, Sicherer SH, Shreffler WG, Noone S, Wanich N, Sampson HA: Tolerance to extensively heated milk in children with cow's milk allergy. J Allergy Clin Immunol 2008;122:342–347.e1–e2.
12 Lemon-Mule H, Sampson HA, Sicherer SH, Shreffler WG, Noone S, Nowak-Węgrzyn A: Immunologic changes in children with egg allergy ingesting extensively heated egg. J Allergy Clin Immunol 2008;122:977–983.e1.
13 Leonard SA, Martos G, Wang W, Nowak-Węgrzyn A, Berin MC: Oral immunotherapy induces local protective mechanisms in the gastrointestinal mucosa. J Allergy Clin Immunol 2012;129:1579–1587.e1.
14 Martos G, Lopez-Exposito I, Bencharitiwong R, Berin MC, Nowak-Węgrzyn A: Mechanisms underlying differential food allergy response to heated egg. J Allergy Clin Immunol 2011;127:990–997.e1–e2.
15 Kim JS, Nowak-Węgrzyn A, Sicherer SH, Noone S, Moshier EL, Sampson HA: Dietary baked milk accelerates the resolution of cow's milk allergy in children. J Allergy Clin Immunol 2011;128:125–131.e2.
16 Leonard SA, Sampson HA, Sicherer SH, Noone S, Moshier EL, Godbold J, Nowak-Węgrzyn A: Dietary baked egg accelerates resolution of egg allergy in children. J Allergy Clin Immunol 2012;130:473–480.e1.
17 Nowak-Węgrzyn A, Groetch M: Let them eat cake. Ann Allergy Asthma Immunol 2012;109:287–288.
18 Henriksen C, Eggesbo M, Halvorsen R, Botten G: Nutrient intake among two-year-old children on cows' milk-restricted diets. Acta Paediatr 2000; 89:272–278.
19 Christie L, Hine RJ, Parker JG, Burks W: Food allergies in children affect nutrient intake and growth. J Am Diet Assoc 2002;102:1648–1651.
20 Flammarion S, Santos C, Guimber D, Jouannic L, Thumerelle C, Gottrand F, Deschildre A: Diet and nutritional status of children with food allergies. Pediatr Allergy Immunol 2011;22: 161–165.
21 Isolauri E, Sutas Y, Salo MK, Isosomppi R, Kaila M: Elimination diet in cow's milk allergy: risk for impaired growth in young children. J Pediatr 1998;132:1004–1009.
22 Delaney AL, Arvedson JC: Development of swallowing and feeding: prenatal through first year of life. Dev Disabil Res Rev 2008;14:105–117.
23 Skypala I: Adverse food reactions – an emerging issue for adults. J Am Diet Assoc 2011;111:1877–1891.
24 Des Roches A, Paradis L, Paradis J, Singer S: Food allergy as a new risk factor for scurvy. Allergy 2006;61: 1487–1488.
25 Palosuo K: Update on wheat hypersensitivity. Curr Opin Allergy Clin Immunol 2003;3:205–209.
26 Perez-Rangel I, Gonzalo-Garijo MA, Perez-Calderon R, Zambonino MA, Corrales-Vargas SI: Wheat-dependent exercise-induced anaphylaxis in elderly patients. Ann Allergy Asthma Immunol 2013;110:121–123.

Assoc. Prof. Anna Nowak-Węgrzyn, MD
Jaffe Food Allergy Institute
Icahn School of Medicine at Mount Sinai
One Gustave L. Levy Place, Box 1198
New York, NY 10029 (USA)
E-Mail anna.nowak-wegrzyn@mssm.edu

Ebisawa M, Ballmer-Weber BK, Vieths S, Wood RA (eds): Food Allergy: Molecular Basis and Clinical Practice.
Chem Immunol Allergy. Basel, Karger, 2015, vol 101, pp 221–226 (DOI: 10.1159/000373907)

Food Allergy: Psychosocial Impact and Public Policy Implications

Hemant P. Sharma[a] · Linda J. Herbert[b]

[a]Department of Pediatrics, George Washington University School of Medicine, and Division of Allergy and
Immunology, Children's National Health System, Washington, D.C., [b]Division of Allergy and Immunology,
Center for Translational Science, Children's National Health System, Washington, D.C., USA

Abstract

Given its increasing prevalence and potential severity, food allergy not only negatively impacts the health and quality of life of affected individuals but also carries a significant economic burden. To address these problems, a community approach including efforts to increase awareness of food allergy among the general public and the implementation of appropriate public policies to keep affected individuals safe is required. This chapter reviews the general public's knowledge and perceptions of food allergy, the disease's psychosocial impact on affected individuals, and the current state and future directions of food allergy public policy. © 2015 S. Karger AG, Basel

Introduction

Food allergy is diagnosed in approximately 1–2% of adults and in 4–8% of children in the United States (U.S.), and comparable prevalence has been observed in other developed countries. Prevalence estimates for general food allergy and peanut allergy diagnosis in children have increased by 18% and 80%, respectively, in the past decade, indicating that a rising number of families are managing food allergies every year [1–3]. There is currently no cure for food allergy, so once an individual is diagnosed, it is necessary to completely avoid the allergen to prevent allergic reactions.

In adults and children, severe allergic reactions, such as anaphylaxis, have the potential to be life-threatening and are regularly treated. As many as 40% of children with food allergy have experienced a severe allergic reaction, and a 2007 review of the National Electronic Injury Surveillance System in the United States reported approximately 30,000 food-related anaphylactic events treated in emergency rooms, 2,000 hospitalizations, and 150 deaths [4, 5]. Thus, the economic impact of food allergy is great; treatment costs an estimated USD 225 million in direct costs and USD 115 million in indirect costs annually [6]. Furthermore, food allergy negatively impacts the quality of life of affected individuals. The health, economic, and quality of life burden of food allergy would be ameliorated if the frequency of unintended allergen exposure and severe allergic reactions were reduced. However, avoiding allergens is challenging due to the prevalence of bulk-manufactured foods, mislabeled ingredients, cross-contamination, and social activities involving food at school, work, restaurants and other public places [7].

Consequently, food allergy management is necessarily a team effort, requiring increased awareness and education of the public and various food industries about food allergies as well as support from the public to implement policies that will enable individuals with food allergy to safely manage their illness. This chapter reviews the general public's knowledge and perceptions of food allergy, the disease's impact on affected individuals, and the current state and future directions of food allergy public policy.

Food Allergy Knowledge and Attitudes

Surveys of food allergy knowledge and attitudes have been conducted among restaurants and reveal inconsistent food allergy knowledge. A minority of surveyed restaurant staff (<50%) receives food allergy training, and despite high confidence in their ability to provide safe meals to food-allergic patrons, many restaurant staff members have misconceptions regarding the impact of cooking an allergen, severity of ingesting minute portions of an allergen, and treatment of an allergic reaction [8, 9]. Indeed, up to 25% of unintentional allergen exposures occur in restaurants, indicating that food-allergic patrons are regularly exposed to allergens [9]. Despite this, restaurant staff members' interest in additional food allergy education is less robust (48–61%) than may be expected, highlighting the need for additional food allergy education [8, 9].

Research on the general public has demonstrated comparable findings regarding food allergy knowledge and attitudes toward public policy. Although individuals without food allergy tend to demonstrate an accurate understanding of the symptoms and severity of an allergic reaction, most do not know the difference between food allergy and food intolerance (49%) or how to treat food allergy (53%), and they report misconceptions about the impact that food allergy can have on quality of life [10, 11]. Furthermore, the data suggest dyssynchrony between the public's belief that policies should be in place to help families manage food allergy and their actual support for these policies. For example, many individuals believe that schools should have a policy to keep food-allergic children safe, yet they also oppose specific school policies such as banning peanuts and tree nuts [10]. Taken together, these data indicate that continued food allergy education of the general public is warranted.

Impact of Food Allergy on Daily Life

The need for public policy is not only a health and economic issue, but also a quality of life issue. Food allergy management is time-consuming and stressful, and it affects multiple domains of life. Food-allergic individuals and parents of food-allergic children must regularly read food labels; prepare meals that are allergen-free; monitor cross-contamination of utensils and cooking/serving dishes; educate restaurant staff, school personnel, and family/friends; plan/prepare for allergen avoidance during air travel and vacations; carry auto-injectable epinephrine; and be knowledgeable about nonfood items that may contain allergens such as vaccines, medications, cosmetics, and toys (e.g., modeling dough, finger paints) [12]. This complex medical regimen may decrease the health-related quality of life of the children, parents, and adults affected by food allergy.

Indeed, studies suggest that food-allergic individuals and their families experience elevated anxiety and distress as well as decreased quality of life. Many parents of food-allergic children report distress regarding the social limitations that result from their children's food allergies [13]. Some parents report that preparations for activities outside of the home are so time-consuming and stressful that they do not participate in these events at all [13, 14]. Additionally, there is some evidence that specific markers of disease severity influence quality of life; parents of food-allergic children who have experienced a severe allergic reaction and/or have multiple food allergies tend to report worse quality of life than parents of peers who have not experienced a severe allergic reaction and who have fewer food allergies [15, 16]. Similarly, among college-age adults with food allergies, a perceived history of anaphylaxis was related to more general anxiety [17]. Food-allergic children also perceive a significant impact on quality of life, potentially even more than that reported by their parents [18].

In addition to general quality of life concerns, preliminary research suggests that children with food allergy are bullied by peers in school. Surveys of over 500 food-allergic children and adults suggest that 24–32% of all food-allergic individuals have experienced food allergy-related bullying or teasing, mostly at school by classmates, and some have even experienced a classmate taunting them with an allergen [19, 20]. Children who were bullied and their parents reported decreased quality of life, even after accounting for the severity of their illness [19]. Collectively, research suggests that public policies that make it easier for food-allergic individuals and their families to safely engage in food allergy management have the potential to vastly improve quality of life.

Current Food Allergy-Related Public Policy

The need for food allergy-related public policy is evidenced by the poor knowledge of the general public regarding food allergy, as well as the health and quality of life impact of the disease. In addition, food-allergic reactions often occur in public places, such as restaurants and schools, further underscoring the need for public policy regarding allergen avoidance and reaction management.

In a registry of individuals with peanut and tree nut allergies, up to 25% of unintentional allergic reactions occurred in restaurants [21]. The implementation of food allergy guidelines in food establishments is variable. In a 2007 survey of 100 restaurant personnel in 100 New York establishments, 58% reported having a plan in place for allergic reactions, and 62% had a plan to provide safe meals [9]. In the U.S., at least two states, Massachusetts and Rhode Island, have adopted laws to make dining at restaurants safer for individuals with a food allergy. In Massachusetts, the law requires the display of a food allergy poster, a food allergy notice on menus, and presence of a trained and certified food protection manager on the restaurant staff [22]. Restaurants in New York City and St. Paul, Minnesota are also required to display food allergy posters [22], and other states are pursuing similar legislation. The U.S. Food and Drug Administration also revised the Food Code in 2009, stating in Section 2-102.11 that food establishments should have a designated employee who is knowledgeable about food allergens, cross-contamination, and reaction symptoms and who is responsible for the food allergy safety training of other employees [23]. The Food Code is used by states and local jurisdictions to regulate food establishments; however, no state has yet adopted the 2009 Code.

In addition to restaurant regulations, public policy has addressed labeling of food allergens. For example, the U.S. Food Allergen Labeling and Consumer Protection Act took effect in 2006 and requires that the labels of foods containing eight major food allergens (milk, egg, fish, shellfish, peanut, tree nuts, wheat, and soy) declare the allergen in plain language [22]. Similar legislation exists in other countries, but there are significant global differences in labeling requirements. For example, mustard, celery, and sesame seed are considered to be allergens for food labeling purposes in the European Union, but not in the U.S. In Australia and New Zealand, the Food Standards Code mandates the labeling of the eight major allergens, as well as sesame seed, but not mustard or celery [24]. In Canada, recent amendments went into effect in 2012, requiring the additional labeling of gluten sources, mustard, and sulfites [25]. Meanwhile, Japan has a different list of allergenic foods that must be declared on food labels [24], and it is the only country to date to forbid precautionary or 'may contain' labels, which are widespread in other countries such as the U.S. and may significantly limit the number of foods that food-allergic individuals may safely ingest.

Public policy has also been directed toward food allergy management in schools. Almost 20% of allergic reactions among children with food allergy occur at school [26], and in a case series of food allergy fatalities among school-aged children, 9 of 32 deaths occurred in school, and most were associated with delayed administration of epinephrine [27]. In 2006, Ontario, Canada, became the first jurisdiction to enact a law (Sabrina's Law) requiring schools to develop policies for the management of students with life-threatening allergies [28]. In the U.S., the Food Allergy and Anaphylaxis Management Act, enacted in 2011, calls for voluntary national guidelines to help schools manage students affected by food allergy and anaphylaxis [22]. In addition to this federal legislation, 15 U.S. states to date have published school food allergy management guidelines [22]. Given that most food allergy fatalities in schools are associated with delayed epinephrine administration, public policy has also focused on access to epinephrine. Almost all U.S. states have passed laws allowing students, with consent, to carry their prescribed epinephrine at school [22]. By early 2013, 12 U.S. states have also passed laws allowing schools to stock 'undesig-

nated' or nonstudent-specific epinephrine autoinjectors [22]. One rationale for such laws is the observation that up to 25% of epinephrine administrations in schools involve students or staff without a previous food allergy diagnosis [29]. Advocacy for federal legislation that would encourage other U.S. states to adopt similar undesignated epinephrine laws is on-going.

Although few studies have evaluated food-allergic reactions during air travel, reports exist of allergic reactions to peanut while in-flight [30]. A recent international survey found that 349 in-flight peanut/tree nut reactions were reported among 3,273 respondents from 11 countries [30]. Policy regarding food allergy management during air travel varies among airline carriers and countries. In the U.S., the management of food-allergic passengers is at each airline's individual discretion. Meanwhile, the Canadian Transportation Agency required Air Canada (but not other Canadian carriers), upon advance request, to implement peanut/tree nut-free buffer zones around allergic passengers [30].

In sum, current policy regarding food allergy management in restaurants, schools, and other public places varies considerably between countries and states within the U.S.

Implications and Future Directions

Food allergies are increasingly prevalent in developed countries and have the potential to be life-threatening. The risks associated with food allergy could be lessened if the general public had adequate knowledge of the condition; however, research to date suggests the general public has knowledge gaps, for example, related to the definition of food allergy and appropriate treatment of reactions. These knowledge deficits have also been observed among food service workers, which is perhaps even more worrisome. Therefore, additional food allergy education is warranted for both the general public and target groups who regularly work with food-allergic individuals. Based on available data, electronic or online education would be the preferred mode of delivery, and on-going research is needed to evaluate the effectiveness of education at improving food allergy-related knowledge, attitudes and behaviors.

Research has also demonstrated that individuals with food allergy may experience impaired quality of life through elevated anxiety, stress, or social isolation. Among children with food allergy, bullying has recently been shown to be prevalent and can negatively impact quality of life. More investigation regarding the effect of food allergy on psychosocial well-being, with the goal of developing and evaluating interventions, is needed.

Various countries have begun to implement policies to ensure the safety of individuals with food allergy in public places, such as schools, restaurants, and airplanes. However, studies are needed to evaluate whether these policies modify attitudes and behaviors, reduce the frequency of food-allergic reactions, and improve quality of life. As the prevalence of food allergy continues to rise, the need to address these education, research, and policy domains will likely be even more pronounced.

References

1 Branum AM, Lukacs SL: Food allergy among U.S. children: trends in prevalence and hospitalizations. NCHS Data Brief 2008;10:1–8.
2 Sicherer SH, Sampson HA: Peanut allergy: emerging concepts and approaches for an apparent epidemic. J Allergy Clin Immunol 2007;120:491–503.
3 Rona RJ, Keil T, Summers C, et al: The prevalence of food allergy: a meta-analysis. J Allergy Clin Immunol 2007;120: 638–646.
4 Gupta RS, Springston EE, Warrier MR, et al: The prevalence, severity, and distribution of childhood food allergy in the United States. Pediatrics 2011;128: e9–e17.
5 Ross MP, Ferguson M, Street D, et al: Analysis of food-allergic and anaphylactic events in the National Electronic Injury Surveillance System. J Allergy Clin Immunol 2008;121:166–171.
6 Patel DA, Holdford DA, Edwards E, et al: Estimating the economic burden of food-induced allergic reactions and anaphylaxis in the United States. J Allergy Clin Immunol 2011;128:110–115.e5.
7 Mandell D, Curtis R, Gold M, et al: Anaphylaxis: how do you live with it? Health Soc Work 2005;30:325–335.
8 Bailey S, Albardiaz R, Frew AJ, et al: Restaurant staff's knowledge of anaphylaxis and dietary care of people with allergies. Clin Exp Allergy 2011;41:713–717.
9 Ahuja R, Sicherer SH: Food-allergy management from the perspective of restaurant and food establishment personnel. Ann Allergy Asthma Immunol 2007;98:344–348.
10 Gupta RS, Kim JS, Springston EE, et al: Food allergy knowledge, attitudes, and beliefs in the United States. Ann Allergy Asthma Immunol 2009;103:43–50.
11 Gupta RS, Kim JS, Barnathan JA, et al: Food allergy knowledge, attitudes and beliefs: focus groups of parents, physicians and the general public. BMC Pediatr 2008;8:36.
12 Kim JS, Sicherer SH: Living with food allergy: allergen avoidance. Pediatr Clin North Am 2011;58:459–470, xi.
13 Springston EE, Smith B, Shulruff J, et al: Variations in quality of life among caregivers of food allergic children. Ann Allergy Asthma Immunol 2010;105:287–294.
14 Bollinger ME, Dahlquist LM, Mudd K, et al: The impact of food allergy on the daily activities of children and their families. Ann Allergy Asthma Immunol 2006;96:415–421.
15 Gupta RS, Springston EE, Kim JS, et al: Food allergy knowledge, attitudes, and beliefs of primary care physicians. Pediatrics 2010;125:126–132.
16 Wassenberg J, Cochard MM, Dunngalvin A, et al: Parent perceived quality of life is age-dependent in children with food allergy. Pediatr Allergy Immunol 2012;23:412–419.
17 Herbert LJ, Dahlquist LM: Perceived history of anaphylaxis and parental overprotection, autonomy, anxiety, and depression in food allergic young adults. J Clin Psychol Med Settings 2008;15: 261–269.
18 van der Velde JL, Flokstra-de Blok BM, Dunngalvin A, et al: Parents report better health-related quality of life for their food-allergic children than children themselves. Clin Exp Allergy 2011;41: 1431–1439.
19 Shemesh E, Annunziato RA, Ambrose MA, et al: Child and parental reports of bullying in a consecutive sample of children with food allergy. Pediatrics 2013; 131:e10–e17.
20 Lieberman JA, Weiss C, Furlong TJ, et al: Bullying among pediatric patients with food allergy. Ann Allergy Asthma Immunol 2010;105:282–286.
21 Sicherer SH, Furlong TJ, Munoz-Furlong A, et al: A voluntary registry for peanut and tree nut allergy: characteristics of the first 5,149 registrants. J Allergy Clin Immunol 2001;108:128–132.
22 FARE: Advocacy, laws and regulations. 2013. www.foodallergy.org/advocacy (accessed March 15, 2013).
23 U.S. Food and Drug Administration: FDA food code. 2009. www.fda.gov/ Food/GuidanceRegulation/Retail FoodProtection/FoodCode (accessed March 15, 2013).

24 Lennard L: Comparison of allergen legislation globally. http://www.allergenbureau.net/resources/legislation (accessed March 15, 2013).
25 Health Canada: Food allergen labeling. 2012. http://www.hc-sc.gc.ca/fn-an/label-etiquet/allergen/index-eng.php (accessed March 15, 2013).
26 Sicherer SH, Mahr T: Management of food allergy in the school setting. Pediatrics 2010;126:1232–1239.
27 Sampson HA, Mendelson L, Rosen JP: Fatal and near-fatal anaphylactic reactions to food in children and adolescents. N Engl J Med 1992;327:380–384.
28 Anaphylaxis Canada: Sabrina's law. www.anaphylaxis.ca/en/resources/sabrinas_law.html (accessed March 15, 2013).
29 Sicherer SH, Furlong TJ, DeSimone J, et al: The US Peanut and Tree Nut Allergy Registry: characteristics of reactions in schools and day care. J Pediatr 2001;138:560–565.
30 Greenhawt M, MacGillivray F, Batty G, et al: International study of risk-mitigating factors and in-flight allergic reactions to peanut and tree nut. J Allergy Clin Immunol Pract 2013;1:186–194.

Hemant P. Sharma, MD, MHS
Division of Allergy and Immunology
Children's National Health System
111 Michigan Avenue, NW, Washington, DC 20010 (USA)
E-Mail hsharma@childrensnational.org

Sharma · Herbert

Ebisawa M, Ballmer-Weber BK, Vieths S, Wood RA (eds): Food Allergy: Molecular Basis and Clinical Practice.
Chem Immunol Allergy. Basel, Karger, 2015, vol 101, pp 227–234 (DOI: 10.1159/000373910)

Worldwide Food Allergy Labeling and Detection of Allergens in Processed Foods

Steve L. Taylor · Joseph L. Baumert

Food Allergy Research and Resource Program, University of Nebraska, Lincoln, Nebr., USA

Abstract

The labeling of allergenic foods is an important public health measure to assist food-allergic consumers in avoiding foods that can cause allergic reactions. The regulatory framework for such labeling depends upon the selection of priority allergenic foods, which vary among countries. Most countries include milk, eggs, fish, crustacean shellfish, peanuts, tree nuts, soybeans, and cereal sources of gluten on the priority allergenic foods list, as recommended by the Codex Alimentarius Commission. However, a variety of other foods appear on the priority lists of some countries but not on others. Sesame seeds, molluscan shellfish, buckwheat, and mustard are identified in two or more countries. In most countries, all ingredients derived from these priority allergen sources must also be declared on labels by source. However, exemptions exist for some ingredients in some countries but not in others. Detection methods are critical for the enforcement of allergen labeling regulations and for the investigation of allergic reactions in the community by public health officials. The development of detection methods has advanced considerably over the past several decades and will be briefly reviewed in this chapter. Because of the emphasis on labeling and the development of detection methods, the ingredient statement on packaged food labels now contains more information than ever before to assist food-allergic consumers. © 2015 S. Karger AG, Basel

Introduction

IgE-mediated food allergies are recognized as an important worldwide public health issue. The prevalence of food allergies and the identity of the most common allergenic foods differ between countries, and avoidance diets remain the primary approach to the prevention of reactions. The ingredient statement on the label of packaged foods is a key source of information for allergic consumers wishing to avoid specific allergenic foods. However, many of the most serious allergic reactions occur in restaurants and other foodservice establishments, where full-label disclosure of ingredients is typically not practiced.

Methods for the detection of allergenic food residues are needed for the regulatory enforcement of labeling regulations. In this chapter, we will review worldwide labeling approaches and briefly comment on detection methods that can be used to enforce those regulations.

Labeling of Allergenic Foods

An excellent and thorough review of worldwide labeling regulations was recently published and is highly recommended as an additional resource [1]. Many countries have implemented laws, regulations or standards for food allergen labeling. These measures typically focus on a list of priority allergenic foods. The foods on such lists vary around the world, leading to key differences in labeling laws and regulations.

Historically, many countries had general food labeling laws and regulations that served to protect food-allergic consumers. These general food labeling laws and regulations required that ingredients deliberately used in the formulations of the foods should be declared on an ingredient list on the package label. However, many exemptions and exceptions existed. The declaration of the sources of some ingredients was not required, and other ingredients were declared using technical terms, e.g. casein, which did not directly reveal the true source. Thus, food-allergic consumers found that allergens were often 'hidden' in packaged food products. Furthermore, they had to learn to identify ingredient terms, such as casein, that indicated the presence of specific allergenic foods.

More clarity in the labeling of allergenic foods began to emerge with guidance from the Codex Alimentarius Commission (CAC), an organization formed jointly by the Food and Agricultural Organization (FAO) and the World Health Organization to develop food standards and guidelines that would be recognized worldwide. The CAC first turned its attention to the labeling of food allergens in 1993 when a working paper on food allergens was developed by the Nordic countries. A FAO Technical Consultation was formed in 1995 and led to the development of a list of priority allergenic foods (table 1) that were adopted by the CAC in 1999. The CAC list of priority allergenic foods serves as guidance to all countries, but individual countries have the option to adopt this list or to modify the list as they might choose.

Since one of us (SLT) was a member of the original 1995 FAO consultation, several comments are appropriate regarding the approaches used by the assembled experts to develop the priority list of allergenic foods that was ultimately adopted by the CAC. In 1995, the level of published information regarding the comparative prevalence of allergies to specific foods was rather limited, largely due to pediatric populations of allergic individuals. Data on adults and on the prevalence of specific food allergies in the general population were lacking. Accordingly, expert judgment was used, in part, to develop the priority list adopted by the CAC in 1999. The main criterion used by the expert panel was comparative prevalence, although the differential severity of certain allergenic foods was also recognized. On this basis, milk, egg, fish, crustacean shellfish, peanut, soybean, tree nuts, and cereal grain sources of gluten were considered priority allergens. The FAO group also considered celiac disease, intolerances, and sensitivity reactions, in addition to IgE-mediated food allergies. Thus, gluten was included because of its association with celiac disease, and sulfites were included because of the documented severity of sulfite-induced asthma.

Subsequently, an International Life Sciences Institute-Europe Task Force on Food Allergy took a more in-depth look at foods that merited placement on the priority allergenic foods list [2]. The criteria used by this group included clinical evidence of an allergic reaction through double-blind, placebo-controlled food challenge and published evidence of severe and/or fatal anaphylactic reactions. Data on prevalence were considered insufficient. This task force determined that the priority list should include milk, egg, fish, crustacean shellfish, peanut, soy, tree nuts, wheat,

Table 1. Priority allergenic food lists

	Codex Alimentarius Commission	U.S.	EU	Canada	Australia/ New Zealand	Japan	Korea
Milk	X	X	X	X	X	X	X
Eggs	X	X	X	X	X	X	X
Peanut	X	X	X	X	X	X	X
Gluten	X		X	X	X		
Wheat	X	X	X	X	X	X[a]	X[b]
Crustacea	X	X	X	X	X	X[a]	X[b]
Fish	X	X	X	X	X		X[b]
Soybean	X	X	X	X	X		X
Tree nuts	X	X	X	X	X		
Sesame seed			X	X	X		
Molluscs			X	X			
Mustard			X	X			
Celery			X				
Lupine			X				
Buckwheat						X	X
Other						X[a]	X[b]

[a] Japan: Shrimp and crab are the only Crustacea on the list. Grains include wheat and buckwheat but not other cereal sources of gluten. Other includes foods that are on a recommended but not required labeling list including salmon, salmon roe, mackerel, abalone, squid, beef, pork, chicken, soybean, orange, kiwi, banana, peach, apple, yam, gelatin, matsutake mushroom and walnut.

[b] Korea: Shrimp and crab are the only Crustacea on the list. Grains include wheat and buckwheat but not other cereal sources of gluten. Other includes peach, pork and tomato.

and sesame seed. Several subsequent groups within International Life Sciences Institute-Europe have continued to develop criteria for the selection of allergenic foods of public health significance [3, 4]. The criteria have since been expanded to include prevalence, severity and potency.

The increase in awareness of the public health significance of food allergies began to occur on a worldwide basis at the same time when CAC was considering the adoption of the priority list of allergenic foods. The priority list released by the CAC in 1999 has been adopted by numerous countries and, as noted in table 1, those 8 foods or food groups are represented on the vast majority of the priority food allergen lists that are recognized by specific countries. However, several countries decided to include additional foods in their priority allergen lists. As thoroughly re-

viewed elsewhere [1], the regulatory framework for the labeling of allergenic foods differs from country to country. The basis for the inclusion of additional foods on the priority lists for specific countries has not been clearly delineated in most cases, and the role of scientific criteria in these judgments appears to be secondary in many cases. Although the World Trade Organization Agreement on the Application of Sanitary and Phytosanitary Measures recognizes the 1999 CAC list, the existence of different priority lists in various parts of the world can lead to trade disputes and consumer confusion.

The first priority list of allergenic foods for the EU was established by the European Parliament and the Council through Directive 2003/89. This list was apparently created from the deliberations of the EU Parliament, but the criteria for inclusion of foods on the list were not clearly stated. In addition to the 8 foods or food groups from the CAC list, this initial EU list included sesame seed, mustard, and celery. Subsequently, the EU priority list of allergenic foods was updated with the release of the European Parliament and the Council through Directive 2007/68. At that time, molluscan shellfish and lupine were added to the EU list of priority allergenic foods. The European Commission apparently used the opinion of the European Food Safety Authority (EFSA) Scientific Panel on Dietetic Products, Nutrition, and Allergies on molluscan shellfish and lupine allergies to reach this decision [5, 6]. For lupine, the decision appeared to be based upon the recognition that some peanut-allergic individuals will experience allergic reactions upon ingestion of lupine.

The U.S. Congress passed the Food Allergen Labeling and Consumer Protection Act (FALCPA) in 2004. FALCPA established a list of priority allergenic foods (table 1) that was quite similar to the 1999 CAC list. The only exception was that FALCPA specifically identified wheat as a cause of food allergies and did not recognize other grain sources of gluten.

In Canada, the original priority allergen list included molluscan shellfish and sesame seeds, in addition to the 8 foods or food groups on the 1999 CAC list. More recently, Canada has added mustard to its list. In Australia and New Zealand, the priority list (table 1) has been stable since its inception but includes sesame seeds as an addition to the 1999 CAC list.

Japan has a rather unique approach to its priority list, with a short mandatory labeling list and a longer recommended labeling list. The mandatory priority list is comprised of wheat, milk, eggs, peanut, buckwheat, and crustacean shellfish (table 1), and crab and shrimp are identified as the only crustacean shellfish of concern. Japan and Korea are the only countries that list buckwheat on their priority allergen lists. Buckwheat is known to cause frequent and occasionally severe allergies in Japan [7]. The recommended priority list in Japan is extensive and includes several molluscan shellfish (abalone, squid), several fish (mackerel, salmon, and salmon roe), several fruits (orange, kiwi, peach, apple, banana), one tree nut (walnut), several meats (pork, chicken, beef), soybean, matsutake mushroom, yam, and gelatin. The basis for the Japanese priority list was a survey of allergy clinics in Japan, where the causative foods of over 1,500 cases of food allergy were compared [8].

As previously noted, many countries simply refer to the 1999 CAC list in their food labeling regulations. However, a few countries (Argentina, Switzerland, Ukraine) have adopted the EU regulatory framework instead [1].

The 1999 CAC priority list includes several food groups – tree nuts, fish and crustacean shellfish. In most countries, fish is used to include all species of finfish. As noted, in Japan, only mackerel and salmon are included on the recommended priority list for allergenic foods. Similarly, most countries include all species of shrimp, crab and lobster among the crustacean shellfish. In Japan, only crab and shrimp are included on the mandatory priority list for allergen labeling, and in several countries, including Canada, the labeling regulations refer only to shellfish and not specifically to crustacean shellfish or molluscan shellfish.

Greater differences occur among various countries in the recognition of various tree nuts as part of the group covered by the allergen labeling regulations. In Europe, the tree nuts group includes walnuts, pecans, cashews, pistachios, almonds, hazelnuts, Brazil nuts, and macadamia nuts. In Canada, these same 8 nuts are listed along with pine nuts. However, the U.S. Congress did not identify specific tree nuts that required mandatory labeling under the provisions of FALCPA. Subsequently, the U.S. Food and Drug Administration drafted a guidance document in October of 2006 that included a very long list of 19 tree nuts that would need to be specifically included on U.S. food labels. Unfortunately, this list includes several foods that are not tree nuts – coconut and litchi.

Ingredient Labeling and Exemptions

The wording of most regulatory approaches indicates that the food and any ingredients derived from those foods must be declared on the ingredient statements of packaged foods. Ingredients derived from allergenic sources vary widely with respect to the amount of protein (allergens) from the allergenic source [9]. Some such ingredients, including casein, whey, and gluten, contain substantial amounts of protein from the allergenic source. A few ingredients, such as fish gelatin, contain substantial protein from the allergenic source, but the protein fraction in the ingredient does not include much of the major allergen from the source [10]. Other ingredients from priority allergenic sources contain low to moderate levels of protein from the source. For example, food-grade lactose may contain as much as 1% milk protein; however, the amount of protein in lactose will depend upon the method of manufacture of this ingredient. Lactose with 1% milk protein likely has sufficient milk allergens to provoke allergic reactions. Still, other ingredients from priority allergenic sources contain no detectable protein or very low levels of detectable proteins. The best examples are highly refined oils from soybeans and peanuts. Other examples include soy lecithin, wheat starch, and several milk-derived flavors (butter oil, butter ester, butter acid, starter distillate).

In a few countries, selected ingredients are exempted from source labeling. The U.S. Congress exempted highly refined oils when it passed FALCPA. The U.S. also set up a regulatory process under FALCPA where food ingredient manufacturers could petition for source labeling exemptions. Recently, the use of specific soy lecithin ingredients manufactured by Solae, LLC (a division of DuPont) as a processing aid for use as a stick-release agent in bakeries has been granted the first source labeling exemption in the U.S. In the EU, the initial directive included an opportunity for companies to petition for source labeling exemptions for specific ingredients derived from the priority allergens. The petitions were evaluated by the EFSA Panel of Dietetic Products, Nutrition and Allergies. Ultimately, based upon the recommendation of the EFSA Panel, several ingredients were exempted from source labeling requirements, although some were exempted only for specific uses (table 2). While the EU appears to have the most source labeling exemptions, the EU does not have a continuing process to seek further exemptions in a manner similar to that of the U.S. Australia and New Zealand have considered the necessity of labeling the fish origin of isinglass, an ingredient used in the clarification of alcoholic beverages, including wines. Isinglass is comprised of collagen derived from fish swim bladders and contains little detectable parvalbumin, the major fish allergen; it is therefore exempt from source labeling in the EU [11]. Currently, Australia and New Zealand are also not requiring the declaration of isinglass on labels of alcoholic beverages.

Advisory Labeling

The existing regulatory frameworks in various countries focus on intentionally added ingredients. However, residues of allergenic foods may also occur adventitiously as the result of common food industry practices, such as the use of shared equipment. Such practices can, on occasion, lead to potentially hazardous levels of allergenic residues. Increasingly, food companies in many countries (U.S., EU, Canada, Australia, New Zealand) are voluntarily providing consumers with advisory labeling statements to alert them to products that are at risk of contamination. Advisory labeling is not required in any country, but it is allowed for voluntary use by food companies in many countries. Many forms of advisory labeling are used worldwide. Some countries mandate certain forms of advisory labeling, while other countries allow the use of a variety of different

Table 2. Ingredients with source-labeling exemption in the EU

Wheat-based glucose syrups, including dextrose, and any products derived from such ingredients.   Wheat-based maltodextrins and any products derived from such ingredients.   Glucose syrups based on barley.   Cereals used for making distillated or ethyl alcohol of agricultural origin for spirit drinks and other alcoholic beverages.
Fish gelatin used as a carrier for vitamin or carotenoid preparations.   Fish gelatin or isinglass used as a fining agent in beer and wine.
Fully refined soybean oil and fat and any products derived from such ingredients.   Natural mixed tocopherols (E306), natural D-alpha tocopherol, natural D-alpha tocopherol acetate, natural D-alpha tocopherol succinate from soybean sources.   Vegetable oils derived from phytosterols and phytosterol esters from soybean sources.   Plant stanol esters produced from vegetable oil sterols from soybean sources.
Whey used for making distillates or ethyl alcohol of agricultural origin for spirit drinks and other alcoholic beverages.   Lactitol.
Nuts used for making distillates or ethyl alcohol of agricultural origin for spirit drinks and other alcoholic beverages.

Adapted from: European Commission. Directive 2007/68/EC, Official Journal of 28 November 2007, L 310, pp 11–14.

forms. For example, Canada uses 'may contain x', while the U.K. uses 'not suitable for x allergy sufferers'. In the U.S., no standard form exists for advisory labeling, but three different formats predominate: (a) 'may contain x', (b) 'manufactured on shared equipment with x' and (c) 'manufactured in shared facility with x'. Many companies who use such advisory labeling do so judiciously and only after assessing the potential risk. For these companies, there will always be some risk of an allergic reaction occurring in a consumer who ignores such labeling. In contrast, other companies appear to use advisory labeling more broadly, even in cases where the risk is virtually nonexistent. Overall, allergic consumers should never be advised to ignore advisory statements on package labels. Physicians should advise food-allergic patients to avoid products with advisory labeling statements because many such products represent an appreciable risk to such consumers.

In Australia, the Allergen Bureau of Australia was voluntarily formed by the food industry in an attempt to curtail the widespread use of advisory labeling. As a result, the Allergen Bureau developed the Voluntary Incidental Trace Allergen Labeling (VITAL) program. Products at potential risk for allergen cross contact from the use of shared equipment or other practices are analyzed to determine the concentration levels of detectable allergen residues. These concentrations are used together with estimated consumption levels for the specific product in a VITAL Calculator (available on-line) to determine the estimated dose of allergenic protein that could be consumed. These doses are then compared to the Reference Doses that have been developed from clinical data on the distribution of individual threshold doses for individuals with specific food allergies. If the estimated consumption dose exceeds the Reference Dose, then advisory labeling is recommended. However, if the estimated consumption dose is below the Reference Dose, then advisory labeling is discouraged. The VITAL program can be reviewed at the website of the Allergen Bureau (www.allergenbureau.net/vital/vital).

Detection of Food Allergen Residues

The increased awareness of the public health implications of food allergies during the 1990s resulted in a need to develop analytical methods to detect residues of allergenic foods to allow enforcement of the labeling regulations described earlier in this chapter. Accordingly, many analytical methods have been developed over the past 20 years [12, 13]. This chapter will include a brief review of quantitative and qualitative immunoassay methods that detect proteins or allergens from food and are the most widely used methods by the food industry and public health authorities. However, polymerase chain reaction methods that detect DNA in food are also used, especially in cases where immunoassays are not available. Furthermore, mass spectrometry methods to detect protein residues are being intensively investigated but have not yet become widely used.

Quantitative Immunoassay Methods

The major quantitative method for the detection of food allergen residues is the enzyme-linked immunosorbent assay (ELISA), which has been widely commercialized. ELISAs allow a quantitative determination of the concentration of allergenic proteins in food products. ELISAs most typically use polyclonal antisera produced against a specific protein (e.g. casein) or a food extract (e.g. peanut). In the case of gluten, monoclonal antibodies are available and used in commercial kits. Commercial ELISA kits have been developed for most of the priority allergenic foods discussed previously, with the exceptions of fish and a few tree nuts (i.e. pecan, pistachio, macadamia nut, pine nut). These assays are highly specific, except in the case of very closely related foods, e.g. pecan would interfere with walnut detection, and pistachio would interfere with cashew detection. ELISAs are also quite sensitive and able to detect residues at low ppm concentrations (µg/g). ELISAs have several disadvantages.

The extraction of the protein residues can be altered by processing, especially by heat processing in dry systems, e.g. baking and deep-fat frying. In most cases, ELISAs detect intact proteins from food and are unable to detect hydrolyzed proteins, which are widespread food ingredients and can retain some allergenicity if incomplete hydrolysis is accomplished. In a few cases, competitive ELISAs have been developed to detect hydrolyzed proteins from specific foods. The only commercial competitive ELISA is for partially hydrolyzed gluten.

Qualitative Immunoassay Methods

Immunoassay methods can also be designed into qualitative lateral flow strips (LFSs), also known as lateral flow immunochromatographic assays or dipsticks. LFSs are widely used by the food industry to assess the cleanliness of shared processing equipment after sanitation. LFSs contain zones where antibodies are affixed to the solid matrix. Swab samples of equipment surfaces are wicked onto the strip and produce visible lines where antigen-antibody interactions occur. LFSs are inexpensive, rapid, and portable, and they do not require instrumentation and are extremely simple to perform. LFSs are specific and sensitive, but the results are qualitative; the usual detection limits are in the range of 5 ppm. Consequently, commercial LFSs are now widely used within the food industry and are available for a wide variety of priority allergenic foods.

Conclusion

A regulatory framework has been developed for labeling of allergenic foods in many parts of the world over the past 15 years. Labeling laws and regulations vary considerably among the various countries of the world, although most countries require the declaration of milk, eggs, fish, crustacean shellfish, peanuts, soybeans, tree nuts, and cereal grain sources of gluten on packaged food products. Additional foods are included on priority lists in various parts of the world. No consistent basis has been developed for generating priority allergen lists, and thus, these lists do not appear to be based solely on a sound scientific basis. Even with the use of scientific information, opinions and actions could differ due to variable weighting of the importance of factors such as prevalence, severity and potency. The worldwide situation is made more complex by the variability in the implementation of requirements to use source labeling for ingredients derived from foods on the priority allergen lists. Some countries provide opportunities for exemptions from source labeling requirements for specific ingredients, and these exemptions are not consistent between countries. However, most countries do use scientific information to reach decisions regarding source labeling exemptions. For the allergic consumer, the widespread use of unregulated advisory labeling also complicates their ability to interpret the risk for specific packaged food products.

Several methods exist for the detection of residues of allergenic foods, allowing public health officials to enforce labeling regulations. These methods can also provide food companies with data on allergen concentrations that are essential to risk assessment and decisions on the voluntary use of advisory labeling options. ELISA methods are currently favored for the analysis of allergen residues because they are specific for the detection of proteins from the allergenic source, sufficiently sensitive to protect allergic consumers, and available in rugged formats that allow quick determination of residue levels within food manufacturing facilities.

References

1   Gendel SM: Comparison of international food allergen labeling regulations. Regul Toxicol Pharmacol 2012;63:279–285.
2   Bousquet J, Bjorksten B, Bruijnzeel-Koomen CA, Huggett A, Ortolani C, Warner JO, Smith M: Scientific criteria and the selection of allergenic foods for product labelling. Allergy 1998;53:3–21.
3   Björkstén B, Crevel R, Hischenhuber C, Lovik M, Samuels F, Strobel S, Taylor S, Wal J-M, Ward R: Criteria for identifying allergenic foods of public health importance. Regul Toxicol Pharmacol 2008;51:42–52.
4   van Bilsen JHM, Ronsmans S, Crevel RWR, Rona RJ, Przyrembel H, Penninks AH, Contor L, Houben GF: Evaluation of scientific criteria for identifying allergenic foods of public health importance. Regul Toxicol Pharmacol 2011;60:281–289.

5   European Food Safety Authority: Opinion of the scientific panel on dietetic products, nutrition and allergies on a request from the commission related to the evaluation of molluscs for labelling purposes. EFSA J 2006;327:1–25.
6   Scientific Panel on Dietetic Products, Nutrition and Allergies: Opinion of the scientific panel on dietetic products, nutrition and allergies on a request from the commission related to the evaluation of lupin for labelling purposes. EFSA J 2005;302:1–11.
7   Akiyama H, Imai T, Ebisawa M: Japan food allergen labeling regulation–history and evaluation. Adv Food Nutr Res 2011;62:139–171.
8   Ebisawa M, Ikematsu K, Imai T, Tachimoto H: Food allergy in Japan. Allergy Clin Immunol Int 2003;15:214–217.
9   Taylor SL, Hefle SL: Hidden triggers of adverse reactions to food. Can J Allergy Clin Immunol 2000;5:106–110.

10 Koppelman SJ, Nordlee JA, Lee PW, Happe RP, Hessing M, Norland R, Manning T, Deschene R, De Jong GA, Taylor SL: Parvalbumin in fish skin-derived gelatin: is there a risk for fish allergic consumers? Food Addit Contam Part A Chem Anal Control Expo Risk Assess 2012;29:1347–1355.
11 Weber P, Steinhart H, Paschke A: Competitive indirect ELISA for the determination of parvalbumins from various fish species in food grade fish gelatins and isinglass with parv-19 anti-parvalbumin antibodies. J Agric Food Chem 2009;57:11328–11334.
12 Hengel AJV, Anklam E, Taylor SL, Hefle SL: Analysis of food allergens. Practical applications; in Yolanda P (ed): Food Toxicants Analysis. Amsterdam, Elsevier, 2007, pp 189–229.
13 Poms RE, Klein CL, Anklam E: Methods for allergen analysis in food: a review. Food Addit Contam 2004;21:1–31.

Prof. Steve L. Taylor, PhD
Food Allergy Research and Resource Program, University of Nebraska
1625 Arbor Drive
Lincoln, NE 68583–0919 (USA)
E-Mail staylor2@unl.edu

Ebisawa M, Ballmer-Weber BK, Vieths S, Wood RA (eds): Food Allergy: Molecular Basis and Clinical Practice.
Chem Immunol Allergy. Basel, Karger, 2015, vol 101, pp 235–252 (DOI: 10.1159/000375106)

The Effects of Food Allergy on Quality of Life

Audrey DunnGalvin[a, b] · A.E.J. Dubois[c] · B.M.J. Flokstra-de Blok[d] · J.O'B. Hourihane[a]

[a]Department of Paediatrics and Child Health and [b]School of Applied Psychology, University College Cork,
Cork, Ireland; Departments of [c]Paediatric Pulmonology and Paediatric Allergy and [d]General Practice,
University Medical Center Groningen, University of Groningen, Groningen, The Netherlands

Abstract

The majority of research on food allergy has been biomedical in orientation, focusing on issues such as the molecular structure of allergens, or aimed at methods of diagnosis. In the last decade, there has been a growing interest in the development of questionnaires that measure the impact of food allergy on health-related quality of life (HRQL). These studies have provided insight into the everyday burden of living with food allergy and have suggested ways that HRQL can be improved. The EuroPrevall project (europrevall@bbsrc.ac.uk) has given great impetus to research in the area of HRQL. In addition to clinical research on the prevalence, mechanisms and causes of food allergy, research output in the area of psycho-social impact has included HRQL measures for all age groups and examination of the socio-economic impact of food allergy. In this chapter, we review the literature on the impact of food allergy on children, teens and their parents; the majority of this data was generated over the life of the EuroPrevall project. We then examine both quantitative and qualitative research findings to provide an in-depth picture of the impact of food allergy on the concerns and everyday lives of children, teens, adults and parents. Research on factors that are related to and impact HRQL is also discussed. There is a strong emphasis throughout the chapter on developmental considerations of food allergy, spanning from infants to adults. We conclude by discussing methodological issues in relation to the measurement of HRQL in relation to food allergy. We offer some recommendations for future research and practice on HRQL so that HRQL measures can reach their full potential in research, practice and policy, with the help of the findings in this review. Overall, the findings suggest that food allergy has a strong impact on HRQL in terms of social, dietary, and psychological factors. 'Rules' and restrictions ostensibly apply to food, but because food is such an integral part of everyday life, these restrictions extend far beyond 'mealtimes'. Therefore, social events are experienced differently and have a different meaning for those living with food allergy, giving rise to feelings of exclusion and difference when compared to those without allergy. Children, teens, and parents need to cope with normal developmental changes as well as with the food allergy, placing them under increased psycho-social stress and leading to adverse effects on HRQL and coping. To address and attempt to alleviate such stressors, both quantitative and qualitative research suggests that targeting uncertainty should be a major goal for health professionals working with children, teens and families with a food allergy. Remarkable similarities in response to food allergy across countries suggest that policies and programmes that address quality of life issues may be relevant to many different populations. An in-depth understanding of the relationship between a diagnosis of food allergy and HRQL, as well as the factors that impact it, will ultimately lead to the promotion of earlier, more effective preventive strategies and interventions that are focused on maximising optimal health development and quality of life. © 2015 S. Karger AG, Basel

Introduction

The growing prevalence of allergic diseases present an increasing challenge for populations and health care systems around the world, and food allergies constitute a notable part of this increase [1–4]. The most common food allergens are peanuts, tree nuts, seafood, eggs, and milk; however, the list is constantly growing [5]. Therefore, food allergy, as a disease burden throughout the world, is becoming a growing public health problem. Food allergy, particularly to peanuts, is the most common cause of anaphylaxis outside hospitals [6], yet other common food causes, such as shellfish, fish, milk, soy, wheat, and eggs, also exist [7]. These foods may not only cause fatal or near-fatal reactions, but they also tend to induce 'persistent sensitivity' in most patients.

Promising new emerging therapies for food allergy, such as oral immunotherapy, may be available in the future [8]. However, the current hallmark of therapy continues to be education of patients and caregivers about avoidance of potential food allergens, early recognition of allergic symptoms, medication for IgE-mediated skin symptoms and early management of anaphylaxis. Anticipatory guidance measures include reading food ingredient labels, concern for cross-contamination, vigilance in a variety of social activities,

and immediate access to an auto-injector [9]. However, avoidance is complicated by the fact that peanuts, nuts, and soy can be found in many foods (e.g. breads, muffins, pastries, biscuits, cereals, soups, ice creams, seasoning, and sauces) and in different forms, such as emulsifiers or thickening agents. Although, the life-threatening nature of anaphylaxis makes prevention the cornerstone of therapy, it also has implications for the health-related quality of life (HRQL) of children, teens, adults and children living with food allergy [10–20].

The conception of health as a dynamic, multi-factor phenomenon that influences physical, psychological, and social functioning has changed the way the impact of any disease is measured. It is now recognised that it is essential to include outcome measures that reflect the patient perspective for evidenced-based decision-making in clinical practice. Perception of HRQL is influenced by the individuality and subjectivity of experience and response, and it may depend on many factors, such as age, gender, context, and culture [21]. Therefore, physiological measures often correlate poorly with functional capacity and well-being [22], and patients with the same clinical criteria often have dramatically different responses. It has become increasingly important, therefore, for researchers and healthcare professionals to understand how the perceptions, experience, and impact of a chronic disease might influence a patient's interpretation and response to it so that we, in turn, can respond more appropriately. Furthermore, involving children as well as adults and parents in research is important because children are increasingly acknowledged to have rights in the determination of medical decisions that affect them [23]. This has encouraged research to be undertaken with children themselves to understand their own views on the impact of a disease on their experiences and relationships.

Although a growing number of families must live and cope with food allergy on a day-to-day basis, it is only in recent years that the socio-emotional impact of food allergy on children, teens, adults and parents has been researched in depth. The EuroPrevall project (europrevall@bbsrc.ac.uk) has given great impetus to research in the area of HRQL. In addition to clinical research on the prevalence, mechanisms and causes of food allergy, research output in the area of psycho-social impact has included HRQL measures for all age groups and examination of the socio-economic impact of food allergy.

HRQL is measured by two major types of instruments, generic and disease-specific. Generic HRQL instruments are not specific to any particular disease and are therefore useful for comparing HRQL across different conditions, whereas disease-specific questionnaires focus on issues pertinent to one disease. However, generic instruments are necessarily more 'general' and therefore less sensitive to the particular problems associated with a particular condition. Disease-specific HRQL questionnaires, which provide an in-depth picture of the day-to-day concerns of patients, are an increasingly important outcome measure, particularly in the context of chronic diseases. They are also capable of capturing small changes in HRQL that may occur as a result of clinical or therapeutic treatment.

Several disease-specific measures have been developed to assess quality of life in children and teens under the aegis of EuroPrevall, including The Food Allergy Quality of Life Questionnaire – Parent Form (FAQLQ-PF; parent-administered for children aged 0–12 years); the Food Allergy Quality of Life Questionnaire – Child/Teen Forms (FAQLQ-CF and FAQLQ-TF, respectively; self-administered to children and teens aged 8–17 years) and the Food Allergy Quality of Life Questionnaire – Adult Form (FAQLQ-AF; ages 18+).

The FAQLQ-PF, FAQLQ-CF, FAQLQ-TF, and FAQLQ-AF were developed and validated in 5 stages: (1) item generation using focus groups containing both children, teens, and parents, expert opinion and literature review; (2) item reduction, using clinical impact and factor analysis; (3) the evaluation of internal and test-retest reliability and construct validity; (4) evaluation of cross-cultural and content validity; and (5) longitudinal validity over several time points [10–20].

HRQL instruments capture the experience and impact of food allergy; however, the manner in which this experience is managed everyday must also be evaluated [24]. Coping has been shown to be related to patient HRQL, and it mediates health behaviour as well as health care utilisation [25], having both short- and long-term impacts. Children with any chronic condition have twice the risk of developing mental health disorders compared to healthy children, even without an accompanying physical disability [26]. Therefore, efforts have increasingly been made to assess coping of children and adolescents with chronic conditions.

In addition to collecting quantitative HRQL data, there is a need to qualitatively explore patients' experiences of what it is like to live with a chronic condition in order to better understand the decisions people make about coping and managing their condition. In the context of research in children, qualitative research also provides an opportunity to tap into the richness of children's thoughts and feelings about themselves, their environments and the world in which they live.

For example, compliance with medical direction is determined, in part, by the person's individual perception of the condition and its management. Although quantitative studies provide consistent, replicable results that can be compared across populations and that are vital to providing reliable and valid outcome data, there are also inherent complexities in studying the experience of living with a disease in the dynamic, interactional process within the family. Lay perceptions of risk may seem irrational to some clinicians but have their own logic and validity from the perspective of those living and coping with food allergy. Qualitative studies were also carried out under EuroPrevall, both in the initial focus groups put in place to generate items for the questionnaires and independently thereafter [27–29].

In this chapter, we review the literature on the impact of food allergy on children, teens and their parents, the majority of which was generated over the life of the EuroPrevall project. We then examine both the quantitative and qualitative research findings to provide an in-depth picture of the impact of food allergy on the everyday lives of children, teens, adults and parents. Research on factors that are related to and impact HRQL is discussed. There is a strong emphasis throughout this chapter on the developmental considerations of food allergy, spanning from infants to adults. We conclude by discussing the methodological issues in relation to the measurement of HRQL due to food allergy. We offer some recommendations for future research and practice on HRQL based on the findings in this review.

Main Body

The Parental Perspective: Quantitative
The impact of a chronic illness on family members varies greatly between families, but it is clear that the family plays a pivotal role in determining how children with chronic conditions adapt to their condition and in how it impacts upon their HRQL [30]. It is generally accepted that children with chronic conditions potentially have lower HRQL because of the additional demands and stressors placed on the children by their condition [31]. In the case of food allergy, like many other chronic conditions, parental HRQL may be affected by the child's diagnosis, as families have to deal with the day-to-day management and emotional strain of the illness, as well as additional costs in terms of time, money and disruption to everyday household routines [32]. Furthermore, parents have valuable insight into the impact of food allergy on the everyday lives of the children.

Therefore, in order to improve care and support for both parents and children, it is necessary to identify and understand the parents' concerns.

The first validated HRQL food allergy-specific measure, the Food Allergy Quality of Life-Parental Burden questionnaire [32], measures the parental burden associated with having a child with a food allergy. Scores in the food-allergic cohort were significantly lower for general health perception, parental distress and worry, and interruptions and limitations in usual family activities, compared to healthy controls.

The FAQLQ-PF is the first disease-specific questionnaire to be published from the EuroPrevall project [10]. The questionnaire is completed by parents on behalf of their children, and to ensure that the measure is developmentally appropriate, it caters to three age groups; 0–3 years (14 items), 4–6 years (26 items) and 7–12 years (30 items). The core questionnaire has 3 sub-scales, which are calculated as the mean of each scale (table 1).

The subscales measure *Food anxiety*, *Social and dietary limitations* and *General emotional impact*; and the total score is calculated as the mean of the 3 subscales. Supplementary sections contain questions on clinical and demographic variables such as parental concern for their child's emotional and physical health, stress levels experienced by the parents and family and the impact on family activities, and expectation of outcome following accidental ingestion of an allergen. The FAQLQ-PF has demonstrated very high reliability and validity (cross-sectional, cross-cultural, longitudinal) [10–14].

In the course of the development and validation of the FAQLQ-PF [10–12], we found a strong impact of food allergy on HRQL in relation to many psycho-social aspects of children's everyday lives. For example, in the initial focus groups put in place to generate items for the FAQLQ-PF, parents suggested that the anxiety associated with the risk of a potential reaction had more profound effects on emotional and so-

General emotional impact	Questions measure psychological phenomena such as feeling different from other children, frustration, control and generalised anxiety stemming from food allergy; my child feels different from other children because of food allergy.
Food anxiety	Questions measure anxiety relating to food; my child is afraid to try unfamiliar foods because of food allergy.
Social and dietary limitations	Questions measure everyday dietary and social restrictions; my child's ability to take part in pre/school events involving food (class parties, treats, lunchtime) is limited by food allergy.

Three factors (general emotional impact; food anxiety; social and dietary limitations) emerged following exploratory and confirmatory factor analysis of the development and validation of the Food Allergy Quality of Life Questionnaire; Parent Form (FAQLQ-PF). Reprinted from DunnGalvin et al. [12].

cial aspects of a child's everyday life than clinical reactivity induced by food intake. The importance of a subscale assessing this aspect of anxiety was subsequently confirmed using clinical impact and factor analytic methodologies. Children were also found to be 'generally anxious', according to the parents; that is, they had anxiety associated with food that was often 'generalised' to non-food situations.

During the longitudinal validation of the FAQLQ-PF [14], we discovered that a food challenge might alleviate anxiety. In our design, we administered the FAQLQ-PF to parents of children 0–12 years before the child underwent a clinically-indicated food challenge, and at 2 months and 6 months post food challenge. Eighty-two children underwent a challenge (42 positive; 40 negative). Although significant differences were found between the positive and negative groups on all subscales and in the total scores at 6 months [F (2, 59) = 6.221, p < 0.003], we found that HRQL significantly improved at the post-challenge time points (all p < 0.05) for both the positive and negative groups. A possible explanation for the improvement in the 'positive' groups (which had long been suspected, but never documented) concerns the impact of uncertainty on the perception of HRQL. 'Living with uncertainty' appears as a

central theme for all age groups with food allergy, including parents [27–29], and will be discussed further throughout this chapter.

Our findings suggest that a food challenge (open or double-blind) may be valuable, not only as an essential diagnostic tool, but as a therapeutic tool. In effect, by providing a sense of certainty, a food challenge may have a positive impact on HRQL, irrespective of outcome. This positive impact may be reinforced by specialist consultation, personalised information and interaction with other children with a food allergy, and other published research on uncertainty regarding chronic disease strengthens this argument [33].

Tracking the impact of food allergy begins at the earliest possible time in the developmental pathway from childhood to adulthood. Findings from the EuroPrevall birth cohort study demonstrated that the impact of a diagnosis of food allergy began early and could be detected over the course of 1 year (unpublished). Iceland (n = 60), the UK (n = 45), Germany (n = 40), Spain (n = 36), the Netherlands (n = 95) and Italy (n = 25) administered the FAQLQ-PF before the infant was diagnosed with food allergy by double-blind, placebo-controlled food challenge and 12 months later. On average, 60% of the infants tested positive for an allergy to at least one food type. We found a similar pattern of responses across countries.

Overall, there were significant differences ($p < 0.05$) between the positive/negative groups over 12 months. In this age group, the subscale measuring *food anxiety* showed the biggest increase in burden, from baseline to 12 months for the positive group. Even at this very young age, it appears that children are reluctant or afraid to try new foods and that they have a lack of variety in their diets. Children's ability to fully take in social events is also adversely impacted, compared to the negative group. Such responses may be due to a projection of parent anxiety, although this in itself is likely to have a profound impact on the children's own perception. We found similar results using the FAQLQ-PF in the US [34].

It is important to also take into account factors related to HRQL that may provide a deeper understanding of the impact and outcomes of a diagnosis of food allergy.

To this end, the FAQLQ-PF was used to examine specific psychological factors that may influence parents' decisions to take part in clinical studies [35]. Parents of food-allergic children in the US were offered investigational oral immunotherapy in a regular outpatient clinic. Forty parents (Group A) declined, and 25 parents (Group B) agreed to take part. Both groups completed the FAQLQ-PF.

Our results showed that parents who perceive that their child is at high risk of dying from food allergy are more likely to enrol their child in an investigational trial in which the child will be given peanut immunotherapy (OR 6.75; CI 3.45–9.73). This is in spite of the fact that the experimental therapy is intensive and has attendant adverse risks such as induction of anaphylaxis, compared to routine clinical practice. The association was independent of the severity of symptoms, experience of anaphylaxis and perception of the impact of food allergy on HRQL. Socio-economic status was not a significant factor.

These findings may be explained by parental concern to avoid potentially life-threatening consequences of accidental ingestion in the often 'uncontrolled' environment of their child's everyday life. This perceived level of threat may be an important factor motivating parents to consent to their children taking part in investigational therapies in a 'controlled' environment, even though this involves a protocol in which reactions are more likely than not to occur in the trial. These findings concur with research on the context of chronic disease [36], which shows that determinants of parental authorisation for involvement of new-born infants in clinical trials include perceptions of risk and benefit to the child.

Age and gender also influence the perception of HRQL. In the course of the development and validation of the FAQLQ-PF, multivariate analysis showed an interaction between sex and age group for *general emotional impact* on HRQL scores [14]. In effect, parents of boys reported higher mean total scores up to the age of 6 years, while parents of girls reported higher mean scores for the 6–12 year age group, particularly for the subscales '*general emotional impact*' and '*food anxiety*'. In addition, boys had higher scores in the 'social and dietary limitations' subscale at all ages.

More recently, we used a time series, case-control design (2 months before challenge, at challenge, 2 months and 6 months following challenge) to investigate if HRQL, as measured by the FAQLQ-PF subscales, changed over time, at what point it changed, and age and gender differences. Furthermore, we investigated the impact of factors related to HRQL and their association with the overall scores of the FAQLQ-PF.

Our research sample consisted of 2 groups of children that differed on a clinical disease-related criterion: a positive (n = 25) and a negative (n = 29) result of a food challenge. Baseline analysis showed that our sample was broadly typical in terms of suspected allergen, reported symptoms and food avoided and in terms of the scores showing a mean HRQL impact, similar to that reported previously in the Irish and US clinic populations [10–20].

Many children live with food allergy for an extended period of time before a diagnosis is confirmed or refuted. It is estimated that 21% of individuals perceive that they, or their child, have a food allergy, compared to the 6% actual prevalence in children [5]. There were no significant differences in scores between the groups at 2 months before challenge and on the day of the challenge, which suggests that the impact of food allergy does not differ between children whose parents perceive that they have food allergy and those who are confirmed as allergic to a particular food.

We found that *food anxiety* and *general emotional impact* showed the least decrease in burden at the 6-month time point for the positive groups, while *social and dietary restrictions* shows the highest decrease in impact. For the negative groups, *general emotional impact* showed the least decrease in impact on HRQL. This suggests that the impact that the emotional 'rules' necessitated by 'being safe' [27–29] may be more difficult to remediate, since they may have a more permanent neural basis, compared to social or dietary restrictions.

Regarding only the positive group, the burden of food allergy, having eased between the *at challenge* to the 2-month time points, again demonstrates an increase in adverse impact at the 6-month time point. This finding is important in several respects. First, it pinpoints the time when both parents and children may need further support on issues such as diet, auto-injectors, risk management, anxiety, and changing developmental and practical challenges. Second, combined with the finding of a strong association with and a significant increase in the impact of variables related to HRQL, it provides a broader view on outcomes. These variables include parental concern over child's physical and emotional well-being, the impact of food allergy on family activities, the *expectation of outcome* [10–20] if a child accidentally ingests an allergen, the level of reassurance given by owning an auto-injector and the level of parental stress. We found, with regards to the level of reassurance provided by owning an auto-injector pen, a significant adverse impact on HRQL occurring sometime between the 2-month to 6-month time points. There is clear consensus in the research literature that auto-injectors are under-used by patients of all ages [6], including parents. The reasons for this have yet to be fully explored.

Attention to subscales, in addition to the overall score for HRQL, is important in order to provide a comprehensive evaluation. For example, we found the strongest burden for *food anxiety* in the 3–6-year age group. Further, we found that females were impacted more negatively in terms of *general emotional impact* compared to males. On the *social and dietary limitations* subscale, the 3–6-year age group again had the highest reported burden, with males being more impacted. *General emotional impact* was highest for the 6–12-year age group, irrespective of gender [34]. We have also consistently found differences between age groups, reinforcing the notion of tracking development in order to accurately assess HRQL at any one point or over time. For example, *general emotional impact* (feeling different, feeling frustrated, and generalised anxiety) has a stronger negative impact in older children. At this point, individual children will have different responses, from strong anxiety to risky behaviour, contributing to the overall score on the subscale. This developmental period corresponds to a broadening of social activities and autonomy. A comparative analysis of subscales may suggest subtle differences in HRQL over time, which may then be targeted for intervention.

The Child, Adolescent and Adult Perspective: Quantitative

In 2009, the first disease-specific HRQL questionnaire for children with food allergy became available. This Food Allergy Quality of Life Questionnaire – Child Form (FAQLQ-CF was demonstrated to be reliable, valid and easy to use in children aged 8–12 years [12]. Because quality of life focuses on the perception of the patients, the questionnaires are usually completed by the patients themselves; this also holds for children. Although the understanding of HRQL is determined by the age, maturity and cognitive development of a child, it has been reported that children 8 years and older are able to understand questions about their HRQL and to give reliable and valid answers [12]. It is, of course, important to take the level of development of the child into account when developing a HRQL questionnaire for children. Therefore, food-allergic children were included in the development phase of FAQLQ-CF. Response categories of the FAQLQ-CF are illustrated by faces (smileys), which is more appropriate for the cognitive development of the child.

The FAQLQ-CF is complementary to the FAQLQ-PF (parent form) because the FAQLQ-PF is completed by the parents of the food-allergic child. Thus, the FAQLQ-PF measures the quality of life of the child according to the parent (proxy-reported). It is known from the literature that children and their parents may differ in their views on and judgments of quality of life [12]. On the other hand, it is obvious that one can only make use of proxy-reported HRQL measures in young children [10]. Recently, the FAQLQ-CF and FAQLQ-PF were simultaneously completed in a sample of 74 food-allergic children (aged 8–12 years) and their parents. It was found that parents reported significantly less impact of food allergy on the quality of life of their child than the children themselves. However, perceived disease severity, as measured with the Food Allergy Independent Measure [15], was comparable for the children and their parents. This may indicate that the parents underestimate the negative impact food allergy has on the quality of life of their child [16].

In addition to the FAQLQ-CF, two other disease-specific HRQL questionnaires have been developed for adolescents (13–17 years) and adults (18 years and older) with food allergy. These questionnaires are also self-completed and have been shown to be reliable and valid instruments for measuring HRQL in food-allergic adolescents and adults, respectively [5, 6]. Research on the longitudinal validation of the FAQLQ-CF, FAQLQ-TF and FAQLQ-AF is underway, but the preliminary results are promising [17].

When looking at food-allergic adolescents, a moderate agreement was found in the impact reported by the adolescents themselves and by their parents. Disagreement was mainly associated with the perceptions and characteristics of the adolescent rather than the perceptions and characteristics of the parent [18]. Therefore, in order to gain as complete a picture as possible of the impact of food allergy on the HRQL of children and teens and to identify areas of disagreement, the proxy forms and self-completed forms should be used together.

In addition to the disease-specific HRQL questionnaires, it is also possible to measure HRQL using generic questionnaires. The advantage of using generic HRQL questionnaires is that they can be used to compare HRQL of different diseases and of the general population [18]. When comparing HRQL of food-allergic children (aged 8–12 years), adolescents (aged 13–17 years) and adults (18 years and older) with age-appropriate samples of the general population, it was found that food-allergic children and adolescents reported fewer limitations in school work or activities with friends due to behavioural problems than children and adolescents from the general population. However, adolescents and adults reported more limitations due to pain, a more impaired perception of overall health, more limitations in social activities and a lower degree of vitality and liveliness than adolescents and adults of the general population. Overall, it was found that generic HRQL of the food-allergic patients was poorer than patients with diabetes mellitus but better than patients with rheumatic arthritis, asthma or irritable bowel syndrome [18]. On the other hand, the disadvantage of generic questionnaires is that they may not adequately focus on HRQL impairments specific for a particular disease [18]. In a recent study, HRQL was measured using the disease-specific questionnaires FAQLQ-CF, FAQLQ-TF and FAQLQ-AF and the generic questionnaires Child Health Questionnaire-Child Form 87 and RAND-36 in the same group of food-allergic patients. The generic questionnaires showed remarkable ceiling effects (percentage of patients giving the maximum score) in a number of domains, whereas the disease-specific questionnaires showed minimal floor or ceiling effects. In addition, the percentage of agreement in identifying the same food-allergic patients with the best or worst HRQL, as measured with the generic and disease-specific questionnaire, was low. Although generic HRQL questionnaires are necessary for comparing the HRQL between different diseases, the disease-specific HRQL questionnaires are important to measure clinically important differences and impairments in HRQL in food-allergic patients [19].

The FAQLQ-AF has been translated and validated in the US and in a number of European countries. In the US, an online version of the FAQLQ-AF was used instead of the conventional paper version. The online version was found to be feasible, consistent and valid in the US. Moreover, when comparing the HRQL scores of US food-allergic patients to those of a comparable sample of Dutch food-allergic patients, a greater impairment in HRQL was found for the US food-allergic patients. As epinephrine auto-injector prescription rates differed remarkably between the two patient groups (but the severity of the reported symptoms were quite similar), prescription of epinephrine auto-injectors and its effect on HRQL are important targets for further research [20]. Another study compared HRQL of food-al-

lergic adults, as measured with the FAQLQ-AF, in seven European countries: Iceland, the Netherlands, Poland, France, Spain, Italy and Greece. The food-allergic adults were recruited through the EuroPrevall project (community survey and outpatient clinic survey). The FAQLQ-AF was shown to be valid and consistent in these European countries, and the HRQL scores were comparable between the seven studied European countries [21]. Also, the FAQLQ-CF has been translated in a number of European countries as part of the EuroPrevall project, but the results on validity and outcomes have not yet been published. In Switzerland, a French version of the FAQLQ-CF has been used to investigate the effect of a didactic game for food-allergic children on HRQL, and a significant improvement in HRQL was found [22, 23].

HRQL instruments are a powerful method for capturing the impact of a diagnosis of food allergy from the patient perspective. However, qualitative methods can be used to explore substantive areas in which little is known or to gain a novel understanding of a particular area. In addition, qualitative methods can be used to obtain intricate details about phenomena such as feelings, thought processes, and emotions that are difficult to extract or learn about through conventional research methods such as quantitative measures. Next, we used the patient's own voices to explore what it is like to live with food allergy in order to better understand the decisions they make regarding management of their condition.

Qualitative Studies on the Impact of Food Allergy on Health-Related Quality of Life

Experience and coping with any chronic disease is an intricate pattern of 'facts' and 'feelings' that are interwoven into a child's developmental pathway from birth to adulthood [27–29]. Coping has not only been shown to be related to patient HRQL, but it also mediates health behaviour (e.g. compliance) and has short- and long-term impacts [26].

We have previously discussed [27] an integrated developmental framework to explain the onset, development and maintenance of food allergy-related cognition, emotions and behaviour. Sixty-two children/teenagers aged 6–15 years took part in 15 age-appropriate focus groups; 52% of the children were female. The parents were also interviewed. All children were physician-diagnosed with IgE-mediated food allergy and had been issued an anapen/epipen. Through qualitative enquiry, a framework for evaluating children with food allergy was developed. Developmentally appropriate techniques, such as vignettes (where children could comment on characters in the third person) and activity books, were designed to stimulate discussion, maintain interest, and minimise threat to the child's self-esteem.

Analyses of the data encompassed precipitating events (stressful events in the children's lives caused by food allergy-related factors), psychological impact (cognitive appraisal and emotional effects) and behavioural consequences or coping strategies. Our findings indicated that experience and coping with food allergy is complex and dynamic, comprising a series of interactive processes (both age-, gender-, and disease-specific) that are embedded in a child's developmental path.

The developmental model is illustrated in figure 1.

Subsequently, we also analysed data from focus groups and interviews held in *Australia (n = 60), the UK (n = 72), Italy (n = 54), Singapore (n = 20), and the US (n = 45)*. The themes that emerged from other countries were strikingly similar to our previous research on the impact of *living with uncertainty*, with *difference,* and with *rules* and the coping strategies that are used (fig. 1). The findings [29] are discussed below using the voices of parents, children, teens and young adults.

The Parent Perspective

The potential impact of food allergy on children's social and emotional impact is a concern for parents in terms of the following:

- Identity:

'*he asked me "when will I be normal" and I was shocked, I didn't realise he felt like that*' (Mother of Jack, age 7, Ireland).

- Confidence:

'*you know, she has to put so much more thought into every social occasion that she's aware of in advance which I think takes away from her confidence*' (Mother of Donna, age 15, Ireland).

- Social integration:

'*it's harder for them the older they get, they just want to fit in with their friends…Danny used to get bullied and now he's very conscious of his allergy…I worry about him and how he's going to cope when he goes to secondary school*' (Mother of Danny, age 10, Ireland).

Children's growing autonomy presents parents with particular challenges;

'*he has alot of new friends now and I worry…but he gives out to me if I mention it when they come over…he's embarrassed about it*' (Father of Peter, age 12, Ireland).
'*If he's gone out for a drink and they've been eating and, you know, like curry, there could be curries, there could be satay and, you know, he's drunk and doesn't know what he's eating, that's my concern – would he be able to look after himself then and give himself an injection*' (Mother of Shane age 19, UK).

A lack of awareness, across a wide range of public settings, negatively impacts both the parents' and children's enjoyment of social occasions.

'*I've had pretty negative experiences, some very negative practice, you know, as soon as they hear they'll say "well it's best if she doesn't eat anything" or "we don't really want to serve her anything", or "the kitchen's too small and there's stuff everywhere*' (Mother of Jenny, age 8, UK).
'*…and they brought a piece of nice fish that had been fried in olive oil and she assured us the fish were fried in olive oil and nothing else in the oil. And when the chips came she started eating them, there was a peanut sitting right in the middle of the chips, so it*

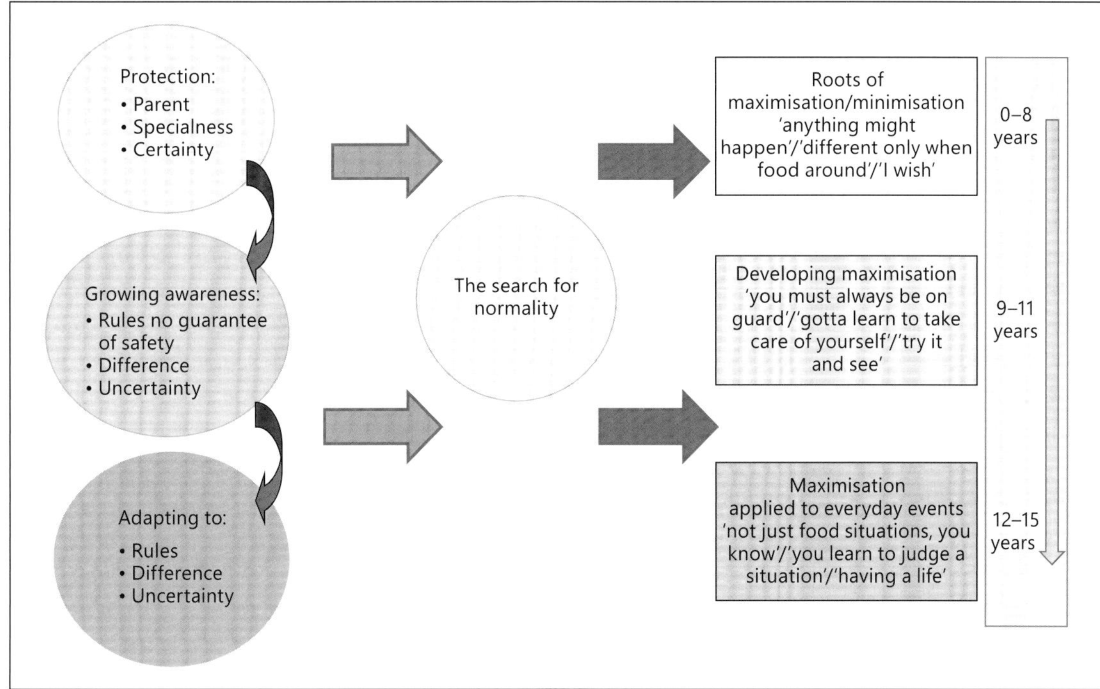

Fig. 1. Because they were diagnosed when infants, young children feel that they are 'the same' as other children, and parents help them to feel normal and protected in their everyday lives. They therefore have an illusory perception of control and certainty. As children become more aware of the rules as restrictive, together with a growing awareness of difference and uncertainty, the search for normality becomes stronger, and children evolve strategies in order to cope. Although the roots of these strategies may be discerned in children in the youngest age group, by adolescence, coping strategies of children become more defined, and in some cases more rigid, and an expanding social world gives further impetus to the search for normality [28].

was just that, God I give up, we were both really depressed by that, you know' (Mother of Emily, age 12, UK).

Living with risk and coping everyday needs to be negotiated carefully, these engender emotions such as confusion, anxiety, uncertainty, frustration and some anger, as the following quotes illustrate:

'I am absolutely terrified that I would buy something with nuts in it by mistake…if anything happened, I would never get over it' (Mother of Jimmy, age 6, Ireland).

'I get confused and anxious trying to get him not to worry too much about it…and then I worry that he's not worried enough' (Mother of Matt, age 10, Ireland).

'You can't have no risk at all you know, even if the child never leaves the house, so you have to deal with risk…we just want a better way' (Mother of Carla, age 10, US).

Parents also struggle with how to support children's independence while controlling their own anxiety and genuine fears of risk.

'I made up reasons for him not to be out and I was very very protective of him and wouldn't let him have the freedom, I was so paranoid that something was going to happen to him' (Mother of Peter, age 13).

'I am so scared for him…when he leaves the house at all for anything…it's always there…sometimes in the background…sometimes strong' (Mother of Jen, age 14, Singapore).

These responses from parents to questions on the impact of food allergy on families' everyday lives illustrate that living with food allergy has direct and indirect effects on emotional adjustment, social interaction, social life, confidence in coping, stress, and overall quality of life. Particular concerns include 'labelling', dietary restrictions, general lack of awareness, and supporting children's growing independence while ensuring their safety.

As we will outline next, children and teens share many of the same experiences, concerns and anxieties as their parents.

Children and Teens

An important transition point occurs when children learn or feel that parents (and therefore the children themselves) cannot conclusively prevent an allergic reaction, after which we see a change in cognition, emotions and behaviour and coping strategies become more differentiated.

To provide an example, *living with uncertainty* is an important concept that affects children's sense of control, beliefs about risk, level of vigilance and confidence in safety. Young children have an illusory perception of control because of parent protection. However, we see the roots of uncertainty in even very young children who are aware of parent anxiety and speak about the possibility of a reaction occurring at any time; *'because you never know what might happen'*. However, always being aware and alert to the possibility of danger is a heavy burden for children in their everyday lives.

'because food is always around it is hard to forget about it' (Becky, age 10, Ireland).
'…I can't just eat something like my friends…or be with people without thinking about what they are eating' (Matt, age 11, Ireland).

Being constantly vigilant also affects children's enjoyment of social events.

'well…it means you can never relax at a party and just enjoy it' (Kevin, age 11, Ireland).

Similar responses were found in the UK, US and Australian data.

'I need to kind of live my life on the risk that something is going to happen or something might never happen' (Kathy, age 16, UK).

Anxiety appears to be particularly strong in the middle childhood years. Even when carefully following the rules, children often cannot pinpoint why a reaction occurred. Older children and teens emphasise the uncertainty of living with food allergy and the consequent feeling of loss of control.

'like sometimes you can't find the cause [of a reaction] …it just happens, you know…not knowing makes you worried and unsure of yourself…when I have a first bite like, if I'm not at home, I think is this it?…will I die?…what can you do?' (Fran, age 12, Ireland).
'sometimes they just joke around and they say "ohh, there's nuts in this"…makes me [sad]…I ask them to stop…and sometimes they don't stop' (Jack, age 10, Australia).

Overall, participants described a low level of awareness and understanding in schools, restaurants, and coffee shops and by friends.

'other kids don't get it…they think it's a bit of a rash…if anything bad happens, I worry they won't know to help me' (Jilly, age 8, Australia).

The experiences described by participants in Ireland, the UK, the US, Singapore and Australia were very similar.

For example, in interviews in Australia (schoolchildren without food allergy) we found only a vague awareness of what food allergy means in terms of symptoms and lifestyle and how to help in an emergency. This finding applied to all age groups.

'I don't know what would happen if he got a reaction… maybe they start having breathing problems, like they start gasping or something…there's nothing about it in the school…the teacher hasn't said anything…yeah we can share food' (Calum, age 12).

This lack of understanding contributes to feelings of uncertainty. Grace (age 13) captured the feelings of many teens when she describes why she feels anxious:

'when I get up in the morning I can't be sure I won't have a reaction that day'.

Uncertainty impinges on developing children's beliefs and subsequent coping strategies. Although being vigilant allows children to feel some form of control, this is undermined by a low understanding and awareness by restaurants, shops, activity camps, schools, peers and the general population, etc. as well as by difficulties in interpreting labels on foods. In Italy, over 75% of children (5–11 years) claim to have a monotonous diet, and school-aged children are significantly less interested in tasting new foods than younger children; 18% of children never attend parties [29].

'The restaurants, hundred percent, even if they say it's nut free I mean you can't tell because they'll be cooking things. If they, say they shove some cashew nuts in a wok, shove the dish out and then my dish goes in there's going to be some bits of the cashew nuts still left' (Sally, age 16, UK).

'I don't usually go to friend's houses, I only go to those that I've known for a long time…in case anything happens' (Kim, age 9, Singapore).

'We don't tend to eat out and if we do me and [brother] will have like chips and garlic bread kind of thing because we just don't trust restaurants' (Cara, age 19, US).

Although their roots may be discerned in children in the youngest age group, by adolescence, children's coping strategies become more defined and in some cases more rigid.

'I don't really want to be in a situation where I'm worried every day about what I eat and have to take all my own food, it's just not worth it, I'm not going to go… So she's making decisions and limiting her own life' (Frances, Mother of Pattie, age 15, UK).

The search for normality [27] becomes clearer when we turn to the coping strategies children use to manage food allergy. For some, normality may mean assurance that they are safe at all times and are accepted and understood by particular friends. For others, it means being able to interact freely and being accepted as normal *'in the real world'*, or it means finding a balance between the two. Coping strategies were found to lie on a maximisation/avoidance to minimisation/risk continuum. They may be emotion-focused or problem-focused, but often they are both. Some are actions, interactions, or cognitions. Their defining quality is that they are used in clusters by particular children, as demonstrated by the responses above.

For example, by *'eating just a little bit'* and seeing how they react, children in the middle age group appear to be trying to determine their own risk thresholds.

'you'd have a small bit now and then and see what happens' (Johnny, age 11).

It may also be a way for children to exert control over uncertain conditions. Older children, particularly teens, appear to take risks as a means of coping in a social situation, counteracting feelings of difference,

'She just wants to be seen as normal, she doesn't want to, like create a fuss and ask in restaurants, you know, is there nuts in that' (Mother of Gillian, age 19, UK).

and because of frustration with labelling.

'When it says "may have traces of nuts" I sometimes still eat them, because it's on everything, that is on absolutely everything and it's like if I can't eat that then what can I eat?…if I actually went by that I wouldn't be able to eat anything' (Gerry, UK, age 15).

Not telling others that you have a food allergy also forms part of the risk cluster of emotions and behaviours, for example, in terms of new relationships.

'why would I tell anyone…it isn't like a cool talent or something' (Jamie, age 14, Ireland).

'Because I remember I went back to this one girl's house and she ate Nutella and I was like, "ach, no". I didn't want to say anything so I just didn't say anything but I was fine, I mean nothing happened...I'm just worried in case if I did kiss her I would have a reaction and "oh no", but nothing happened' (David, age 19, UK).

Research shows that adolescents with severe allergies are at particularly high risk of severe and fatal anaphylactic reactions [37]. The factors contributing to these reactions are unclear, as there has been no systematic research into the attitudes and experiences of this group. The observed high rates of morbidity and mortality may be due to a combination of limited allergen avoidance and poor emergency management amongst adolescents. As stated earlier, there is agreement in the research literature that auto-injectors are under-used by patients of all ages; however, the reasons for this must be fully explored in order to inform improvements to clinical practice. Because auto-injectors are central to emergency management, ensuring their correct use is a priority for clinicians. To do so, clinicians need to understand how and why adolescents respond in the way they do, taking into account the social context and the developmental transitions of adolescence.

In the developmental model, taking risks with medication is termed 'minimisation'.

'I try to "forget" the stupid pen, but Mum makes me get it' (Danny, age 10, Ireland).

'you would remember it in the usual situations...it's just that if it's something out of the ordinary, you know or like if you are going somewhere with friends that isn't like a restaurant, that's ok then, isn't it?' (Julie, age 15, UK).

'I hate bringing [the pen] because you can't hide it and it reminds me of being allergic' (Tom, age 16, US).

These responses clearly demonstrate that, although children are aware that they should bring the auto-injector with them at all times, there are many barriers to full compliance. In many cases, this knowledge does not generalise to non-'usual' occasions or activities.

Taken together, these findings suggest that children, teens and families living with food allergy need to cope with normal developmental changes as well as with their condition, placing them under increased psycho-social stress, leading to possible maladaptive coping strategies and consequent risk. Taking the example of auto-injectors, which are central to emergency management. To ensure compliance, clinicians and other health professionals need to understand how and why adolescents respond in the way they do, taking into account the social context, developmental pathways, and transitions of adolescence.

The remarkable similarity in the responses from different countries suggests the cross-cultural validity of our disease-specific developmental model, which may help in the identification, assessment and initial management of food allergy-specific emotional and behavioural problems.

Discussion

In this chapter, we reviewed the literature on the impact of food allergy on children, teens, parents and adults. Overall, the findings suggest that food allergy has a strong impact on HRQL in terms of social, dietary, and psychological factors. 'Rules' and restrictions ostensibly apply to food, but because food is such an integral part of everyday life, these restrictions extend far beyond 'mealtimes'. Therefore, social events are experienced differently and have a different meaning for those living with food allergy, giving rise to feelings of exclusion and difference, compared to those without allergy. Children, teens, and parents need to cope with the normal developmental changes and as well as with the food allergy, placing them under increased psycho-social stress, leading to adverse effects on HRQL and coping.

Outcomes research, including the development and use of HRQL questionnaires, has been key in altering the culture of clinical practice and health care research by changing how we assess the end results of health care services, including clinical and therapeutic interventions, evaluation and health policy.

However, there are important methodological issues in relation to the use of HRQL measures. First, questionnaires should be primarily generated according to patient concerns, reflect the patient perspective and be reliable and valid for the population in which they are being used. Second, in order to create as complete a picture as possible of the HRQL of children and teens, self-reports as well as proxy measures should be used whenever possible. Third, disease-specific questionnaires are more sensitive measures; however, generic measures may be used when comparing two different diseases. Fourth, questionnaires must be developmentally appropriate; and finally, subscales should be taken into account when evaluating an individual or sample population.

For example, in relation to the last two points, the subscales suggested subtle differences in HRQL over time in relation to both developmental age and child gender, which may suggest optimum times for intervention.

It is also vital that health professionals working in the field of food allergy understand how and why children, teens, parents and adults respond in the way that they do, taking into account the social context, developmental pathways, and transition points. An important reason for choosing any method lies in the nature of the research problem. Qualitative methods may be more suitable for measuring the individuality and subjectivity of experience and response in-depth or to gain a novel understanding of a particular area. In addition, they may often obtain the intricate details about phenomena such as feelings, thought processes, and emotions, which are difficult to extract or learn about through more conventional research methods, such as questionnaires. In the context of research in children, qualitative research also provides an opportunity to tap into the richness of children's thoughts and feelings about them-

selves, their environments and the world in which they live. However, it is important to state that qualitative methods must be subject to the same standards of reliability and validity as quantitative methods.

Using both qualitative and quantitative methods in HRQL studies can be complementary and can enrich the overall findings. For example, *uncertainty* appears as a central theme in many of the studies presented here, and the stressors in living with a food allergy were perceived to be uncontrollable to a greater or lesser extent. Stressors that impact the perception of HRQL and that are linked to uncertainty include labelling, auto-injector use, diagnosis, transition points, and lack of general awareness in restaurants, shops, schools, and social venues. However, although all children acknowledge the 'uncertainty' of food allergy to some extent, some older children and adolescents spoke about 'informing others' and 'raising awareness' as a way of improving the experience of 'living with uncertainty', whereas others emphasise that there is 'no point'. Therefore, the perception of controllability of the same stressor, and hence HRQL, may vary from child to child, depending on factors such as the attitude of the parents and prior experiences.

In a similar manner, uncertainty around 'labelling' and thresholds for severe to mild reactions has direct and indirect effects on emotional adjustment, social interaction and social life, and, by inducing a state of uncertainty, may result in poor HRQL, leading to anxiety/generalised avoidance or risky behaviours in children and young people.

Improving HRQL

To address and attempt to alleviate such stressors, both quantitative and qualitative research suggests that alleviating uncertainty should be a major goal for health professionals working with children, teens and families. Remarkable similarities in the responses to food allergy across countries suggest that policies and programmes that address quality of life issues may be relevant to many different populations.

Greater support and clear information is important at the time of diagnosis and at the different transition points along the development pathway. Specifically, parents have suggested that greater emphasis is needed on the social and emotional aspects of food allergy, on knowing 'what to expect', and on enhancing the self-management skills of children and their families [27–29].

Transition points are a source of stress and uncertainty, particularly for parents of food-allergic children. Whether the child has already attended a nursery or entered an infant/primary school is a new trigger of anxiety because the parent is required to hand over responsibility and control to a third party, and parents need to put strategies in place to cope with this. As children grow and become more aware of their differences and as their social world expands, parents worry that children may take risks in order to 'fit-in' with other children. Keeping children safe, while helping them to be independent and self-reliant, can be a challenging balancing act. Going to secondary school is a transition point that tests parents' resources, increases uncertainty, and intensifies anxiety in parents. Our findings show that perception of HRQL and coping strategies result from a cumulative history of interactive processes (both age- and disease-specific) that are embedded in a child's developmental pathway; therefore, the goal of an intervention should be to promote a stable growth dynamic by including issues that are food allergy-specific as well as age- and context-specific.

Elements of an intervention designed to help achieve this goal include identifying and labelling feelings; understanding the difference between feelings and behaviours; reducing stress; self-talk; using steps for problem-solving and decision-making; managing conflict; body-awareness; and practical aspects such as label reading, auto-injector use, etc. The intended outcomes should include positive coping strategies (behavioural and emotional) that lead to improved psycho-social adaptation to growing up and living with food allergy and improved quality of life and well-being. The development and validation of a psycho-educational intervention for parents, children, teens and schools is currently underway by the Cork Research Group in collaboration with the UK, the Netherlands and the US. In focus groups and interviews, children, teens and parents stressed that education at a societal level was also necessary to inform others of the realities of food allergy so that there might be an increase in awareness and consequent understanding.

Early and accurate diagnosis is also important, since, as discussed, perceived allergy has a similar impact as confirmed allergy. There are now new diagnostic tools that can accurately predict what the outcome of a food challenge would be [35]. The authors' findings have implications for a potentially more cost-effective method of determining food allergy, which will ultimately help provide better care to food-allergic patients and improve HRQL.

Stress engendered by 'labelling' and by uncertainty around thresholds is also germane, and the emphasis to date has been on hazard control rather than risk assessment. However, precautionary labelling, which was initially welcomed by allergic consumers, has been devalued through perceived over-use and inconsistent application. Parents and families living with food allergy dislike precautionary labelling because they are uncertain about the basis of its use, it considerably reduces their food choices, and it has adverse effects on nutritional status. Consumers are therefore faced with a dilemma. In an on-going worldwide study under the aegis of Food Allergy Research and Resource Program (www.farrp.org/) on the effects of labelling on the concerns of the allergic consumer, we are investigating the acceptability by stakeholders (parents, young people, clinicians, producers) of alternative approaches, with the ultimate aim of improving the sense of control and hence HRQL in parents and patients.

Conclusion

The majority of research on food allergy has been bio-medical in orientation, focusing on issues such as the molecular structure of allergens, or aimed at methods of diagnosis. In the last decade, there has been a growing interest in the development of questionnaires to measure the impact of food allergy on HRQL. These studies have provided an insight into the everyday burden of living with food allergy and have suggested ways that HRQL can be improved.

To conclude, we suggest that there are important questions that must be answered so that HRQL measures can reach their full potential in research, practice and policy.

These questions include the following:

- What are the correlates of HRQL (e.g. anxiety, compliance, risk perception, coping behaviours), and how may they impact the perception of health and health reporting?
- Which variables are causally related to HRQL status, and which variables are the effects of HRQL status?
- What developmental processes are involved in particular emotional and behavioural outcomes?

Such questions are relevant for the interpretation and usefulness of HRQL measures in clinical practice (e.g. treatment choices for certain patient groups and individual patients), health policy (e.g. the allocation of healthcare funds), the development of psycho-educational interventions (the precise targeting of information) and research (the causal direction of factors related to HRQL).

A broader understanding of HRQL will ultimately lead to the promotion of earlier, more effective preventive strategies and interventions that are focused on maximising optimal health development and quality of life.

References

1 Jackson KD, Howie LD, Akinbami LJ: Trends in Allergic Conditions among Children: United States, 1997–2011. NCHS Data Brief, no 121. Hyattsville, MD, National Center for Health Statistics, 2013.

2 Rona R, Keil T, Summers C: The prevalence of food allergy: a meta-analysis. J Allergy Clin Immunol 2007;120:638–646.

3 Sicherer SH, Sampson HA: 9. Food allergy. J Allergy Clin Immunol 2006; 117(2 suppl):S470–S475.

4 Decker WW, Campbell RL, Manivannan V, Luke A, St Sauver JL, Weaver A, Bellolio MF, Bergstralh EJ, Stead LG, Li JT: The etiology and incidence of anaphylaxis in Rochester, Minnesota: a report from the Rochester Epidemiology Project. J Allergy Clin Immunol 2008;122: 1161–1165.

5 Sicherer SH, Muñoz-Furlong A, Godbold JH, Sampson HA: US prevalence of self-reported peanut, tree nut, and sesame allergy: 11-year follow-up. J Allergy Clin Immunol 2010;125:1322–1326.

6 Branum AM, Lukacs SL: Food allergy among US children: trends in prevalence and hospitalizations. NCHS Data Brief, no 10. Hyattsville, MD, National Center for Health Statistics, 2008.

7 Sampson HA: Update on food allergy. J Allergy Clin Immunol 2004;113:805–819.

8 Wang J, Sampson HA: Food allergy: recent advances in pathophysiology and treatment. Allergy Asthma Immunol Res 2009;1:19–29.

9 Tole JW, Lieberman P: Biphasic anaphylaxis: review of incidence, clinical predictors, and observation recommendations. Immunol Allergy Clin North Am 2007;27:309–326.

10 Sampson HA, Mendelson L, Rosen JP: Fatal and near-fatal anaphylactic reactions to food in children and adolescents. N Engl J Med 1992;327:380–384.

11 Van der Velde JL, Flokstra-de Blok BMJ, Vlieg-Boerstra BJ, Oude Elberink JNG, Schouten JP, DunnGalvin A, Hourihane JO, Duiverman EJ, Dubois AEJ: Test-retest reliability of the Food Allergy Quality of Life Questionnaires (FAQLQ) for children, adolescents and adults. Qual Life Res 2009;18:245–251.

12 DunnGalvin A, Flokstra-de Blok BMJ, Burks AW, Dubois AEJ, Hourihane JO: Food allergy QoL questionnaire for children aged 0–12 years: content, construct and cross cultural validity. Clin Exp Allergy 2008;38:977–988.

13 DunnGalvin A, Cullinane C, Daly D, Flokstra-de Blok B, Dubois A, Hourihane JO: Longitudinal validity and responsiveness of the Food Allergy Quality of Life Questionnaire – Parent Form in children 0–12 years following positive and negative food challenges. Clin Exp Allergy 2010;40:476–485.

14 Soller L, Hourihane JO, DunnGalvin A: The impact of oral food challenge tests on food allergy health-related quality of life. Allergy 2014;69:1255–1257.

15 Flokstra-de Blok BMJ, DunnGalvin A, Vlieg-Boersta BJ, Oude Elberink JNG, Duiverman EJ, Hourihane JO, Dubois AEJ: Development and validation of a self-administered Food Allergy Quality of Life Questionnaire for children. Clin Exp Allergy 2009;39:127–137.

16 Flokstra-de Blok BMJ, DunnGalvin A, Vlieg-Boerstra BJ, Oude Elberink JNG, Duiverman EJ, Hourihane JO, Dubois AEJ: Development and validation of the self-administered Food Allergy Quality of Life Questionnaire for adolescents. J Allergy Clin Immunol 2008;122:139–144.e1–e2.

17 Flokstra-de Blok BMJ, van der Meulen GN, DunnGalvin A, Vlieg-Boerstra BJ, Oude Elberink JNG, Duiverman EJ, Hourihane JO, Dubois AEJ: Development and validation of the Food Allergy Quality of Life Questionnaire-Adult Form. Allergy 2009;64:1209–1217.

18 de Blok BMJ, Vlieg-Boerstra BJ, Oude Elberink JNG, Duiverman EJ, DunnGalvin A, Hourihane JO, Cornelisse-Vermaat JR, Frewer L, Mills C, Dubois AEJ: A framework for measuring the social impact of food allergy across Europe: a EuroPrevall state of the art paper. Allergy 2007;62:733–737.

19 Pinczower GD, Bertalli NA, Bussmann N, Hamidon M, Allen KJ, DunnGalvin A, Hourihane JO, Gurrin LC, Tang MLK: The effect of provision of an adrenaline auto-injector on quality of life in children with food allergy. J Allergy Clin Immunol 2013;131:238–240.

20 DunnGalvin A, Keena A, Hourihane JO, Koman E, Raver E, Frome H. Adams M: Validation of the Food Allergy Quality of Life Questionnaire-Parent Form (FAQLQ-PF) in an American sample of children between 0–12 years. Allergy, submitted.

21 DunnGalvin A, Cullinane C, Daly DA, Flokstra-de Blok BMJ, Dubois AEJ, Hourihane J: Longitudinal validity and responsiveness of the Food Allergy Quality of Life Questionnaire-Parent Form in children 0–12 years following positive and negative food challenges. Clin Exp Allergy 2010;40:476–485.

22 Velde JL, Flokstra de Blok BM, Vlieg-Boerstra BJ, Oude Elberink JN, DunnGalvin A, Hourihane JO, Duiverman EJ, Dubois AE: Development, validity and reliability of the food allergy independent measure (FAIM). Allergy 2010;65:630–635.

23 Eiser C, Morse R: A review of measures of quality of life for children with chronic illness. Arch Dis Child 2001;84:205–211.

24 Dixon SD, Stein MT: Encounters with children: pediatric behavior and development, ed 4. Philadelphia, Mosby Elsevier, 2006.

25 Curry SL, Russ SW: Identifying coping strategies in children. J Clin Child Psychol 1985;14:61–69.

26 Eisenberg N, Fabes RA, Guthrie IK: Coping with stress: the roles of regulation and development; in Wolchik SA, Sandler IN (eds): Handbook of Children's Coping: Linking Theory and Intervention. New York, Plenum, 1997, pp 41–70.

27 Donaldson D, Prinstein MJ, Danovsky M, Spirito A: Patterns of children's coping with life stress: Implications for clinicians. Am J Orthopsychiatry 2000;70:351–359.

28 DunnGalvin A, Gaffney A, Hourihane JO: Developmental pathways in food allergy: a new theoretical framework. Allergy 2009;64:560–568.

29 DunnGalvin A, Sheik A, Polloni L, Muraro A, Hourihane JO: Pathways to anxiety and risk in food allergy. JACI, submitted.

30 DunnGalvin A, Hourihane JO: Developmental aspects of HRQL in food related chronic disease; in The International Handbook of Behaviour, Diet and Nutrition. US, Springer, 2011.

31 Brouwers MC, Kho ME, Browman GP, Burgers JS, Cluzeau F, Feder G, Fervers BÃ, Graham ID, Grimshaw J, Hanna SE, Littlejohns P, Makarski J, Zitzelsberger L: AGREE II: advancing guideline development, reporting and evaluation in health care. CMAJ 2010;182:E839–E842.

32 Cohen BL, Noone NS, Munoz-Furlong A, Sicherer SH: Parental burden in food allergy. J Allergy Clin Immunol 2004;114:1159–1163.

33 Wassenberg J, Cochard MM, DunnGalvin A, Ballabeni P, Flokstra-de Blok BM, Newman CJ, Hofer M, Eigenmann PA: Parent perceived quality of life is age-dependent in children with food allergy. Pediatr Allergy Immunol 2012;23:412–419.

34 Stewart JL, Mishel MH: Uncertainty in childhood illness: a synthesis of the parent and child literature. Sch Inq Nurs Pract 2000;14:299–319.

35 DunnGalvin A, Chang W, Laubach S, Steele P, Dubois A, Burks W, Hourihane JO: Profiling families enrolled in food allergy immunotherapy studies. Pediatrics 2009;124:e503–e509.

36 DunnGalvin A, Daly D, Cullinane C, Stenke E, Keeton D, Erlewyn-Lajeunesse M, Roberts G, Lucas J, Hourihane JO: Highly accurate prediction of food challenge outcome using routinely available clinical data. J Allergy Clin Immunol 2011;127:633–639.e1–e3.

37 Rothmier JD, Lasley MV, Shapiro GG: Factors influencing parental consent in pediatric clinical research. Pediatrics 2003;111:1037–1041.

Audrey DunnGalvin, MSc, PhD, Reg. Psychol.
School of Applied Psychology
University College Cork
Cork City, Co. Cork (Ireland)
E-Mail a.dunngalvin@ucc.ie

Ebisawa M, Ballmer-Weber BK, Vieths S, Wood RA (eds): Food Allergy: Molecular Basis and Clinical Practice.
Chem Immunol Allergy. Basel, Karger, 2015, vol 101, pp 253–262 (DOI: 10.1159/000373911)

Prevention of Food Allergy

Teresa Tsakok[a] · George Du Toit[a, b] · Gideon Lack[a]

[a]Department of Paediatric Allergy, Guy's and St. Thomas' NHS Foundation Trust, London, and [b]MRC and
Asthma UK Centre in Allergic Mechanisms of Asthma, King's College London, King's Health Partners,
London, UK

Abstract

Despite a trend towards delayed weaning, food allergies (FAs) have increased in the past few decades and are now considered a public health concern, resulting in significant morbidity as well as occasional mortality. Whilst genetic factors are clearly important in the development of FA, a rise in FAs has occurred over a short period of time and is therefore unlikely to be due to germ-line genetic changes alone. Thus, it seems plausible that one or more environmental exposures may, via epigenetic changes, result in the interruption of the 'default immunologic state' of tolerance to foods. Strategies are therefore required for the prevention of FA: *primary prevention* seeks to prevent the onset of IgE-sensitisation; *secondary prevention* seeks to interrupt the development of FA in IgE-sensitised children; and *tertiary prevention* seeks to reduce the expression of 'end-organ' allergic disease in children with established FA. This chapter will outline the major findings in this field, with the aim of equipping the clinician with an evidence-based approach to a burgeoning yet poorly understood clinical problem. We also highlight the methodological challenges hindering the interpretation of existing FA studies. Fortunately, there are now robust studies underway, the results of which are expected to guide public health recommendations with respect to how and when to introduce major allergenic foods to children, regardless of allergic risk.

© 2015 S. Karger AG, Basel

Introduction

Food allergy (FA) is now considered a public health concern, affecting 3–6% children in the developed world [1, 2] and resulting in significant morbidity as well as occasional mortality. Known risk factors for the development of allergy include family history, male sex (at least in childhood), ethnicity and genetic polymorphisms. Whilst genetic factors are clearly important in the development of FA, the rise in FA has occurred over a short period of time and is therefore unlikely to be due to germ-line genetic changes alone. Thus, it seems plausible that one or more environmental exposures may, via epigenetic changes, result in the interruption of the 'default immunologic state' of tolerance to foods. Strategies are therefore required for the prevention of FAs: *primary prevention* seeks to prevent the onset of IgE-sensitisation; *secondary prevention* seeks to interrupt the development of FA in IgE-sensitised children; and *tertiary prevention* seeks to reduce the expression of 'end-organ' allergic disease in children with established FA.

Methodological Challenges

Although cautious conclusions and recommendations may be drawn about allergy prevention via dietary means, it is notable that numerous methodological limitations affect the many studies informing the field (summarised in table 1). In terms of defining FA, the majority of papers discussed in this chapter used surrogate sensitisation markers such as skin prick tests and IgE level determination, as opposed to the gold standard of double-blind, placebo-controlled food challenges.

Onset of Sensitisation and Food Allergy

Since it remains unclear as to when prevention strategies should be implemented, it is important to determine whether sensitisation occurs in utero. This possibility is suggested by the early clinical presentation of IgE-mediated FAs. In a large population-based sample of 12-month-old infants in Australia [3], the prevalence of challenge-proven peanut allergy (PA) was 3.0% (95% CI 2.4–3.8), of raw egg allergy was 8.9% (95% CI 7.8–10.0), and of sesame allergy was 0.8% (95% CI 0.5–1.1). Likewise, non-IgE-mediated food-induced immunological reactions such as cow's milk protein (CMP)-induced colitis may present in infancy [4]. Although it has been suggested that food and aeroallergens may be transmitted via the placenta [5], two large birth cohort studies [6, 7] were unable to demonstrate measurable food-specific IgE in cord blood, even in children subsequently developing FAs or sensitisation.

Maternal Diet (During Pregnancy and/or Breastfeeding) and the Prevention of Food Allergy

Manipulation of the maternal diet during pregnancy and/or breastfeeding has not consistently been shown to exert protective effects on the development of FA. Furthermore, such strategies carry the risk of nutritional compromise for both the mother and child. One cross-sectional study [8] evaluated the relevant route of peanut exposure in the development of PA. Peanut consumption in the mother and amongst all household members was quantified, and the median weekly household peanut consumption for patients with PA was significantly increased (18.8 g; n = 5,133) compared to control subjects without allergy (6.9 g, n = 5,150) and high-risk control subjects (1.9 g, n = 5,160; p < 0.0001). Furthermore, a dose-response relationship was observed between environmental (non-oral) peanut exposure and the development of PA. Although peanut consumption during pregnancy was increased in the mothers of children with PA, this relationship was no longer significant after adjustment for household exposure. Likewise, the Avon Longitudinal Study of Parents and Children study [6] showed no effect of maternal peanut consumption during pregnancy or lactation on the development of immunologic or clinical reaction to peanuts by 4–6 years of age.

Complementary Infant Feeding and the Prevention of Food Allergy

The World Health Organization (WHO) recommends that the term 'weaning' be replaced by the term 'complementary feeding', which

Table 1. Examples of methodological issues known to complicate the interpretation of studies aimed at the prevention of food allergy

Issue	Explanation	Recommended approach
Study design	The majority of studies are observational, not interventional.	Randomised controlled trials
Reverse causality	Early signs of suspected allergic disease (such as eczema or a presumed allergic reaction) will result in altered feeding patterns.	Randomised controlled trials
Randomisation	There are necessary ethical restraints that limit randomisation to dietary interventions other than breastfeeding.	Breastfeeding should be encouraged. Studies should randomise within the breastfed group.
Blinding of dietary interventions	Blinding of specific dietary interventions may not be possible due to safety concerns or practical limitations, e.g. breastfeeding or formula odour.	It may not be possible, or safe, to have a placebo arm to infant nutritional studies.
Determination of food allergy	Few studies make use of Oral Food Challenges (OFCs) for the diagnosis of food allergy.	Aim to perform OFCs in all participants. For children who do not undergo OFCs, a priori diagnostic algorithms are required.
Surrogate markers	Eczema, rhinitis and asthma are often used as surrogate markers of food allergy.	Same as above
Natural history of food allergy	Tolerance is anticipated for many food allergies in the first decade of life.	Account for natural remission and onset of food allergy before assessing for a study effect.
Allergy diagnosis	Many studies use generic terms such as 'allergy' or 'atopy'. Definitions and diagnostic criteria for each of these conditions are open to great variability.	Consensus with respect to the diagnosis of common allergic disorders is required.
Determination of diet	The determination of food consumption is usually by retrospective Food Frequency Questionnaires, which are prone to many forms of bias and may not include important variables (allergen processing, sequence of ingestion, concomitant breastfeeding, etc.).	Use should be made of prospective food diaries that have been validated for context, language and consistency.
Definitions: weaning	Use of the term 'weaning' is not consistent and is usually limited to only the introduction of solid foods.	Adopt the WHO term 'complementary feeding', which incorporates any nutrient-containing food or liquid other than breast milk that is given to young children.
High-risk markers	Many studies are aimed at high-risk atopic populations.	Ideally, studies should include entire study populations (i.e. both low and high-risk). At-risk populations should be defined a priori.
Separation of specific effects when interventions are combined	Multiple interventions are often studied at different time points.	Preliminary proof-of-concept studies need to separate out the effects of each intervention.
Introduction of complementary feeding is associated with multiple variables	The early cessation of breastfeeding and introduction of complementary feeding has been associated with cultural, socioeconomic and other factors.	Regression analysis should control for as many relevant confounders as possible.
Monitoring adherence	Monitoring of adherence to interventions, particularly dietary interventions, is difficult.	Better tools for monitoring dietary adherence are required.

encompasses any nutrient-containing food or liquid other than breast milk. Studies in this field have traditionally considered weaning to be the introduction of solids, but the allergenic potential of liquid foods may be no different. Valuable lessons may thus become apparent when including studies assessing all foods, irrespective of 'medium'. Numerous specialist organisations offer advice on feeding at-risk infants; whilst there is consensus that breast milk remains unchallenged as the milk of choice, advice differs with respect to duration of exclusive breastfeeding and avoidance of other common food allergens.

In 2003, a review [9] of 132 studies reported that breastfeeding was protective of atopic diseases but not of FA. However, in a more recent review by Muraro et al. [10], exclusive breastfeeding for at least 4 months was associated with a lower cumulative incidence of cow's milk allergy until 18 months of age. Brew et al. [11] combined data from two large cohorts, including subjects with a gestational age of >36 weeks and at least one parent with wheeze or asthma (n = 882). Breastfeeding was a risk factor for sensitisation to cow's milk, peanuts, and eggs at 8 years. Although some evidence suggests that exclusive breastfeeding for 3 months may protect against the development of allergy, prolonged exclusive breastfeeding beyond 3 months of age has not been shown to consistently protect against the development of FA or atopy.

Kramer et al. [12] performed a WHO-commissioned systematic review of the effects of exclusive breastfeeding for 6 months versus exclusive breastfeeding for 3–4 months followed by mixed breastfeeding (complementary liquid or solid foods with continued breastfeeding) to 6 months. Although FA outcomes were not assessed, there was no significant reduction in risk of atopic outcomes amongst infants who were exclusively breastfed for 6 months, compared with those who were exclusively breastfed for 3–4 months followed by mixed feeding. It is therefore surprising that the WHO recommendations use the justification of reduction in atopy to support exclusive breastfeeding for the first 6 months of an infant's life.

Only two randomised studies have evaluated the effects of CMP formula vs. exclusive breastfeeding on the subsequent development of FA and atopy. Lucas et al.'s [13] randomised interventional study of premature infants (n = 777) compared the effects of human breast milk, standard preterm formula and nutrient-enriched preterm formula. Interestingly, at 18 months, there was no overall difference in the incidence of food-allergic reactions between dietary groups. Similarly, de Jong et al. [14] found that early high-dose exposure to CMP was not associated with an increase in sensitisation or allergy to CMP in children up to 5 years old. A recent case-control within a cohort study [15] asked mothers to keep prospective food diaries for their infants during their first year of life, and these mothers reported that infants diagnosed with FA by 2 years old were introduced to solids earlier (<16 weeks) and were less likely to be receiving breast milk when CMP was introduced. This supports the current American Academy of Paediatrics' recommendations [16] and the European Society of Paediatric Gastroenterology, Hepatology and Nutrition advice [17] to avoid introducing solids before 4–6 months of age. It also supports the American Academy of Paediatrics' recommendations that breastfeeding should continue whilst solids are introduced into the diet and that breastfeeding should ideally continue for 1 year or longer [16].

Some observational studies demonstrate an increased risk for the development of FA in breastfed infants. Using retrospective questionnaires, Paton et al. [18] found that of 15,142 children, a strong allergic reaction to peanuts and other nuts was reported in 487 (3.2%) and 307 (3.9%) of the children, respectively. Those who were exclusively breastfed were more likely to have a parent-reported nut allergy (OR 1.43; 1.21–1.69; p < 0.001), whilst nut allergy was less likely in children only fed food/fluid other than breast milk (OR 0.63; 0.45–0.89; p = 0.009) and in those who were both breastfed and given other food/fluid (OR 0.83; 0.70–0.98; p = 0.025).

Since 1975, there has been a significant trend in developed countries towards the later introduction of solid foods. The proportion of UK infants given solids by 8 weeks of age has fallen: 49% in 1975, 24% in 1980 and 1985, and 19% in 1990 [19]. It is notable that this decrease to a third of the original value has coincided with a three-fold increase in childhood allergy [20]. However, Tarini et al. [21] performed a review of evidence for the relationship between early (<4 months) introduction of solids and the development of allergic disease. They concluded that there was insufficient data to suggest that the early introduction of solids alone was associated with an increased risk of FA, asthma or allergic rhinitis.

Although exclusive breastfeeding does not have proven effects on the prevention of allergy, numerous studies have examined the protective effects of different types of formulas – especially CMP-hydrolysates as substitutes for breast milk where the mother is unable or reluctant to breast-feed. Osborn et al.'s [22] Cochrane review found no evidence to support feeding with a hydrolysed formula for the prevention of allergy compared to exclusive breastfeeding. For high-risk infants unable to be completely breastfed, they found limited evidence that prolonged feeding with a hydrolysed formula compared to with a cow's milk formula reduced infant and childhood allergy and infant cow's milk allergy. The general consensus amongst reviews is that the use of hydrolysed milk formula in at-risk infants offers at least some protection against allergic disease, in particular, eczema. These findings are reflected in the recommendations of specialist allergy organisations [23–29].

The German Infant Nutritional Interventional study [30, 31] and the Melbourne Allergy Cohort Study [32] are two of the largest studies on this topic, but whilst the German Infant Nutritional Interventional study was unable to clearly define the end-point of FA by food challenge or by sensitisation, the Melbourne Allergy Cohort study found no group difference at age 2 years for either FA or eczema.

Soy has long been used as a CMF alternative, but Osborn et al.'s [33] Cochrane review concluded that the use of soy formulas could not be recommended for the prevention of allergy or food intolerance in at-risk infants. Notably, no study demonstrated an increase in soy allergy. There is also no evidence to support the use of other mammalian milks for the prevention of FA.

Combined Maternal and Infant Dietary Measures and the Prevention of Food Allergy

Two randomised studies have adopted a multi-intervention approach. In Zeiger et al.'s [34] study of 165 mother/infant pairs, participants were randomised to either a prophylactic group (maternal avoidance of cow's milk, egg, and peanut during the last trimester of pregnancy and lactation; infant's diet free from cow's milk for ≤1 year, egg for ≤2 years, and peanut and fish for ≤3 years) or a control group (standard feeding practice). The findings demonstrated a significant reduction in cow's milk sensitisation and eczema before the age of 2 years but no significant reduction in FA, food sensitisation, serum IgE levels or atopic disease at 7 years of age.

Arshad et al.'s [35] study of 120 infants randomised participants to either a prophylactic group (breastfed with mother on a low-allergen diet or given an extensively hydrolysed formula and house dust mite reduction) or a control group (following standard UK Department of Health advice). The findings demonstrated a preventive effect on asthma, atopic dermatitis, rhinitis, and atopy. Study powering did not allow for the assessment of FA at 8 years of age, but earlier transient effects were noted.

Routes of Sensitisation

Until recently, preventive strategies have focused on oral exposure to foods. However, exposure to food allergens may also occur via aerosolised allergens (e.g. fish and milk cooking vapours) or via the skin. Data from the Avon Longitudinal Study of Parents and Children birth cohort [6] (n = 13,971) showed a positive association between PA and eczema, an even greater association with an oozing or crusting skin rash, and increased use of peanut oil-containing skin preparations in children with PA. Such observations support the concept of transcutaneous sensitisation, particularly via abraded skin. The molecular basis for the increased skin permeability seen in some eczema patients was recently discovered to be loss-of-function or missense mutations in the gene encoding filaggrin (FLG). This protein has been recognised as the strongest genetic contributor to eczema and is important for epidermal differentiation, desquamation, and barrier function [36–39]. Given that low-dose exposure to environmental food proteins on table-tops, hands, and dust can occur [40], it is thought that such food proteins may penetrate the disrupted skin barrier and be taken up by Langerhans cells, leading to Th2 responses and IgE production by B cells [37].

Brown et al.'s case-control study [41] demonstrated that FLG loss-of-function mutations showed a strong and significant association with PA in peanut challenge-positive patients (OR 5.3; 2.8–10.2; p = 3.0×10^{-6}); they then replicated these findings in a separate group of children with PA (OR 1.9; 1.4–2.6; p = 5.4×10^{-5}). The association of FLG mutations with PA remained significant (p = 0.0008) after controlling for coexistent eczema.

Oral Tolerance Induction

No interventional studies have examined the potential role of oral tolerance induction to foods in childhood. Ecological data suggests that countries in which peanuts are consumed throughout pregnancy and early childhood (e.g. in Africa, Asia and the Middle East) enjoy low rates of PA compared to Western, industrialised societies such as in the UK and USA; here, PA is high, despite peanut avoidance during pregnancy and infancy [42–44]. However, differential atopic predisposition due to genetic and environmental factors could explain these differences. In a cross-sectional study by Toit du et al. [45], amongst Israeli (n = 5,615) and UK (n = 5,171) Jewish children, the prevalence of PA was ten-fold higher in the UK (1.85%) than in Israel (0.17%, p < 0.001). This study also found that peanuts are introduced earlier, eaten more frequently and in larger quantities in Israel than in the UK. Such findings raise the question of whether early introduction of peanut during infancy, rather than avoidance, would prevent the development of PA.

A recent study by Joseph et al. [46] found that early feeding (<4 months of age) of any complementary food (solid food and/or cow's milk) was associated with a reduced risk of peanut sensitisation at age 2–3 years in children with a parental atopic history; however, food challenges were not done to confirm true allergy.

Data from Poole et al.'s [47] large prospective cohort study (n = 1,612) suggested that delaying the introduction of cereal grains until after 6 months might increase the risk of wheat allergy. By contrast, Saarinen et al.'s [48] observational study found no difference in the cumulative incidence of fish and citrus allergy at 3 years of age between children introduced to fish early or late.

Recent studies have suggested that it may be beneficial to introduce egg in small amounts, either in baked goods or cooked (scrambled, hard-boiled, fried, or poached), at an early age. Nwaru et al. [49] demonstrated an increased risk of egg sensitisation at age 5 years if egg was introduced at >10.5 months. Koplin et al. [50] reported that later introduction of egg was associated with higher rates of egg allergy, with an adjusted odds ratio of 3.4 for egg introduction at >12 months (95% CI 1.8–6.5) compared with introduction at 4–6 months. Interestingly, introduction of cooked egg was more protective than egg in baked goods. Lastly, Palmer et al.'s recent randomised controlled trial [51] randomised infants to receive a daily spoonful of powered egg or powered rice at between 4 and 8 months old. Egg allergy (based here on both food challenge and SPT) was lower in the egg group than in the control group (RR 0.65; 0.38–1.11); however, this difference was not significant (p = 0.11).

Unpasteurised Milk, Probiotics and Prebiotics

Observational studies suggest that consumption of unpasteurised milk may reduce the prevalence of allergic sensitisation and disease. Although the subject of several studies on allergy prevention [52, 53], there are safety concerns regarding unpasteurised milk, and this cannot therefore be recommended for the prevention of FA. Although some studies show that the use of probiotics [54] (and in one study a mixture of both pro- and prebiotics [55]) reduces eczema, these effects are not consistent in all studies and are not associated with a reduction in sensitisation to foods or FAs. Currently, neither prebiotics nor probiotics can be recommended as a strategy to prevent FA or other allergic diseases.

Nutritional Supplements

Ecological observations note that the geographical distribution of allergy prevalence is linked to regional dietary practices [56]. In recent years, there has been a focus on the role of vitamins, antioxidants, fruits, and vegetables, as well as fatty acids on the prevention or treatment of allergies. Studies investigating fatty acids have yielded conflicting results [57–61], and observational studies examining the effect of vitamin D supplementation during infancy [62–64] suggest an increased rate of sensitisation and allergy, but it has been reported that this is only true when administered in a water-soluble vehicle [65]. Ecological observations imply that increased intake of antioxidant-rich fresh fruit and vegetables is associated with a decreased prevalence of FA in certain European countries [56], whilst preliminary studies suggest that foods rich in trace elements may confer protection against allergy outcomes [66]. There are also data to support an association between obesity and allergic sensitisation to foods [67]. Although the role of nutritional supplements for the prevention of allergy is interesting, further randomised interventional studies are required.

Conclusions

The natural history of FA suggests 'plasticity' within the developing immune system, since common FAs such as egg and milk allergy are often outgrown. Indeed, the switch from a state of allergy to tolerance may even occur during the first few years of life. Turcanu et al. [68] demonstrated that the resolution of PA was accompanied by a shift from a Th2 polarisation of cytokine production to a Th1-skewed, allergen-specific immune response. These findings are encouraging, as they raise the possibility that immune responses are susceptible to prevention strategies.

Conventional wisdom holds that early exposure to allergenic food proteins during pregnancy, lactation, or infancy leads to FA; therefore, prevention strategies should aim to eliminate allergenic food proteins during these periods of 'immunologic vulnerability', especially in high-risk subgroups. However, the evidence does not support this finding, and indeed there are data suggesting that environmental food allergen exposure leads to allergic sensitisation and that early consumption of food antigens may induce tolerance. There is some evidence to support the use of dietary interventions in high-risk pregnant and/or lactating women, especially for the prevention of atopic eczema. Such interventions may, however, compromise maternal and foetal nutrition. Exclusive breastfeeding for at least the first 3 months of life offers some protection against allergic disease in high-risk infants; however, the protective effect of exclusive breastfeeding beyond 4 months of age remains uncertain. For high-risk infants who are not exclusively breastfed, or where supplementation of breastfeeding is required, the use of hydrolysed formula may offer some protection against the development of eczema and allergic disease, including FA. The findings of studies investigating dietary interventions such as fatty acids, antioxidants, pre- and probiotics and vitamin supplementation are unconvincing, inconsistent or not adequately tested. Furthermore, there are safety concerns surrounding some of these interventions.

Future studies will need to overcome the methodological challenges highlighted in this chapter, many of which are unique to this field of research. Furthermore, superior markers are required to identify high-risk populations, as not all children who develop FA are born to atopic families. With current advances in the field of gene-environment interactions, it may also be that future studies need to focus their interventions on specifically-defined groups of children, where genotyping has identified them as being at risk of (or protected from) specific environmental exposures.

Finally, in order for significant advances to be made in the field of FA prevention, strategies will need to be put to the test using rigorous study design methodologies.

References

1 Sicherer SH, Sampson HA: 9. Food allergy. J Allergy Clin Immunol 2006; 117:S470–S475.
2 Rona RJ, Keil T, Summers C, Gislason D, Zuidmeer L, Sodergren E, et al: The prevalence of food allergy: a meta-analysis. J Allergy Clin Immunol 2007;120: 638–646.
3 Osborne NJ, Ukoumunne OC, Wake M, Allen KJ: Prevalence of eczema and food allergy is associated with latitude in Australia. J Allergy Clin Immunol 2012; 129:865–867.
4 Toit du G, Meyer R, Shah N, Heine RG, Thomson MA, Lack G, et al: Identifying and managing cow's milk protein allergy. Arch Dis Child Educ Pract Ed 2010;95:134–144.
5 Vance GH, Lewis SA, Grimshaw KE, Wood PJ, Briggs RA, Thornton CA, et al: Exposure of the fetus and infant to hens' egg ovalbumin via the placenta and breast milk in relation to maternal intake of dietary egg. Clin Exp Allergy 2005;35:1318–1326.
6 Lack G, Fox D, Northstone K, Golding J; Avon Longitudinal Study of Parents and Children Study Team: Factors associated with the development of peanut allergy in childhood. N Engl J Med 2003;348: 977–985.
7 Arshad SH, Kurukulaaratchy RJ, Fenn M, Matthews S: Early life risk factors for current wheeze, asthma, and bronchial hyperresponsiveness at 10 years of age. Chest 2005;127:502–508.
8 Fox AT, Sasieni P, Toit du G, Syed H, Lack G: Household peanut consumption as a risk factor for the development of peanut allergy. J Allergy Clin Immunol 2009;123:417–423.
9 van OJ, Kull I, Borres MP, Brandtzaeg P, Edberg U, Hanson LA, et al: Breastfeeding and allergic disease: a multidisciplinary review of the literature (1966–2001) on the mode of early feeding in infancy and its impact on later atopic manifestations. Allergy 2003;58:833–843.
10 Muraro A, Dreborg S, Halken S, Host A, Niggemann B, Aalberse R, et al: Dietary prevention of allergic diseases in infants and small children. Part III: Critical review of published peer-reviewed observational and interventional studies and final recommendations. Pediatr Allergy Immunol 2004;15:291–307.
11 Brew BK, Kull I, Garden F, Almqvist C, Bergstrom A, Lind T, et al: Breastfeeding, asthma, and allergy: a tale of two cities. Pediatr Allergy Immunol 2012;23: 75–82.
12 Kramer MS, Kakuma R: The optimal duration of exclusive breastfeeding: a systematic review. Adv Exp Med Biol 2004; 554:63–77.
13 Lucas A, Brooke OG, Morley R, Cole TJ, Bamford MF: Early diet of preterm infants and development of allergic or atopic disease: randomised prospective study. BMJ 1990;300:837–840.
14 de Jong MH, Scharp-Van Der Linden VT, Aalberse R, Heymans HS, Brunekreef B: The effect of brief neonatal exposure to cows' milk on atopic symptoms up to age 5. Arch Dis Child 2002;86:365–369.

15 Grimshaw KEC, Maskell J, Oliver EM, Morris RCG, Foote KD, Mills ENC, et al: Introduction of complementary foods and the relationship to food allergy. Pediatrics 2013;132:e1529–e1538.

16 Greer FR, Sicherer SH, Burks AW: Effects of early nutritional interventions on the development of atopic disease in infants and children: the role of maternal dietary restriction, breastfeeding, timing of introduction of complementary foods, and hydrolyzed formulas. Pediatrics 2008;121:183–191.

17 Agostoni C, Decsi T, Fewtrell M, Goulet O, Kolacek S, Koletzko B, et al: Complementary feeding: a commentary by the ESPGHAN Committee on Nutrition. J Pediatr Gastroenterol Nutr 2008;46:99–110.

18 Paton J, Kljakovic M, Ciszek K, Ding P: Infant feeding practices and nut allergy over time in Australian school entrant children. Int J Pediatr 2012;2012:675724.

19 Department of Health: Weaning and the Weaning Diet. Report of the Working Group on the Weaning Diet of the Committee on Medical Aspects of Food Policy, no 45. London, HMSO, 1994.

20 Asher MI, Montefort S, Bjorksten B, Lai CK, Strachan DP, Weiland SK, et al: Worldwide time trends in the prevalence of symptoms of asthma, allergic rhinoconjunctivitis, and eczema in childhood: ISAAC Phases One and Three repeat multicountry cross-sectional surveys. Lancet 2006;368:733–743.

21 Tarini BA, Carroll AE, Sox CM, Christakis DA: Systematic review of the relationship between early introduction of solid foods to infants and the development of allergic disease. Arch Pediatr Adolesc Med 2006;160:502–507.

22 Osborn DA, Sinn J: Formulas containing hydrolysed protein for prevention of allergy and food intolerance in infants. Cochrane Database Syst Rev 2006;4:CD003664.

23 Host A, Koletzko B, Dreborg S, Muraro A, Wahn U, Aggett P, et al: Dietary products used in infants for treatment and prevention of food allergy. Joint Statement of the European Society for Paediatric Allergology and Clinical Immunology (ESPACI) Committee on Hypoallergenic Formulas and the European Society for Paediatric Gastroenterology, Hepatology and Nutrition (ESPGHAN) Committee on Nutrition. Arch Dis Child 1999;81:80–84.

24 Host A, Halken S, Muraro A, Dreborg S, Niggemann B, Aalberse R, et al: Dietary prevention of allergic diseases in infants and small children. Pediatr Allergy Immunol 2008;19:1–4.

25 Committee on Toxicity of Chemicals in Food, Consumer Products and the Environment: Peanut Allergy. Department of Health, 1998.

26 Fifty-Fourth World Health Assembly: Provisional Agenda Item 13.1.1. Global Strategy for Infant and Young Child Feeding: The Optimal Duration of Exclusive Breastfeeding. Geneva, World Health Organisation, 2001.

27 Fiocchi A, Assa'ad A, Bahna S: Food allergy and the introduction of solid foods to infants: a consensus document. Adverse Reactions to Foods Committee, American College of Allergy, Asthma and Immunology. Ann Allergy Asthma Immunol 2006;97:10–20.

28 Gartner LM, Morton J, Lawrence RA, Naylor AJ, O'Hare D, Schanler RJ, et al: Breastfeeding and the use of human milk. Pediatrics 2005;115:496–506.

29 Prescott SL, Tang ML: The Australasian Society of Clinical Immunology and Allergy position statement: summary of allergy prevention in children. Med J Aust 2005;182:464–467.

30 Berg von A, Koletzko S, Grubl A, Filipiak-Pittroff B, Wichmann HE, Bauer CP, et al: The effect of hydrolyzed cow's milk formula for allergy prevention in the first year of life: the German Infant Nutritional Intervention Study, a randomized double-blind trial. J Allergy Clin Immunol 2003;111:533–540.

31 Berg von A, Koletzko S, Filipiak-Pittroff B, Laubereau B, Grubl A, Wichmann HE, et al: Certain hydrolyzed formulas reduce the incidence of atopic dermatitis but not that of asthma: three-year results of the German Infant Nutritional Intervention Study. J Allergy Clin Immunol 2007;119:718–725.

32 Lowe AJ, Hosking CS, Bennett CM, Allen KJ, Axelrad C, Carlin JB, et al: Effect of a partially hydrolyzed whey infant formula at weaning on risk of allergic disease in high-risk children: a randomized controlled trial. J Allergy Clin Immunol 2011;128:360–365.

33 Osborn DA, Sinn J: Soy formula for prevention of allergy and food intolerance in infants. Cochrane Database Syst Rev 2006;4:CD003741.

34 Zeiger RS, Heller S: The development and prediction of atopy in high-risk children: follow-up at age seven years in a prospective randomized study of combined maternal and infant food allergen avoidance. J Allergy Clin Immunol 1995;95:1179–1190.

35 Arshad SH, Bateman B, Sadeghnejad A, Gant C, Matthews SM: Prevention of allergic disease during childhood by allergen avoidance: the Isle of Wight prevention study. J Allergy Clin Immunol 2007;119:307–313.

36 Brown SJ, McLean WH: Eczema genetics: current state of knowledge and future goals. J Invest Dermatol 2009;129:543–552.

37 Dubrac S, Schmuth M, Ebner S: Atopic dermatitis: the role of Langerhans cells in disease pathogenesis. Immunol Cell Biol 2010;88:400–409.

38 Palmer CN, Irvine AD, Terron-Kwiatkowski A, Zhao Y, Liao H, Lee SP, et al: Common loss-of-function variants of the epidermal barrier protein filaggrin are a major predisposing factor for atopic dermatitis. Nat Genet 2006;38:441–446.

39 Smith FJ, Irvine AD, Terron-Kwiatkowski A, Sandilands A, Campbell LE, Zhao Y, et al: Loss-of-function mutations in the gene encoding filaggrin cause ichthyosis vulgaris. Nat Genet 2006;38:337–342.

40 Perry TT, Conover-Walker MK, Pomes A, Chapman MD, Wood RA: Distribution of peanut allergen in the environment. J Allergy Clin Immunol 2004;113:973–976.

41 Brown SJ, Asai Y, Cordell HJ, Campbell LE, Zhao Y, Liao H, et al: Loss-of-function variants in the filaggrin gene are a significant risk factor for peanut allergy. J Allergy Clin Immunol 2011;127:661–667.

42 Frank L, Marian A, Visser M, Weinberg E, Potter PC: Exposure to peanuts in utero and in infancy and the development of sensitization to peanut allergens in young children. Pediatr Allergy Immunol 1999;10:27–32.

43 Hill DJ, Hosking CS, Heine RG: Clinical spectrum of food allergy in children in Australia and South-East Asia: identification and targets for treatment. Ann Med 1999;31:272–281.

44 Levy Y, Broides A, Segal N, Danon YL: Peanut and tree nut allergy in children: role of peanut snacks in Israel? Allergy 2003;58:1206–1207.

45 Toit du G, Katz Y, Sasieni P, Mesher D, Maleki SJ, Fisher HR, et al: Early consumption of peanuts in infancy is associated with a low prevalence of peanut allergy. J Allergy Clin Immunol 2008; 122:984–991.

46 Joseph CL, Ownby DR, Havstad SL, Woodcroft KJ, Wegienka G, MacKechnie H, et al: Early complementary feeding and risk of food sensitization in a birth cohort. J Allergy Clin Immunol 2011;127:1203–1210.

47 Poole JA, Barriga K, Leung DY, Hoffman M, Eisenbarth GS, Rewers M, et al: Timing of initial exposure to cereal grains and the risk of wheat allergy. Pediatrics 2006;117:2175–2182.

48 Saarinen UM, Kajosaari M: Does dietary elimination in infancy prevent or only postpone a food allergy? A study of fish and citrus allergy in 375 children. Lancet 1980;1:166–167.

49 Nwaru BI, Erkkola M, Ahonen S, Kaila M, Haapala AM, Kronberg-Kippila C, et al: Age at the introduction of solid foods during the first year and allergic sensitization at age 5 years. Pediatrics 2010; 125:50–59.

50 Koplin JJ, Osborne NJ, Wake M, Martin PE, Gurrin LC, Robinson MN, et al: Can early introduction of egg prevent egg allergy in infants? A population-based study. J Allergy Clin Immunol 2010;126: 807–813.

51 Palmer DJ, Metcalfe J, Makrides M, Gold MS, Quinn P, West CE, et al: Early regular egg exposure in infants with eczema: a randomized controlled trial. J Allergy Clin Immunol 2013;132:387–392.e1.

52 Perkin MR, Strachan DP: Which aspects of the farming lifestyle explain the inverse association with childhood allergy? J Allergy Clin Immunol 2006;117: 1374–1381.

53 Waser M, Michels KB, Bieli C, Floistrup H, Pershagen G, Mutius von E, et al: Inverse association of farm milk consumption with asthma and allergy in rural and suburban populations across Europe. Clin Exp Allergy 2007;37:661–670.

54 Boyle RJ, Tang MLK: The role of probiotics in the management of allergic disease. Clin Exp Allergy 2006;36:568–576.

55 Kukkonen K, Savilahti E, Haahtela T, Juntunen-Backman K, Korpela R, Poussa T, et al: Probiotics and prebiotic galacto-oligosaccharides in the prevention of allergic diseases: a randomized, double-blind, placebo-controlled trial. J Allergy Clin Immunol 2007;119:192–198.

56 Heinrich J, Holscher B, Bolte G, Winkler G: Allergic sensitization and diet: ecological analysis in selected European cities. Eur Respir J 2001;17:395–402.

57 Peat JK, Mihrshahi S, Kemp AS, Marks GB, Tovey ER, Webb K, et al: Three-year outcomes of dietary fatty acid modification and house dust mite reduction in the Childhood Asthma Prevention Study. J Allergy Clin Immunol 2004;114: 807–813.

58 Kull I, Bergstrom A, Lilja G, Pershagen G, Wickman M: Fish consumption during the first year of life and development of allergic diseases during childhood. Allergy 2006;61:1009–1015.

59 Almqvist C, Garden F, Xuan W, Mihrshahi S, Leeder SR, Oddy W, et al: Omega-3 and omega-6 fatty acid exposure from early life does not affect atopy and asthma at age 5 years. J Allergy Clin Immunol 2007;119:1438–1444.

60 Anandan C, Nurmatov U, Sheikh A: Omega 3 and 6 oils for primary prevention of allergic disease: systematic review and meta-analysis. Allergy 2009; 64:840–848.

61 Palmer DJ, Sullivan T, Gold MS, Prescott SL, Heddle R, Gibson RA, et al: Effect of n-3 long chain polyunsaturated fatty acid supplementation in pregnancy on infants' allergies in first year of life: randomised controlled trial. BMJ 2012;344: e184.

62 Hypponen E, Sovio U, Wjst M, Patel S, Pekkanen J, Hartikainen AL, et al: Infant vitamin d supplementation and allergic conditions in adulthood: northern Finland birth cohort 1966. Ann N Y Acad Sci 2004;1037:84–95.

63 Milner JD, Stein DM, McCarter R, Moon RY: Early infant multivitamin supplementation is associated with increased risk for food allergy and asthma. Pediatrics 2004;114:27–32.

64 Wjst M: Another explanation for the low allergy rate in the rural Alpine foothills. Clin Mol Allergy 2005;3:7.

65 Kull I, Bergstrom A, Melen E, Lilja G, van Hage M, Pershagen G, et al: Early-life supplementation of vitamins A and D, in water-soluble form or in peanut oil, and allergic diseases during childhood. J Allergy Clin Immunol 2006;118: 1299–1304.

66 Shaheen SO, Newson RB, Henderson AJ, Emmett PM, Sherriff A, Cooke M: Umbilical cord trace elements and minerals and risk of early childhood wheezing and eczema. Eur Respir J 2004;24:292–297.

67 Visness CM, London SJ, Daniels JL, Kaufman JS, Yeatts KB, Siega-Riz AM, et al: Association of obesity with IgE levels and allergy symptoms in children and adolescents: results from the National Health and Nutrition Examination Survey 2005–2006. J Allergy Clin Immunol 2009;123:1163–1169.

68 Turcanu V, Maleki SJ, Lack G: Characterization of lymphocyte responses to peanuts in normal children, peanut-allergic children, and allergic children who acquired tolerance to peanuts. J Clin Invest 2003;111:1065–1072.

George Du Toit, MD
Department of Paediatric Allergy
Guy's and St. Thomas' NHS Foundation Trust
Westminster Bridge Road
London SE1 7EH (UK)
E-Mail george.dutoit@gstt.nhs.uk

Ebisawa M, Ballmer-Weber BK, Vieths S, Wood RA (eds): Food Allergy: Molecular Basis and Clinical Practice.
Chem Immunol Allergy. Basel, Karger, 2015, vol 101, pp 263–269 (DOI: 10.1159/000373913)

Educational Programmes in Food Allergy

Claudia Kugler[a] · Knut Brockow[a] · Johannes Ring[b]

[a]Department of Dermatology and Allergy Biederstein, Technische Universität München, München, Germany;
[b]Christine-Kühne Center for Allergy Research and Education (CK-CARE), Davos, Switzerland

Abstract

About 17% of German children and adolescents suffer from at least one of the following atopic illnesses: allergic rhinoconjunctivitis, atopic eczema or asthma. Consistent professional therapy is necessary to limit the health-related risks and improve these medical conditions. The consequences of a diagnosis often mean an additional task for the parents of diseased children, where they have to act simultaneously as an educator and therapist for their children. Structured educational programmes were developed for a few diseases such as asthma and atopic eczema in order to prepare parents and affected children to accept this important responsibility. Moreover, a structured programme for anaphylaxis is being developed. These proposals aim not only to transfer knowledge about the disease but also to effectively support self-reliant treatment and emotional coping with the disease as well as its collateral strain.   © 2015 S. Karger AG, Basel

Introduction

Food hypersensitivity reactions represent an increasing problem in the daily practice of many physicians, especially allergists, dermatologists and paediatricians. The clinical symptoms range from nausea, vomiting and abdominal symptoms, urticaria, and dyspnoea and upper respiratory symptoms to the full-blown picture of anaphylaxis and anaphylactic shock. In addition, eczema can be elicited by foods, for example, T helper 1-mediated systemic allergic contact eczema or – more commonly – atopic eczema. The most common diseases associated with food hypersensitivity are anaphylaxis and atopic eczema. Therefore, the following chapter focuses on educational programmes on these two diseases.

Individual Dietetic Treatment of Food Allergy

During the treatment of food hypersensitivity, avoidance is the most important principle in all steps of management. This requires a thorough and detailed allergy diagnosis and – in many cases – the help of an experienced nutritionist. Avoidance may be difficult when basic foods or hidden food allergens are involved. Age has to also be considered in dietary recommendations, which are clearly different for infants, children and adults.

Once the diagnosis of food hypersensitivity is established, a nutritionist with allergological experience should always be consulted to give therapeutic advice. In Germany, dieticians or nutritionists are generally authorised to conduct these interviews. They discuss the individual situation with the patient or parents in order to elaborate a detailed diet plan, taking into consideration the diagnostic results together with the child's preferences and dislikes. The nutritionist also recommends methods to integrate the new dietetic needs into common cooking habits and into everyday life. The overall aim of the consultation is to enforce the elimination of the food trigger and to contribute to a balanced diet as well as to a high quality of life. In addition, the nutrition expert may add to the diagnostic process by analysing the patient's medical history, elaborating the nutrition protocol, advising diagnostic elimination diets, and performing oral food provocation together with the physician where required [1].

During the consultation, the patient receives detailed information identifying appropriate and inappropriate foods. Lists of food producers can also be very helpful to provide recent ingredient lists of compound foods [2].

Therapeutic elimination diets over a long period can cause nutrient deficiencies. Hence, the nutritionist is supposed to control nutrient intake and ensure that the nutrients, which might not be or might be insufficiently provided due to the elimination diet, are supplied as needed. If a diet is not possible, supplemental nutritional products should be provided.

For patients with diagnosed food hypersensitivity, individual therapeutic advice cannot be replaced by educational group programmes [2]. However, for chronic or chronically relapsing diseases, educational group programmes are an excellent additional option for patients and affected families to increase quality of life and confidence in dealing with the illness in their daily life [3].

Structured Educational Group Sessions for Patients and Families with Atopic Eczema or Anaphylaxis

According to the Federal Survey of Children's and Adolescents' State of Health (bundesweiter Kinder- und Jugendgesundheitssurvey) in Germany, about 17% of German children and adolescents suffer from at least one of the following atopic illness: allergic rhinoconjunctivitis, atopic eczema or asthma [4]. Consistent, professional therapy is necessary to limit the health-related risks and to improve the medical condition. The consequences of the diagnosis often mean an additional task for the parents of the diseased children, and they have to simultaneously act as an educator and therapist for their children.

Structured educational programmes were developed for a few diseases such as asthma and atopic eczema in order to prepare parents and affected children to accept this important responsibility. Moreover, a structured programme for anaphylaxis is being developed. These proposals aim not only to transfer knowledge about the disease but also to effectively support self-reliant treatment and emotional coping with the disease as well as its collateral strain [5].

Corresponding educational programmes that cover the whole spectrum of the respective illness are planned to be offered nationwide and to be standardised by specially qualified trainers (physicians, psychologists, pedagogues, dieticians, medical expert staff and nursing staff). So far, the reimbursement of costs by health insurance companies has not been uniformly regulated [6].

Educational Programmes for Atopic Eczema

Educational Programmes for the Control of Atopic Eczema in Children and Adolescents (According to 'Arbeitsgemeinschaft Neurodermitis-Schulung')
Atopic eczema commonly begins in childhood, affecting at least 10–20% of young children. Atopic eczema is less common among adults, and the actual prevalence amounts to 1.5–3% in Germany. Within the last five decades, the disease's prevalence has increased significantly. While during the 1950s and 1960s, atopic eczema was prevalent in 2–3% of children between birth and school

enrolment, it now affects four- to six-times more children. The reasons for this increase are controversial and focus primarily on changes in general living conditions [7].

Up to now, atopic eczema has not been completely curable, meaning a huge emotional burden for the young patients and their families. In particular, the chronic, relapsing progression of the illness, along with intense itching and insomnia, are big challenges for the family.

With the support of the Federal Ministry for Health and statutory health insurance companies, the effectiveness of ambulant educational programmes for atopic eczema was tested by means of an interdisciplinary trial. Pursuant to the trial's outcome, the Central Federal Association of the Health Insurance Funds have recommended the reimbursement of costs for conducting educational programmes on atopic eczema since 2007. In these kinds of programmes, the participation of physicians, psychologists/psychotherapists and dieticians is obligatory, whilst in other countries, like Great Britain and the Netherlands, the programmes are held by nursing staff [3, 5] (table 1).

In 2006, Staab et al. published the results of a large randomised trial including three age groups in a controlled German multicentre study referring educational programmes for atopic eczema. To study the effect of the educational programme, approximately 1,000 patients who had been assessed or their parents were enrolled after a qualifying period of 1 year [8].

Parents with children suffering from atopic eczema aged 0–7 years and 8–12 years as well as adolescents aged 13–18 years were evaluated. The inclusion criteria included a severity of eczema of more than 20 points according to the scoring of atopic eczema scale (SCORAD). In all age groups, a significant improvement of eczema severity could be attested 6–12 months after having been trained in ambulant educational programmes on atopic eczema. The programme for ambulant education of parents, children and adolescents consisted of

six sessions, each lasting 2 hours. An interdisciplinary team (physician, psychologist and dietician) trained the parents and caregivers of at most 6 patients. The courses were normally held once a week to enable the participants to apply what they had learned to their daily life in the interim [8].

According to the SCORAD, the improvement in severity of eczema was more substantial in the educated groups 1 year after the training programme compared to the groups still waiting for training sessions. Significant improvements regarding quality of life were also determined in the investigated parameters.

The content of the outpatient educational programmes comprised information on treatment options depending on the stages of the disease, practical exercises for everyday life (e.g. techniques for applying cream), possible triggers and their avoidance, suitable measures for the prevention of eruptions of eczema, relaxation techniques, strategies for dealing with psychosocial strain in chil-

Table 1. Contents of an educational programme in atopic eczema (eczema school)

Medical content
    Clinical symptoms, aetiology, pathophysiology
Treatment
    Basic emollient therapy, non-corticosteroid topicals, glucocorticosteroids, topical immunosuppressives, antiseptics, complications, alternative approaches
Individual trigger factors and avoidance
    Inhalant allergens (aero-allergens) – house dust mites (Dermatophagoides pteronyssinus and D. farinae), animal dander, tree and grass pollens
    Irritants like wool or synthetic clothing
    Climate – extremes of temperature and humidity
Psychosocial situation
    Self-perception, itch-scratch cycle, avoidance of scratching, improving of efficacy, coping with stress, relaxation techniques, training of social competence
Nutrition
    Balanced diet in childhood
    Diagnostic and therapeutic diets
    Declaration regulations
    Recommendations and tricks for recipes

dren and parents, discussion of familial burdens caused by the illness and handling of the itching as well as elaboration of scratching alternatives.

Referring to diet, information on child-oriented nutrition and diagnosis of food allergies was added. Nutrition was presented as the fourth unit and was moderated by specially-qualified dieticians.

A possible connection between disease and food hypersensitivity might seem assured according to current data but has to be regarded individually and treated in a different manner. Food hypersensitivity that might affect the course of the illness in patients with atopic eczema is essentially due to an IgE-mediated allergy to basic food, a pollen-associated food allergen or a pseudo-allergy [9–15].

Usually, it is the patients' great hope to improve the development of the disease by adapting nutrition and to reduce psychological stress by active engagement. This attitude often results in malnutrition and strong emotional distress in the persons concerned because of non-specific diets, which burden the family's situation in addition to the chronic illness [16, 17].

Group sessions are no alternative to individual consultation. In a 90-minute group session, profound questions cannot be answered individually. Nevertheless, by choosing the right topics, such as healthy nutrition in childhood, and by discussing the correct procedure for diagnosed food intolerance, the right foundation can be created, and non-specific diets can be prevented.

Educational Programmes for the Management of Atopic Eczema in Adults ('Arbeitsgemeinschaft Neurodermitis-Schulung für Erwachsene')
Epidemiological data with respect to atopic eczema in adulthood are not available to the same extent as that in childhood [17].

There are also investigations regarding the effectiveness of group sessions, in general, for adult patients affected by atopic eczema.

In 2001, Coenraads et al. examined 46 young adults aged 18–24 years within a multidisci-

plinary educational programme and reported a significant improvement in disease severity according to the SCORAD as well as an improvement in psychological variables in the groups being trained in educational programmes compared to those receiving routine treatment [5].

A survey of Ehlers et al. (1995) compared, within a randomised controlled study, 135 adult patients who were offered autogenic training, behaviour therapy, dermatological education and a combination programme of all these items to a group receiving routine treatment. In the group participating in the combination program, a significant improvement of atopic eczema severity was demonstrated [6].

Following the example of the Educational Programs for Parents and Adolescents (Eltern und Jugendlichenschulungen), an educational programme for adult patients was established. The content, duration and scope of the educational courses were defined in several consensus meetings. The evaluation study is currently being carried out, and upon positive outcome, the assumption of the costs can be negotiated with the health insurance companies by means of a framework agreement.

An additional inclusion criterion is chronically existing atopic eczema with moderate to severe symptoms. The training team consists of dermatologists, dieticians, psychologists and pedagogues and optionally of nurses and medical expert staff. Adult educational programmes have a different emphasis, as in adulthood, fewer allergies to basic food but more pollen-associated food allergies exist [18].

In addition, the number of hours divided between medical and psychological content was shifted to favour more psychological education.

Referring to nutrition, the correlation between (pollen-associated) [19] food allergies and increased eczema severity as well as the subject of allergy prevention is discussed with the participants. The latest improvements include parental atopy prevention with respect to nutrition that is presented to affected patients who want to have children. In total, the nutritional part of the adult educational programme is clearly substantially reduced in comparison to that of the educational programme for parents and amounts to only 30 minutes.

Educational Program for Anaphylaxis Patients and Families

Anaphylaxis is a serious form of an immediate, life-threatening allergic reaction. In most cases, anaphylaxis occurs outside of medical offices or hospitals. Within the first 3 years, the national registry for anaphylaxis at the Berlin Charité reported 1,452 severe anaphylactic reactions. In 1,177 cases, adults were affected; and in 275 cases, children were affected. Insect venom and medications were the most common causes of anaphylaxis in adults, whereas in children, food, mostly peanuts and nuts, were the triggers. According to investigations within German-speaking countries registered with the national registration agency, two-thirds of all anaphylactic shocks in children were caused by peanut or nut allergies. Of concern, only 10% of the anaphylaxis patients made use of the recommended emergency kits, and one-third of the affected persons repeatedly suffered anaphylactic reactions [20, 21].

Improved allergen prevention and immediate therapy can prevent fatalities. After having suffered from anaphylaxis, patients are equipped with an emergency kit that includes an adrenalin auto-injector for self-therapy. Frequently, knowledge and instructions with respect to application and self-therapy are insufficient in patients. Educational programmes for anaphylaxis seem to be necessary to guarantee the avoidance of trigger factors as far as possible as well as the application of emergency therapy [13, 22].

Hence, a nationwide standardised and evaluated training programme for the management of anaphylaxis has been developed by the Committee for Anaphylaxis Training and Education (Arbeitsgemeinschaft Anaphylaxietraining und Edukation) [23].

This training programme is intended for allergic persons who have suffered an anaphylaxis as well as for high-risk patients, their families and caregivers who receive an adrenalin auto-injector.

In group sessions, patients and parents or legal guardians are trained interactively and with constant reference to the personal situation regarding the fundamental principles of anaphylaxis management, self-treatment in the case of emergency, trigger prevention and ways of coping with anxiety or conflict situations. The individual situation of each patient and potential supporting measures are taken into consideration. Functional demonstration and exercise in the use of adrenaline auto-injectors as well as coaching in trigger avoidance strategies represent the main contents of the training programme. The elaboration of the educational programme was conducted primarily because of the patient requirements and without financial support. In order to realise these programmes entirely, health insurance companies will have to cover the costs.

Thus, in these programmes, patients or the parents of affected children are supposed to be educated on how to avoid relevant allergens in order to reduce the risk of suffering an anaphylactic shock without excessively reducing life quality. Furthermore, they learn that it is important to develop strategies for coping with anxiety in the case of emergency. Additionally, persons suffering from an allergy are expected to always carry the prescribed emergency kit. The correct use of the emergency kit is also instructed within the training programme. The trainer transfers comprehensive information but also provides practical advice regarding allergies [24].

In the training courses of Arbeitsgemeinschaft Anaphylaxietraining und Edukation, allergists (dermatologists, paediatricians, pulmonary specialists, ear-nose-and-throat physicians), nutritionists with allergological experience, psychologists and optionally nurses and medical expert staff teach basic knowledge of anaphylaxis, allergen avoidance strategies and practical measures for managing emergencies on two evenings (3 hours each).

The fact that anaphylactic shock can be fatal within minutes emphasises the importance of educating affected patients and parents of at-risk children. Regarding fatal food allergy, the mean time interval from eating the trigger to death is 30 minutes. Individuals allergic to insect venom die after a mean of 15 minutes, whereas persons allergic to medications die after 5 minutes.

Therefore, at-risk patients are expected to permanently carry emergency medication and to be trained in handling it correctly. In the event that there is no physician available right away, special adrenalin auto-injectors are to be applied. These injectors provide basic life support whenever an anaphylactic reaction can be foreseen. However, even in these cases, profound education and training are essential. In addition, patients often are uncertain about how to use emergency medication and do not know the correct order of application. Due to anxiety and ignorance, auto-injectors frequently are not applied at all [9, 19].

Allergen avoidance plays an important part in the training programmes for anaphylaxis. The nutritional part of the training's content focuses on allergen avoidance. As a minimum amount of the trigger food can cause severe reactions, an educational unit of 20–45 minutes is dedicated to nutritional allergen avoidance on the second day of the educational training.

Declared lists of ingredients offer substantial support for allergen avoidance. However, lists of ingredients need to be re-examined at every purchase, as manufacturers can change the recipe of the products at any time. Attention is to be paid to the fact that food constituents might be characterised in terms that cannot be automatically identified as an allergen (e.g. the term lactalbumin, which is relevant for cow milk allergy sufferers, or ovalbumin, which is relevant for hen's egg

allergy sufferers). Hidden allergens in food constitute a problem for food allergy sufferers. The European Union reacted to this circumstance with a corresponding directive that has been effective since November 2003. Subsequently, the product identification has been amended EU-wide and has eliminated many exceptions within food legislation. The most allergenic foods and some foods causing intolerances must be specified according to EU-directive 2000/13/EG, appendix IIIa. These so-called major allergens (amounting to a number of 14) cover the majority of food allergens and have to be listed on the labelling of groceries. The mentioned regulation for product identification refers to the labelling on the packaging of ready-to-use food.

Until now, groceries handed out loosely to the customer at the counters of bakeries, butchers and canteens have not been included in the regulation. Commencing on 12/14/2014, an upcoming regulation will change this in favour of allergy sufferers. At this point, ingredients must also be declared on bulk food. At present, there exists no threshold values in Germany or the EU that oblige the producer to list the allergenic components that are subject to labelling. There is also no obligation for the producer to specify allergens that were not intended to be added to the grocery. That is why manufacturers on occasion use the term 'may contain traces of X,Y' (X,Y standing for allergen, e.g. hazelnut) for reasons of product liability. If this declaration is only applied preventively, since appropriate measures for restricting cross-contamination would increase the cost of production, consumer protection will not be responsibly fulfilled.

In the future, caregivers (educators and teachers) will also be invited to attend educational programmes, and children shall be trained independently. For this reason, working groups have been established within the committee to determine the content and structure of these specific educational programmes.

References

1 Niggemann B, Sielaff B, Beyer K, Binder C, Wahn U: Outcome of double-blind, placebo-controlled food challenge tests in 107 children with atopic eczema. Clin Exp Allergy 1999;29:91–96.

2 Kugler C: Ernährungstherapie bei atopischem Ekzem; in Reese I, Schäfer C (eds): Ernährungstherapie in der Allergologie, ed 2. Auflage, München, Dustri-Verlag Dr. Karl Feistle, 2012.

3 Staab D, von Rueden U, Kehrt R, Erhart M, Wenninger K, Kamtsiuris P, Wahn U: Evaluation of parental training program for the management of childhood atopic eczema. Pediatr Allergy Immunol 2002;13:84–90.

4 Schmitz R, Atzpodien K, Schlaud M: Prevalence and risk factors of atopic diseases in German children and adolescents – findings from the German Health Interview and Examination Survey for Children and Adolescents (KiGGS). Pediatr Allergy Immunol 2012; 23:716–723.

5 Coenraads PJ, Span L, Jaspers JP, Fidler V: Intensive patient education and treatment program for young adults with atopic eczema. Hautarzt 2001;52:428–433.

6 Ehlers A, Stangier U, Gieler U: Treatment of atopic eczema: a comparison of psychological and dermatological approaches to relapse prevention. J Consult Clin Psychol 1995;63:624–635.

7 Schäfer T, Krämer U, Behrendt H, Ring J: Epidemiologie des atopischen Ekzem. Allergo J 2003;12:430–438.

8 Staab D, Diepgen TL, Fartasch M, Kupfer J, Lob-Corzilius T, Ring J, Scheewe S, Scheidt R, Schmid-Ott G, Schnopp C, Szczepanski R, Werfel T, Wittenmeier M, Wahn U, Gieler U: Age-related structured educational programmes for the management of atopic dermatitis in children and adolescents: multi-center, randomised controlled trial. BMJ 2006; 332:933–938.

9 Arkwright PD, Farragher AJ: Factors determining the ability of parents to effectively administer intramuscular adrenaline to food allergic children. Pediatr Allergy Immunol 2006;17:227–229.

10 Ellman LK, Chatchatee P, Sicherer SH, Sampson HA: Food hypersensitivity in two groups of children and young adults with atopic eczema evaluated a decade apart. Pediatr Allergy Immunol 2002;13:295–298.

11 Eng PA, Ferrari G: IgE-mediated food allergies in Swiss infants and children. Swiss Med Wkly 2007;13:137–157.

12 Fuglsang G, Madsen C, Halken S, Jorgensen M, Ostergaard PA, Osterballe O: Adverse reaction to food additives in children with atopic symptoms. Allergy 1994;49:31–37.

13 Ring J: Allergy in Practice. Berlin, Heidelberg, New York, Springer, 2005.

14 Worm M, Ehlers I, Sterry W, Zuberbier T: Clinical relevance of food additives in adult patients with atopic eczema. Clin Exp Allergy 2000;30:407–414.

15 Zuberbier T, Edenharter G, Worm M, Ehlers I, Reimann S, Hantke T, Roehr CC, Bergmann KE, Niggemann B: Prevalence of adverse reactions to food in Germany – a population study. Allergy 2004;59:338–345.

16 Osterballe M, Hansen TK, Mortz CG, Host A, Bindslev-Jensen C: The prevalence of food hypersensitivity in an unselected population of children and adults. Pediatr Allergy Immunol 2005; 16:567–573.

17 Ring J: Neurodermitis – Atopisches Ekzem, ed 1. Stuttgart, Georg Thieme Verlag, 2011.

18 Gutgesell C, Schäkel K, Fuchs T, Neumann C: Nahrungsmitteladditiva sind kein Schubfaktor der atopischen Eczema bei Erwachsenen. Allergologie 1997;20:519–521.

19 Breuer K, Wulf A, Constien A, Tetau D, Kapp A, Werfel T: Birch pollen-related food as a provocation factor of allergic symptoms in children with atopic eczema/eczema syndrome. Allergy 2004; 59:988–994.

20 Hompes S, Beyer K, Köhli A, Scherer K, Lange L, Rietschel E, Reese T, Worm M: Anaphylaxie im Kindes-und Jugendalter. Kinder und Jugendmedizin 2009;9: 393–399.

21 Hompes S, Köhli A, Nemat K, Scherer K, Lange L, Rueff F, Rietschel E, Reese T, Szepfalusi Z, Schwerk N, Beyer K, Hawranek T, Niggemann B, Worm M: Provoking allergens and treatment of anaphylaxis in children and adolescents data from the anaphylaxis registry of German-speaking countries. Pediatr Allergy Immunol 2011;22:568–574.

22 Ring J, Brockow K, Duda D, Eschenhagen T, Fuchs T, Huttegger I, Kapp A, Klimek L, Müller U, Niggemann B, Pfaar O, Przybilla B, Rebien W, Rietschel E, Ruëff F, Schnadt S, Tryba M, Worm M, Sitter I, Schultze-Werninghaus G: Akuttherapie anaphylaktischer Reaktionen. Leitlinie der Deutschen Gesellschaft für Allergologie und Klinische Immunologie (DGAKI), des Ärzteverbandes Deutscher Allergologen (ÄDA), der Deutschen Gesellschaft für Pädiatrische Allergologie und Umweltmedizin (GPA) und der Deutschen Akademie für Allergologie und Umweltmedizin (DAAU). Allergo J 2007;16:420–434.

23 Ring J, Beyer K, Dorsch A, Biedermann T, Fischer J, Friedrichs F, Gebert N, Gieler U, Grosber M, Jakob T, Klimek L, Kugler C, Lange L, Pfaar O, Przybilla B, Reese I, Rietschel E, Schallmayer S, Schnadt S, Szczepanski R, Worm M, Brockow K: Anaphylaxis school. Allergo J 2012;2:96–102.

24 Joshi P, Katelaris CH, Frankum B: Adrenaline (epinephrine) autoinjector use in preschools. J Allergy Clin Immunol 2009;124:383–384.

Dipl. oec. troph. Claudia Kugler
Department of Dermatology and Allergy Biederstein
Technische Universität München
Biedersteinerstrasse 29, DE–80802 München (Germany)
E-Mail claudia.kugler@lrz.tum.de

Acknowledgments

Motohiro Ebisawa, the main editor of the volume, would like to express his sincere appreciation to Dr. Makoto Nishino, Sagamihara National Hospital, Sagamihara, Kanagawa, Japan, for his assistance.

The editors would like to thank Professor Paul Rösch and Dr. Christian Seutter von Loetzen, Lehrstuhl Biopolymere und Forschungszentrum für Bio-Makromoleküle, Universität Bayreuth, Bayreuth, Germany, for providing the cover illustration. The meaning and importance of the 2S albumin-type peanut allergen Ara h 6 are explained in the paper by Lehmann K, Schweimer K, Reese G, Randow S, Suhr M, Becker WM, Vieths S, Rösch P entitled 'Structure and stability of 2S albumin type peanut allergens: implications for the severity of peanut allergic reactions' [Biochem J 2006;395:463–472]. The figure has been created using the pdb file 1w2q using Pymol (The PyMOL Molecular Graphics System, Version 1.2r3pre, Schrödinger, LLC).

Author Index

Subject Index